MEDICO-LEGAL TRAPS IN NOT-SO COMMON PAIN SYNDROMES

CONCERNS, ASPECTS & CONSIDERATIONS

SERIES EDITORS

Dr. Ravinder Singh Channey

Ph.D., D.Sc.(Med) Journalist)

Ripudaman Singh Channey

B.Pharm, M.B.A. (Pharma Management)

MEDICO-LEGAL TRAPS IN NOT-SO COMMON PAIN SYNDROMES

CONCERNS, ASPECTS & CONSIDERATIONS

First Edition 2025.

For the use only of a Registered Medical Practionar or a Hospital, or a Laboratory.

Printed and Published by

CUSTOMED

D-71, Hauz Khas, New Delhi-110 016.

customedgroup.com

info@customedgroup.com

ISBN: 9798284603284

DISCLAIMER

The authors, publisher, and printer of "Medico-Legal Traps in Not - So - Common Pain Syndromes" have made every effort to ensure that the information presented in this book is accurate, up-to-date, and in line with current medical and legal standards at the time of publication. However, the field of pain management and medico-legal issues is constantly evolving, and new developments may occur that are not reflected in this book.

This book is intended for educational and informational purposes only. It is not a substitute for professional medical advice, diagnosis, or treatment. The techniques and approaches discussed in this book should only be performed by licensed healthcare professionals in accordance with local, regional, and national laws, guidelines, and best practices. It is the responsibility of each reader to ensure compliance with all applicable legal, ethical, and professional standards within their jurisdiction before applying any of the techniques described herein.

Neither the authors, publisher, nor printer can be held liable for any direct, indirect, incidental, or consequential damages, including but not limited to injury, malpractice claims, legal actions, or any other legal disputes arising from the use or misuse of the information contained in this book. Readers are strongly advised to consult with appropriate legal and medical professionals for personalized guidance related to their specific circumstances.

By using this book, readers acknowledge and agree that the authors, publisher, and printer assume no responsibility or liability for any outcomes associated with the use of the material presented.

This disclaimer is applicable internationally and covers all legal jurisdictions.

Dedication

To the patients whose pain defies pattern,
To the clinicians who refuse to dismiss the undiagnosed,
And to the professionals who must defend every decision they make -
This book is dedicated to your courage, your scrutiny, and your relentless pursuit of answers in a world where pain speaks louder in court than it does at the bedside.

Dr. Ravinder Singh Channey

Ripudaman Singh Channey

PREFACE

Pain may be universal, but its interpretations are anything but. From whispered complaints in a clinic to thunderous debates in a courtroom, pain doesn't just demand attention - it demands answers. And in today's litigious world, the wrong answer could cost more than your reputation - it could cost your career. Welcome to *Medico-Legal Traps in Not - So - Common Pain Syndromes*, the world's first guidebook to navigate the minefield where medicine meets the law.

This isn't just a book; it's a survival kit - crafted over a decade of blood, sweat, and late-night caffeine marathons. Covering *"120 not - so - common pain syndromes with over 600 potential medico-legal traps with thumb rule considerations"*, it peels back the layers of diagnostic dilemmas, treatment puzzles, and legal booby traps that make pain one of the most misunderstood and mismanaged fields.

Each syndrome is dissected with clinical precision - offering a "bird's-eye overview", a "deep dive into symptoms", and "pearls and oysters" that transform hindsight into foresight. Need quick takeaways? The "thumb rule considerations" act as guardrails to keep you on track, and the "bottom-line statements" deliver distilled wisdom - short, sharp, and lawsuit-proof.

But this book doesn't stop at being a clinician's confidant. It's equally indispensable for "hospitals", "health educators", lawyers and advocates", and even "law colleges", making it the Swiss Army knife of pain management and legal preparedness. Whether you're dissecting a case in a lecture hall or defending one in a courtroom, this guide ensures you don't just show up - you show up ready.

So brace yourself. With "123 syndromes", countless clinical nuances, and a legal landscape that changes faster than social media trends, this isn't just another textbook. We present your armor in a battlefield where pain has the final say - unless, of course, you've read this book first.

Series Editors

Dr. Ravinder singh Channey

Ripudaman Singh Channey

January 2025

Contents

Q

R

S

ABDOMINAL ANGINA

Abdominal angina is postprandial pain that occurs in mesenteric vascular occlusive disease when blood flow to the colon is unable to meet visceral demands. This is similar to intermittent claudication in peripheral vascular disease or angina pectoris in coronary artery disease.

Tayama S, Sakamoto T, Taguchi E, Sawamura T, Koyama J, Ogawa H, Nakao K. Successful stenting to superior mesenteric artery (SMA) after endovascular aneurysm repair (EVAR) of abdominal aorta. J Cardiol Cases. 2010 Oct;2(2):e78-e82.

Clinical Description

The typical clinical presentation of abdominal angina is severe pain out of proportion to the physical exam. The patient usually complains of severe abdominal pain that starts after eating a meal. In most cases, the pain gradually subsides after a few hours. Because the pain is so severe, most people develop a fear of eating and hence lose weight. One should always ask about a history of smoking, claudication, and hyperlipidemia. On physical exam, marked weight loss is obvious. The abdomen is often soft, and there are no peritoneal signs. An abdominal bruit may be heard in some patients. One may also find features of peripheral vascular disease with diminished pulses in the leg. The digital rectal exam is usually guaiac negative.

Abdominal angina is rare and has a high mortality rate. It is more common in females and the elderly. The problem with diagnosis is that the symptoms are often vague and no work up is ever done. The average age of those affected is slightly older than 60 years although it has been reported in young individuals. Females outnumber males by approximately 3 to 1. Because of the few cases, there are no large series to determine which population is most at risk. Outside the United States, there are few cases of abdominal angina reported.

Ischemia of the intestine results from an imbalance of oxygen supply to and oxygen consumption by the GI tract. A decrease in blood flow results from the decreased size of mesenteric vessels. Atherosclerotic disease is the most common cause of abdominal angina. It frequently involves ostia of the mesenteric vessels. In most people, it is occlusion of the superior mesenteric artery that is responsible for the abdominal symptoms. Risk factors for superior mesenteric artery atherosclerosis include smoking and hyperlipidemia

Pearls & Oysters

Duplex ultrasonography is used for follow-up. The blood flow velocities are measured regularly to ensure that restenosis is not occurring. Even with treatment, a morbidity rate of 30% has been reported. The most common complications of surgery or an endovascular procedure include a hematoma, pseudoaneurysm, and thrombosis followed by bowel infarction. It is vital to tell the patient to stop smoking.

Once discharged from the hospital, the patient should be told to consume several small meals rather than one large meal. This practice requires less blood flow in the mesenteric vessels. If the surgery is not a success, the symptoms will appear immediately. A number of patients with failed surgery end up having massive bowel resection and end up with a short gut.

Bottom Line Statement

The presentation of abdominal angina can be non-specific, but if the diagnosis is delayed, the disorder carries high morbidity and mortality. Thus, the disorder is best managed by an interprofessional team that includes a general surgeon, vascular surgeon, gastroenterologist, emergency department physician, radiologist, and operative and ICU nurses. Even after treatment, patients need to be monitored to ensure that there is no recurrence. Graft thrombosis and occlusion may lead to bowel ischemia and necessitate the need for emergent surgery.

Medico-Legal Traps

Failure to Recognize Early Symptoms

- Abdominal angina often presents with non-specific symptoms like postprandial pain, which can be easily overlooked. If physicians fail to recognize these early signs, particularly in high-risk individuals (elderly, smokers, or those with hyperlipidemia), delayed diagnosis could lead to catastrophic outcomes.
- **Thumb Rule Consideration:** Always consider abdominal angina in patients with unexplained postprandial pain and risk factors like smoking or vascular disease.

Delayed Diagnosis

- The vague presentation of abdominal angina often results in delayed diagnosis, increasing the risk of bowel ischemia. Failure to promptly order diagnostic tests such as duplex ultrasonography or CT angiography can worsen patient outcomes.

- **Thumb Rule Consideration:** Act quickly with diagnostic imaging in patients with postprandial pain and vascular risk factors to prevent complications from delayed treatment.

Inadequate Postoperative Monitoring

- After procedures like stenting or surgical intervention, patients need close monitoring for complications like restenosis, thrombosis, or bowel infarction. Failing to follow up could result in life-threatening outcomes.
- **Thumb Rule Consideration:** Ensure regular post-op imaging (e.g., duplex ultrasound) and close follow-up to detect any signs of restenosis or graft thrombosis early.

Failure to Inform and Educate the Patient

- Patients should be clearly instructed about lifestyle changes, such as smoking cessation and eating smaller meals, to reduce the risk of recurrence. Failure to provide this education can lead to poor outcomes and legal repercussions.
- **Thumb Rule Consideration:** Always educate patients on the necessary lifestyle adjustments and the warning signs of recurrence or surgical failure.

Neglecting Interprofessional Collaboration

- Managing abdominal angina involves multiple specialties, including vascular surgery, gastroenterology, and radiology. Lack of coordination among the healthcare team can result in suboptimal care.
- **Thumb Rule Consideration:** Involve an interprofessional team in managing abdominal angina, with clear communication and documentation of collaborative care to ensure optimal treatment.

Failure to Adjust Dietary Recommendations Postoperatively

- Patients who undergo surgery for abdominal angina should be advised to eat smaller, frequent meals to reduce the demand for blood flow. Failure to give these dietary recommendations can lead to worsening symptoms.
- **Thumb Rule Consideration:** Advise patients to consume smaller meals postoperatively to reduce the burden on mesenteric blood flow and prevent recurrence of symptoms.

REFERENCES

- Tayama S, Sakamoto T, Taguchi E, Sawamura T, Koyama J, Ogawa H, Nakao K. Successful stenting to superior mesenteric artery (SMA) after endovascular aneurysm repair (EVAR) of abdominal aorta. J Cardiol Cases. 2010 Oct;2(2):e78-e82.

- Mosselveld P, van Werkum MH, Menting TP, Pieters AMMJ, Müller METM, Bosch FH. A case of progressive abdominal angina. Neth J Med. 2018 Jul;76(5):255.
- Melas N, Haji Younes A, Lindberg R, Magnusson P. A case of extreme weight loss due to mesenteric ischemia and antiphospholipid syndrome. Clin Case Rep. 2018 Jun;6(6):1055-1059.
- Talledo Ó, Torres L, Valenzuela H, Calle A, Mena MA, De La Peña Ó, Lizarzaburu D. [Persistent abdominal pain caused by superior mesenteric artery and celiac trunk dissection that does not respond to conservative treatment]. Rev Gastroenterol Peru. 2017 Jul-Sep;37(3):262-266.
- Barret M, Martineau C, Rahmi G, Pellerin O, Sapoval M, Alsac JM, Fabiani JN, Malamut G, Samaha E, Cellier C. Chronic Mesenteric Ischemia: A Rare Cause of Chronic Abdominal Pain. Am J Med. 2015 Dec;128(12):1363.e1-8.
- Mensink PB, Moons LM, Kuipers EJ. Chronic gastrointestinal ischaemia: shifting paradigms. Gut. 2011 May;60(5):722-37.
- Naganuma T, Fujino Y, Mitomo S, Basavarajaiah S, Nakamura S. One-year follow-up optical coherence tomography after endovascular treatment with a new-generation zotarolimus-eluting stent for chronic mesenteric ischemia. Hellenic J Cardiol. 2017 May-Jun;58(3):233-235.

ACCESSORY NAVICULAR PAIN SYNDROME

An accessory navicular is a large accessory ossicle that can be present adjacent to the medial side of the navicular bone. The accessory navicular bone presents as a sesamoid in the posterior tibial tendon, in articulation with the navicular or as an enlargement of the navicular itself.

Raymond T., Morrissy and Stuart L.Weinstein Lovell, Winter's Padiatric Orthopaedics. United States: Lippincot William's Wilkin Publication, 2005.

Clinical Description

An accessory navicular bone is located posterior to the posteromedial tuberosity of the tarsal navicular bone. The tibialis posterior tendon inserts into the navicular bone. Tibialis posterior is an inverter of the foot, assists in the plantar flexion of the foot at the ankle and also has a major role in supporting the medial arch of the foot. This can be compromised where there exists an abnormal insertion of the tendon into the accessory navicular bone and result in a loss of suspension of the tibialis posterior tendon.

The presence of a type I or II accessory navicular is also a cause of Posterior Tibial tendinopathy as the insertion of the tibialus posterior tendon onto the accessory navicular is more proximal. Leverage of the malleolus on the tibialus posterior tendon is reduced increasing stress on the tendon. The calcaneal pitch angle is also reduced in patients with a symptomatic accessory navicular than in normal subjects.

Most of the time it is asymptomatic and found incidentally on radiographs, although medial side foot pain (accessory navicular syndrome) is the most common presenting feature of accessory navicular bone. The pain is aggravated by walking, running and weight-bearing activities. When large, it can protrude medially and cause friction against footwear.

Pearls & Oysters

For patients who have failed conservative care or who have recurrent symptoms, surgery can be considered. Surgical intervention requires an excision of the accessory navicular and reattachment of the posterior tibial tendon to the navicular. Oftentimes, this is the only procedure necessary. However, if there are other deformities, such as a flat foot or forefoot that is abducted, other procedures may be required.

Bottom Line Statement

A type I accessory navicular is rarely symptomatic. Where symptoms do appear, type I usually responds well to conservative management. Patients with Type II have an increased risk of injury and onset is usually insidious or as a result of trauma. It fails to respond to conservative treatment when severe and fusion of the accessory navicular to the navicular may successfully relieve pain without disrupting the tibialis posterior tendon insertion. With Type III, excising the accessory navicular is indicated over excising the navicular prominence.

Medico-Legal Traps

Failure to Diagnose Symptomatic Accessory Navicular

- Many patients with an accessory navicular bone are asymptomatic, but when symptoms such as medial foot pain or swelling arise, failure to consider accessory navicular syndrome can delay treatment. Missed diagnoses, especially in active individuals or athletes, can lead to prolonged discomfort and functional impairment.
- **Thumb Rule Consideration:** Always consider accessory navicular syndrome in patients presenting with unexplained medial foot pain, especially if aggravated by weight-bearing activities.

Inadequate Conservative Management

- Conservative treatments, such as immobilization, orthotics, or physical therapy, are often the first line of management. Failing to provide adequate conservative care or not allowing sufficient time for these methods to work can lead to premature surgical intervention or prolonged patient discomfort.
- **Thumb Rule Consideration:** Prioritize conservative treatment options like immobilization, custom orthotics, and physical therapy, and ensure an adequate trial period before considering surgery.

Delayed Surgical Intervention in Refractory Cases

- Some patients with Type II or Type III accessory navicular may fail conservative care and require surgical intervention. Delaying surgery in patients with persistent symptoms can result in worsened outcomes, increased pain, and further tendon degeneration.
- **Thumb Rule Consideration:** For patients with Type II or Type III accessory navicular who do not respond to conservative treatments, timely surgical intervention should be considered to prevent long-term damage.

Failure to Address Concomitant Deformities

- In some cases, the presence of accessory navicular may be accompanied by other foot deformities, such as flatfoot or forefoot abduction. Failing to recognize and treat these associated deformities during surgery can lead to poor outcomes or recurrent symptoms.
- **Thumb Rule Consideration:** Always assess for associated deformities like flatfoot or forefoot abduction in patients with symptomatic accessory navicular, and address these issues if necessary during surgery.

Inadequate Postoperative Care

- Surgical excision of the accessory navicular and tendon reattachment require proper postoperative rehabilitation. Failing to provide adequate rehabilitation, including immobilization and physical therapy, can lead to complications like weakened tendon function or recurrent pain.
- **Thumb Rule Consideration:** Ensure comprehensive postoperative care, including immobilization and structured rehabilitation, to optimize recovery and prevent recurrent symptoms or tendon dysfunction.

REFERENCES

- Radiopedia Accessory navicular Available:https://radiopaedia.org/articles/accessory-navicular-2?lang=us (accessed 8.6.2022)
- Golano P., 'The anatomy of the navicular and periarticular structures.' Foot Ankle Clinics, 2004, March, vol. 9, p. 1-23.
- Kiter E., Erdan N., Karatosun V., Gunall I., 'Tibialis posterior tendon abnormalities in feet with accessory navicular bone and flatfoot'. Acta orthopaedica Scandinavia, 1999, December, vol. 70, p. 618-621
- Kulkarni. G.S. Textbook of orthopedics and trauma.India: Jaypee Brother Publication, 1999
- Kidner FC. The prehallux (accessory scaphoid) in its relation to flat-foot. J Bone Joint Surg 1929 : II : 831
- A. Bernaerts, F.M. Vanhoenacker, S. Van de Perre, A.M. De Schepper, P.M. Parizel1 Accessory navicular bone: Not Such a normal variant. JBR–BTR, 2004, 87 (5) page 250-252
- Prichausuk S, Sinphurmsukskul O: Kinder Procedure for symptomatic accessory navicular and its relation to pes planus, Foot Ankle 16:500,1995
- Kidner FC. Pre-hallux in relation to flatfoot. JAMA 1933; 101: 1539-42.
- Kulkarni. G.S. Textbook of orthopedics and trauma.India: Jaypee Brother Publication, 1999.</ref><ref name="p7">Kidner FC. The prehallux (accessory scaphoid) in its relation to flat-foot. J Bone Joint Surg 1929 : II : 831.

ACHILLES BURSITIS

Achilles tendon bursitis is inflammation of the fluid-filled sac (bursa) located either between the skin of the back of the heel and the Achilles tendon (called posterior Achilles tendon bursitis) or in front of the attachment of the Achilles tendon to the heel bone (called anterior Achilles tendon bursitis or retromalleolar bursitis).

Fauci, Anthony (2010). Harrison's Rheumatology, Second Edition. McGraw-Hill Professional Publishing; Digital Edition. p. 271.

Clinical Description

The Achilles tendon is the tendon that attaches the calf muscles to the heel bone. Bursitis is painful inflammation of a bursa (a flat, fluid-filled sac that provides cushioning and reduces friction in areas where skin, muscles, tendons, and ligaments rub over bones).

Posterior Achilles tendon bursitis occurs mainly in young women but can develop in men. Walking in a way that repeatedly presses the soft tissue behind the heel against the stiff back support of a shoe can cause or aggravate the bursitis. Shoes that taper sharply inward toward the posterior heel (such as high-heeled shoes or pumps) can cause or worsen an enlargement of the bone of the back of the heel (called pump bump or Haglund deformity), which contributes to posterior Achilles tendon bursitis.

Anterior Achilles tendon bursitis (also called Albert disease or retromalleolar bursitis) can be caused by any condition that puts extra strain on the Achilles tendon. Injuries to the heel (such as those caused by stiff or poorly fitting shoes) and diseases (such as rheumatoid arthritis and gout) can also cause it.

Posterior Achilles tendon bursitis

Early symptoms of posterior Achilles tendon bursitis may include redness, pain, and warmth at the back of the heel. Later, the top layer of skin may wear away. After several months, a bursa, which looks like a raised, red or flesh-colored area (nodule) that is tender and soft, forms and becomes inflamed. If posterior Achilles tendon bursitis becomes chronic, the bursa may become hard and scarlike.

Anterior Achilles tendon bursitis

When the bursa becomes inflamed after an injury or gout, symptoms of anterior Achilles tendon bursitis usually develop suddenly. When the bursitis develops because of other disorders, symptoms develop gradually. Pain, swelling, and warmth develop at the back of the heel. People have difficulty walking and wearing shoes. A minimally red, swollen, tender spot develops on the back of the heel. When the inflamed bursa enlarges, the swelling spreads sideways to both sides of the heel.

Pearls & Oysters

For both posterior and anterior Achilles tendon bursitis, warm or cold compresses, NSAIDs, and injections of a corticosteroid/anesthetic mixture into the inflamed bursa can temporarily relieve the pain and inflammation. The doctor is careful not to inject the mixture into the tendon. After this treatment, the person should rest.

For posterior Achilles tendon bursitis, treatment is aimed at reducing the inflammation and adjusting the foot's position in the shoe to relieve pressure and motion on the back of the heel. Foam rubber or felt heel pads can be placed in the shoe to eliminate pressure by elevating the heel. Placing protective gel padding over the painful bursa or stretching the back part of the shoe and placing padding around the inflamed bursa may help. A backless shoe may be worn until inflammation lessens. Sometimes a special shoe, such as a running shoe designed to stabilize the midsole heel, devices placed in the shoe (orthoses), or both can help to control abnormal foot and heel motion contributing to the posterior heel irritation. Other shoes have padding that reduces irritation to the posterior heel and Achilles tendon.

If these treatments are not effective, part of the heel bone may need to be surgically removed.

Bottom Line Statement

A good clinical practise includes evaluation of the tendon, bursa and calcaneum by, careful history, inspection of the region for bony prominence and local swelling as well as palpation of the area of maximal tenderness. Biomechanical abnormalities, joint stiffness and proximal soft tissue tightening can exacerbate an anatomical predisposition to retrocalcaneal bursitis, they warrant correction when present.

Plain radiographs of the calcaneus may reveal a Haglund deformity (increased prominence of the posterosuperior aspect of the calcaneus). However, on weight-bearing lateral radiographs, the retrocalcaneal recess often appears normal even in patients with retrocalcaneal bursitis, limiting its usefulness in making this diagnosis. Radiographs may be used as a diagnostic measure to support a clinician's diagnosis of retrocalcaneal bursitis. Individuals with retrocalcaneal bursitis may have an absence of the normal radiolucency (ie, blunting) that is seen in the posteroinferior corner of the Kager fat pad, known as the retrocalcaneal recess or bursal wedge. This may occur with or without an associated erosion of the calcaneus.

Magnetic resonance imaging (MRI) may demonstrate bursal inflammation, but this modality probably does not offer much more information than that found by careful physical examination. Theoretically, MRI could help the physician to determine whether the inflammation is within the subcutaneous bursa, the subtendinous bursa, or even within the tendon itself; however, such testing is generally not necessary.

Medico-Legal Traps

Failure to Diagnose Achilles Bursitis Early

- Achilles bursitis, particularly posterior Achilles tendon bursitis, often presents with pain, swelling, and redness in the heel, which can be confused with other heel disorders. Misdiagnosing or failing to recognize early symptoms can delay appropriate treatment, leading to chronic pain or complications such as Haglund deformity.
- **Thumb Rule Consideration:** Always consider Achilles bursitis in patients presenting with heel pain, especially those with a history of ill-fitting shoes or foot deformities, and conduct a thorough clinical evaluation to confirm.

Inappropriate Use of Corticosteroid Injections

- While corticosteroid injections can relieve bursitis pain, improper technique, such as injecting the mixture into the Achilles tendon itself rather than into the bursa, can lead to tendon weakening or rupture. This can result in significant complications and potential litigation.
- **Thumb Rule Consideration:** Be cautious with corticosteroid injections, ensuring the mixture is injected only into the bursa and not the tendon to avoid complications such as tendon rupture.

Failure to Address Biomechanical Abnormalities

- Patients with Achilles bursitis often have underlying biomechanical issues, such as joint stiffness or foot malalignment, which can exacerbate the condition. Failure to address these abnormalities during treatment can result in recurrent bursitis and ongoing pain.
- **Thumb Rule Consideration:** Assess for and correct biomechanical abnormalities, such as joint stiffness or improper foot alignment, to prevent recurrence and optimize patient outcomes.

Neglecting Proper Footwear Adjustments

- One of the key contributing factors to posterior Achilles bursitis is improper footwear, particularly shoes that aggravate the heel. Failing to advise patients on appropriate shoe modifications or orthotic use can lead to persistent symptoms and worsening of the condition.
- **Thumb Rule Consideration:** Recommend footwear modifications, including orthotics, heel pads, or backless shoes, to reduce pressure on the heel and prevent recurrence of bursitis symptoms.

Delayed or Inadequate Surgical Intervention

- In cases where conservative treatment fails, surgery may be necessary to remove part of the heel bone or correct deformities. Delaying necessary surgical intervention or performing incomplete surgeries can result in prolonged pain or recurrence of symptoms.
- **Thumb Rule Consideration:** Consider timely surgical intervention for patients with chronic or recurrent Achilles bursitis that does not respond to conservative measures, ensuring the procedure addresses both the bursa and any underlying deformities.

REFERENCES

- Brinker MR, Miller MD. The adult foot. Fundamentals of Orthopaedics. Philadelphia, Pa: WB Saunders Co; 1999:342-63.
- McGee DJ. Lower leg, ankle, and foot. Orthopedic Physical Assessment. 2nd ed. Philadelphia, Pa: WB Saunders Co; 1992:448-515.
- Snider RK, ed. Foot and ankle. Essentials of Musculoskeletal Care. 2nd ed. Rosemont, Ill: American Academy of Orthopedic Surgeons; 1997:366-489.
- Young JL, Olsen NK, Press JM. Musculoskeletal disorders of the lower limbs. In: Braddom RL, ed. Physical Medicine and Rehabilitation. Philadelphia, Pa: WB Saunders Co; 1996:783-812.
- Lyman J, Weinhold PS, Almekinders LC. Strain behaviour of the distal Achilles tendon: Implications for insertional Achilles tendinopathy. Am J Sports Med 2004; 32(2):457-61.
- Brukner P, Khan Karim. Clinical Sports Medicine. Ch.32. 3rd edition.
- van Sterkenburg MN, Muller B, Maas M, Sierevelt IN, van Dijk CN. Appearance of the weight-bearing lateral radiograph in retrocalcaneal bursitis. Acta Orthop. Jun 2010;81(3):387-90. [Medline].
- Ly JQ, Bui-Mansfield LT. Anatomy of and abnormalities associated with Kager's fat Pad. AJR Am J Roentgenol. Jan 2004;182(1):147-54.

ACUTE INTERMITTENT PORPHYRIA

Acute intermittent porphyria is a rare autosomal dominant disease characterized by a deficiency of hydroxymethylbilane synthase (HMBS). It presents with abdominal pain, nausea, vomiting, peripheral neuropathy, and seizures. Treatment for acute attacks is intravenous heme. Definitive treatment is an orthotopic liver transplant.

Wang B, Rudnick S, Cengia B, Bonkovsky HL. Acute Hepatic Porphyrias: Review and Recent Progress. Hepatol Commun. 2019 Feb;3(2):193-206.

Clinical Description

'Porphyria' has been derived from the ancient Greek word porphura, meaning purple. Porphyrins are precursors of heme, an essential component of hemoglobin. Each subunit of hemoglobin is a globular protein containing an embedded heme group that contains one iron atom, capable of binding one oxygen molecule. The heme synthesis pathway is a multi-step process that involves a specific enzyme at every step. Thus, porphyrias are distinct clinical syndromes, which arise due to deficiency or defect in a particular enzyme needed for a specific step of the heme synthesis pathway. Although these syndromes have conventionally been classified depending on the predominant system involved (cutaneous vs. neurohepatic), significant overlap occurs, and many porphyrias present with mixed symptoms.

The clinical presentation, severity, and prognosis of individual porphyrias depend on which enzyme is deficient and the corresponding heme precursor or porphyrin accumulation. Acute intermittent porphyria (AIP) ranks as the most common and severe form of acute porphyria. Other acute porphyrias include hereditary coproporphyria (HCP), variegate porphyria (VP), and 5-aminolevulinic acid (ALA) dehydratase deficiency porphyria (Doss porphyria).

Similar to the majority of porphyrias, AIP shows an autosomal dominant pattern of inheritance. Acute porphyrias like AIP characteristically demonstrate acute episodes of neurovisceral symptoms but may not manifest fully for a long time. AIP manifests as episodes of abdominal pain, neuropathies, and constipation, but, unlike most other porphyrias, patients with AIP do not develop a cutaneous rash. The primary enzymatic defect in AIP is the deficiency of porphobilinogen-deaminase, also called hydroxymethylbilane synthase (HMBS), the third enzyme in heme synthesis. The acute attacks of AIP are a result of the uncontrolled upregulation of the ALA synthase enzyme. The diagnosis of AIP gets delayed due to nonspecific symptoms and similarities with other diseases. The only cure is orthoptic liver transplantation.

Pearls & Oysters

Systemic arterial hypertension and chronic kidney disease - Reports exist of the prevalence of up to 30% of these closely linked disorders in patients with AIP. End-stage renal disease (ESRD) is a life-threatening complication in AIP patients with chronic active disease. Muscle denervation is another major pathologic complication.

Some patients after acute attacks have residual deficits such as foot/wrist drop or wasting of the intrinsic muscles of hands.

Hepatocellular carcinoma (HCC): This is the most deadly long-term complication of AIP. Results of studies performed over the last 3 to 4 decades have shown a remarkably increased incidence of HCC in AIP patients compared with the general population. A Swedish study showed that the risk for HCC in AIP is increased 80 times after the age of 50 years. It is worthwhile to know that AIP-associated HCC is typically free from the usual preceding comorbidities such as Hepatitis B or C infection.

Bottom Line Statement

Clinicians should suspect acute intermittent porphyria should in patients with abdominal pain, and symptoms or signs suggestive of neuropsychiatric morbidity. A patient with a purely medical ailment often ends up with the surgeons due to recurrent acute abdomen and may undergo unnecessary surgeries. Thus, the surgical team should be aware of this non-surgical cause of severe acute abdomen and maintain a high index of suspicion in a patient with recurrent attacks or one who presents with additional neuropsychiatric symptoms.

Interprofessional involvement of the primary care physician, nurse practitioner, metabolic/genetic disease expert, hematologist, biochemist, pharmacist, nursing, and the surgeon is essential to diagnose the disease early to limit the long-term complications of the patient. Lastly, the involvement of clinical geneticists for genetic counseling regarding the conception of a child by a patient with AIP is paramount to discuss the risk of acquisition, prenatal testing, and other aspects of prevention and/or early identification of AIP carrier state in the offspring. Nursing will be responsible for heme therapy administration and should monitor therapy progress as well as any adverse reactions, and inform the clinician should there be an issue. Pharmacists should verify dosing, as well as perform medication review to scan both for drug interactions, as well as drugs that can precipitate porphyria attacks, reporting any concerns to the team physicians managing the case. Open communication and collaboration between interprofessional members of the team are essential if one wants to avoid the high morbidity of this disorder.

Medico-Legal Traps

Failure to Recognize Acute Intermittent Porphyria (AIP) Early

- AIP presents with vague symptoms such as abdominal pain, nausea, vomiting, and neuropsychiatric symptoms, which are easily mistaken for more common conditions. Misdiagnosis or delayed diagnosis can lead to inappropriate treatments, such as unnecessary surgeries or delayed administration of life-saving heme therapy.
- **Thumb Rule Consideration:** Always consider AIP in patients with unexplained acute abdomen and neuropsychiatric symptoms, particularly when the patient has a history of recurrent episodes.

Improper Management of Acute Attacks

- Mismanagement of acute AIP attacks, including failure to promptly administer intravenous heme or inappropriate use of medications that can precipitate attacks, can worsen the patient's condition, leading to severe complications such as seizures or permanent neurological damage.
- **Thumb Rule Consideration:** Administer intravenous heme promptly during acute attacks and review medications carefully to avoid those that could trigger a porphyria attack.

Overlooking the Need for Genetic Counseling

- AIP is an autosomal dominant disorder, meaning there is a significant risk of transmission to offspring. Failure to refer patients for genetic counseling could result in missed opportunities for early diagnosis or prevention in family members.
- **Thumb Rule Consideration:** Ensure that all patients diagnosed with AIP are referred for genetic counseling to discuss the risk of transmission, prenatal testing, and early identification of the carrier state in offspring.

Neglecting Long-Term Monitoring for Complications

- AIP is associated with serious long-term complications such as systemic arterial hypertension, chronic kidney disease, and hepatocellular carcinoma (HCC). Failure to monitor patients for these complications can lead to delayed detection and poorer outcomes.
- **Thumb Rule Consideration:** Establish long-term monitoring for AIP patients, especially for hypertension, renal function, and hepatocellular carcinoma, to mitigate the risks of serious complications.

Inadequate Interprofessional Collaboration

- AIP requires a multidisciplinary approach involving specialists such as geneticists, hematologists, pharmacists, and surgeons. Failure to ensure proper interprofessional collaboration can result in fragmented care, leading to mismanagement of acute attacks or inadequate long-term care.
- **Thumb Rule Consideration:** Foster strong interprofessional collaboration between geneticists, hematologists, surgeons, and pharmacists to ensure comprehensive care and prevent complications in AIP management.

REFERENCES

- Wang B, Rudnick S, Cengia B, Bonkovsky HL. Acute Hepatic Porphyrias: Review and Recent Progress. Hepatol Commun. 2019 Feb;3(2):193-206.
- Pischik E, Kauppinen R. An update of clinical management of acute intermittent porphyria. Appl Clin Genet. 2015;8:201-14.
- Fontanellas A, Ávila MA, Berraondo P. Emerging therapies for acute intermittent porphyria. Expert Rev Mol Med. 2016 Nov 02;18:e17.
- Szlendak U, Bykowska K, Lipniacka A. Clinical, Biochemical and Molecular Characteristics of the Main Types of Porphyria. Adv Clin Exp Med. 2016 Mar-Apr;25(2):361-8.
- Roveri G, Nascimbeni F, Rocchi E, Ventura P. Drugs and acute porphyrias: reasons for a hazardous relationship. Postgrad Med. 2014 Nov;126(7):108-20.
- Ramanujam VS, Anderson KE. Porphyria Diagnostics-Part 1: A Brief Overview of the Porphyrias. Curr Protoc Hum Genet. 2015 Jul 01;86:17.20.1-17.20.26.
- Cerbino GN, Gerez EN, Varela LS, Melito VA, Parera VE, Batlle A, Rossetti MV. Acute intermittent porphyria in Argentina: an update. Biomed Res Int. 2015;2015:946387.
- Puy H, Gouya L, Deybach JC. Porphyrias. Lancet. 2010 Mar 13;375(9718):924-37.
- Chen B, Solis-Villa C, Hakenberg J, Qiao W, Srinivasan RR, Yasuda M, Balwani M, Doheny D, Peter I, Chen R, Desnick RJ. Acute Intermittent Porphyria: Predicted Pathogenicity of HMBS Variants Indicates Extremely Low Penetrance of the Autosomal Dominant Disease. Hum Mutat. 2016 Nov;37(11):1215-1222.

ADDUCTOR TENDINITIS

Longstanding (chronic) adductor-related groin pain syndrome is a widely common problem for athletes in many sports activities which often drastically reduces player activity and performance. The first choice in therapeutic treatment is conservative therapy.

Biol Sport. 2021 Mar; 38(1): 45–63.

Clinical Description

Adductor-related groin pain syndrome (GPS), is a common problem for athletes in several sports, often reducing the players' activity when chronic. Indeed, its yearly incidence in football (soccer) of 10–18% continues to increase due to many risk factors such as high loads and short recoveries. It is important to note that the majority of injury surveillance studies in football are based on the so called "time loss concept".

The GPS has a multifactorial etiopathogenesis and the adductor tendinopathy is a common, but not easily recognizable cause of longstanding GPS (i.e. chronic adductor-related GPS) especially in athletes. This could be due to an extremely complex hip anatomy with several structures interacting and contributing to its functioning.

The muscles involved in the hip joint adduction movement are: gracilis (the only bi-articular muscle of the group), adductor brevis, adductor longus, adductor magnus, pectineus and obturator externus (all mono-articular muscles). Longstanding adductor-related GPS can be classified as an overuse condition of an adductor muscle tendon (in the majority of cases located at the adductor longus), which leads to disrepair and further degeneration. This is a common injury in many sports activities, especially in those with sudden cutting/changes of direction and/or high mechanical loads, as they transmit both horizontal and cutting forces to the symphysis during athletic activity.

Pearls & Oysters

Despite appropriate physiotherapy management, some patients with this condition do not improve adequately. When this occurs, the treating physiotherapist or doctor can advise on the best course of management. This may include investigations such as an X-ray, ultrasound, CT scan or MRI, pharmaceutical intervention, corticosteroid injection, autologous blood injection or referral to appropriate medical authorities who can advise on any intervention that may be appropriate to improve the condition. A review with a podiatrist may be indicated for the prescription of orthotics in patients with abnormal foot biomechanics. In very rare cases surgical intervention may be considered.

Bottom Line Statement

Adductor-related GPS is a frequent problem in athletes practicing a wide range of sports such as football/soccer, hockey or athletics. For example, in football, adductor-related GPS accounts for 16–18% of all football injuries with an incidence of time loss injury equal to 1.0–1.1 injury/1000 hours of exposure. The first-choice in therapeutic treatment is conservative therapy, and surgical treatment should be considered only if conservative treatment fails. Despite the significant incidence of adductor-related GPS in sports, there are relatively few studies validating the various types of conservative treatment in literature. For instance, there are no studies regarding the use of extra-corporal shock wave therapy, which is widely used in tendinopathies.

Medico-Legal Traps

Failure to Diagnose Adductor Tendinitis Early

- Adductor tendinitis, particularly in athletes, is often underdiagnosed due to its vague presentation and complex hip anatomy. Misdiagnosis or delayed recognition can prolong the injury, leading to chronic groin pain and reduced athletic performance, which can result in medico-legal claims for mismanagement.
- **Thumb Rule Consideration:** Always consider adductor tendinitis in athletes with groin pain, particularly those involved in sports with high mechanical loads and frequent directional changes, and ensure timely and accurate diagnostic imaging.

Inadequate Conservative Treatment

- Conservative therapy, including physiotherapy and rest, is the first line of treatment for adductor tendinitis. Failing to provide adequate conservative management or prematurely escalating to more invasive treatments without a proper trial of conservative options can lead to suboptimal outcomes and legal repercussions.
- **Thumb Rule Consideration:** Prioritize conservative treatments, such as physical therapy, rest, and gradual return to activity, ensuring that these measures are fully explored before considering more invasive interventions like injections or surgery.

Premature Surgical Intervention

- Surgical intervention is rarely necessary for adductor tendinitis and should only be considered when conservative treatments fail. Premature surgery without exhausting less invasive options may lead to complications and potential legal disputes.
- **Thumb Rule Consideration:** Recommend surgery for adductor tendinitis only after thorough and unsuccessful conservative management, and ensure the patient is well-informed about the risks and benefits of surgery.

Neglecting to Address Biomechanical Factors

- Biomechanical abnormalities, such as improper foot alignment or gait issues, often contribute to the development of adductor tendinitis. Failing to address these underlying factors, such as not involving a podiatrist for orthotic prescription, may result in recurrence of the condition and patient dissatisfaction.
- **Thumb Rule Consideration:** Always assess for and address biomechanical factors like abnormal foot biomechanics, and involve a podiatrist early for orthotics or gait correction to prevent recurrence.

Inadequate Monitoring and Follow-up

- Longstanding adductor tendinitis requires careful follow-up to ensure the effectiveness of conservative treatments and to monitor for any need for escalation of care. Failing to provide ongoing monitoring can lead to worsening symptoms and missed opportunities for intervention, resulting in legal exposure.
- **Thumb Rule Consideration:** Ensure regular follow-up with patients undergoing conservative treatment for adductor tendinitis, monitoring progress and adjusting treatment plans as needed to prevent long-term complications.

REFERENCES

- Khan KM, Cook JL, Bonar F, Harcourt P, Astrom M. Histopathology of common tendinopathies. Update and implications for clinical management. Sports Med. 1999;27:393–408
- Ebonie Rio; Dawson Kidgell; G Lorimer Moseley; Jamie Gaida; Sean Docking; Craig Purdam; Jill Cook, Changing the Way we Think About Tendon Rehabilitation A Narrative Review Br J Sports Med. 2016;50(4):209-215.
- Brukner et al (2012). Brukner & Khan's clinical sports medicine (4th ed.), 559. Australia: McGraw Hill Education.
- Cook JL1, Purdam CR. Is tendon pathology a continuum? A pathology model to explain the clinical presentation of load-induced tendinopathy. Br J Sports Med. 2009 Jun;43(6):409-16.
- Holmich P, Uhrskou P, Ulnits L, et al: Effectiveness of active physical training as treatment for long-standing adductor-related groin pain in athletes: Randomised trial. Lancet 353: 439-443, 1999

ANKYLOSING SPONDYLITIS

Ankylosing spondylitis (AS) is a chronic, inflammatory disease of the axial spine. Chronic back pain and progressive spinal stiffness are the most common features of this disease. Involvement of the spine, sacroiliac joints, peripheral joints, digits, and entheses are characteristic. Impaired spinal mobility, postural abnormalities, buttock pain, hip pain, peripheral arthritis, enthesitis, and dactylitis are all commonly associated with ankylosing spondylitis.

Proft F, Poddubnyy D. Ankylosing spondylitis and axial spondyloarthritis: recent insights and impact of new classification criteria. Ther Adv Musculoskelet Dis. 2018 Jun;10(5-6):129-139.

Clinical Description

Ankylosing spondylitis (AS) is a chronic, inflammatory disease of the axial spine that can manifest with various clinical signs and symptoms. Chronic back pain and progressive spinal stiffness are the most common features of the disease. Involvement of the spine and sacroiliac (SI) joints, peripheral joints, digits, entheses are characteristic of the disease. Impaired spinal mobility, postural abnormalities, buttock pain, hip pain, peripheral arthritis, enthesitis, and dactylitis ("sausage digits") are all associated with AS.

Extraskeletal organs may also be affected by this disease. The most common extraarticular manifestations of AS include inflammatory bowel disease (up to 50%), acute anterior uveitis (25% to 35%), and psoriasis (approximately 10%). AS is also associated with an increased risk of cardiovascular disease. The cause of this increased risk has been postulated to be due to the systemic inflammation evident in AS. Pulmonary complications are also associated with AS, as diminished chest wall expansion and decreased spinal mobility predispose patients to a restrictive pulmonary pattern.

Finally, AS predisposes people to at least a two-fold increased incidence of vertebral fragility fractures. These patients are also at increased risk of atlantoaxial subluxation, spinal cord injury, and, rarely, cauda equina syndrome.

Pearls & Oysters

The possibility of vertebral fracture should always be considered in patients with ankylosing spondylitis (AS), even after minor trauma. Patients with AS are at increased risk of vertebral fracture and subluxation, especially of the cervical spine. Therefore, these patients are more susceptible to neurologic compromise.

Prevention of disease morbidity can be achieved with exercise, physical therapy, tailored pharmacologic intervention, and regimented follow-up appointments with providers.

Bottom Line Statement

Ankylosing spondylitis (AS) is a systemic disorder that can affect many organ systems and hence an interprofessional team approach is recommended to avoid the morbidity.

Rheumatologist to evaluate and manage the acute symptoms and address any coexisting spondyloarthropathies.

Gastroenterologist to assess for inflammatory bowel disease.

Ophthalmologist to assess for anterior uveitis.

Cardiologist to assess for heart block or valvular involvement.

Physical therapy to help with function.

Neurologist to assess for nerve compression syndromes.

Pharmacist to monitor for drug interactions and dependence on analgesics.

Nurse to educate the patient on the management of daily living activities.

There are many reports indicating that an interprofessional approach to ankylosing spondylitis can improve function, lower pain and increase the quality of life.

Medico-Legal Traps

Failure to Diagnose Ankylosing Spondylitis (AS) Early

- Ankylosing spondylitis often presents with non-specific symptoms like chronic back pain and stiffness, which can be mistaken for more common musculoskeletal conditions. Failure to diagnose AS early can delay proper treatment, leading to irreversible spinal damage and complications such as vertebral fractures or nerve compression syndromes.
- **Thumb Rule Consideration:** Always consider AS in patients with chronic back pain, particularly if it is inflammatory in nature (worse in the morning or with rest) and involves reduced spinal mobility or sacroiliac joint pain.

Neglecting to Assess and Treat Extra-Articular Manifestations

- AS can affect multiple organ systems, including the eyes, cardiovascular system, and gastrointestinal tract. Failure to recognize and manage these extra-articular manifestations, such as uveitis or inflammatory bowel disease, can lead to severe complications, vision loss, or life-threatening conditions.

- **Thumb Rule Consideration:** Ensure a multidisciplinary approach that includes regular assessment for uveitis, inflammatory bowel disease, and cardiovascular risks in patients with AS to prevent extra-articular complications.

Inadequate Monitoring for Vertebral Fractures and Spinal Injuries

- Patients with AS are at higher risk for vertebral fractures, even after minor trauma, due to reduced bone density and spinal rigidity. Failing to monitor for these fractures, especially in the cervical spine, can lead to serious complications, including spinal cord injury and neurological deficits.
- **Thumb Rule Consideration:** Always suspect vertebral fractures in AS patients following trauma, no matter how minor, and conduct appropriate imaging and neurologic evaluations to prevent permanent damage.

Overlooking Pulmonary and Cardiovascular Complications

- AS is associated with restrictive pulmonary disease due to limited chest expansion and increased risk of cardiovascular complications from systemic inflammation. Failure to monitor for these conditions can result in missed diagnoses of serious comorbidities like heart disease or lung complications.
- **Thumb Rule Consideration:** Regularly assess chest expansion and respiratory function, and screen for cardiovascular risk factors in patients with AS to detect and manage these complications early.

Inadequate Long-Term Management and Lack of Interprofessional Collaboration

- AS requires long-term management involving multiple specialists, including rheumatologists, physical therapists, gastroenterologists, and ophthalmologists. Failing to engage an interprofessional team or to provide regimented follow-up can result in poor disease control, increased morbidity, and patient dissatisfaction.
- **Thumb Rule Consideration:** Implement an interprofessional care plan for AS patients, ensuring consistent follow-up with relevant specialists, and maintain regular assessments to address systemic and skeletal complications.

REFERENCES

- Bridgewood C, Watad A, Cuthbert RJ, McGonagle D. Spondyloarthritis: new insights into clinical aspects, translational immunology and therapeutics. Curr Opin Rheumatol. 2018 Sep;30(5):526-532.
- Watad A, Cuthbert RJ, Amital H, McGonagle D. Enthesitis: Much More Than Focal Insertion Point Inflammation. Curr Rheumatol Rep. 2018 May 30;20(7):41.
- Mahmoudi M, Garshasbi M, Ashraf-Ganjouei A, Javinani A, Vojdanian M, Saafi M, Ahmadzadeh N, Jamshidi A. Association between rs6759298 and Ankylosing Spondylitis in Iranian Population. Avicenna J Med Biotechnol. 2018 Jul-Sep;10(3):178-182.
- van den Berg R, Jongbloed EM, de Schepper EIT, Bierma-Zeinstra SMA, Koes BW, Luijsterburg PAJ. The association between pro-inflammatory biomarkers and nonspecific low back pain: a systematic review. Spine J. 2018 Nov;18(11):2140-2151.
- Wang R, Ward MM. Epidemiology of axial spondyloarthritis: an update. Curr Opin Rheumatol. 2018 Mar;30(2):137-143.
- Aloush V, Dotan I, Ablin JN, Elkayam O. Evaluating IBD-specific antiglycan antibodies in serum of patients with spondyloarthritis and rheumatoid arthritis: are they really specific? Clin Exp Rheumatol. 2019 Jan-Feb;37(1):32-36.
- Rabelo CF, Baptista TSA, Petersen LE, Bauer ME, Keiserman MW, Staub HL. Serum IL-6 correlates with axial mobility index (Bath Ankylosing Spondylitis Metrology Index) in Brazilian patients with ankylosing spondylitis. Open Access Rheumatol. 2018;10:21-25.
- Rahbar MH, Lee M, Hessabi M, Tahanan A, Brown MA, Learch TJ, Diekman LA, Weisman MH, Reveille JD. Harmonization, data management, and statistical issues related to prospective multicenter studies in Ankylosing spondylitis (AS): Experience from the Prospective Study Of Ankylosing Spondylitis (PSOAS) cohort. Contemp Clin Trials Commun. 2018 Sep;11:127-135.

ANCONEUS EPITROCHLEARIS

The discrepancy regarding the AEM starts by its nomenclature. In 1866, it was termed the anconeus sextus muscle by Gruber; unlike the fourth and fifth anconeus muscles, which are treated as variations of the triceps brachii muscle, the AEM is considered a variation of the flexor carpi ulnaris. It is also called the anconeus internus, the epitrochleo-olecranonis, and the epitrochleocubital. The clinical signs of this syndrome are sensory loss or hypoesthesia in the fourth and fifth digits and loss of strength in finger abduction.

Chalmers J. Unusual causes of peripheral nerve compression. Hand (N Y). 1978;10:168-175.

Clinical Description

The anconeus epitrochlearis, which is found in 1–34% of individuals, was first described by Gruber in 1866. Gruber investigated the presence of the anconeus epitrochlearis muscle using 100 cadavers. He found the muscle in 26 males and eight females and that it was bilateral in 15 males and four females The anconeus epitrochlearis (AE) is an anomalous accessory muscle known to compress the ulnar nerve at the elbow leading to classical symptoms of cubital tunnel syndrome. The prevalence of this anomalous muscle is estimated to be 3% to 34% based on cadaveric and imaging studies and is often found bilaterally. Classically, this muscle was described as an extension of the medial head of the triceps and often presents in conjunction with an enlarged medial triceps muscle. In fact, prior reports show AE shortening with elbow extension and relaxation with passive elbow extension suggesting it to be an extension of the medial head of the triceps. In contrast to the triceps, this muscle is innervated by a branch of the ulnar nerve.

Pearls & Oysters

The major complications associated with anconeus epitrochlearis fall into two categories:

(1) iatrogenically induced complications resulting from persistent and overaggressive treatment of "resistant golfer's elbow" and

(2) the potential for permanent neurological deficits resulting from prolonged untreated entrapment of the ulnar nerve.

Failure of the clinician to recognize an acute inflammatory or infectious arthritis of the elbow may result in permanent damage to the joint and chronic pain and functional disability.

Bottom Line Statement

Cubital tunnel syndrome is compression of the ulnar nerve about the elbow and is the second most common compressive neuropathy after carpal tunnel syndrome, affecting up to 5.9% of the population. The AE has long been thought to be a compressive force on the ulnar nerve and the clinical implications are not well known. When present, the AE muscle occupies more space than the typically present Osborne fascia. Patients with cubital tunnel syndrome and an AE accessory muscle improve after release of this muscle. Prior case reports have hypothesized that ulnar neuropathy associated with an AE muscle may be dynamic and have different characteristics than idiopathic cubital tunnel syndrome including a more rapid progression, younger age of presentation, and shorter duration of symptoms. Others have suggested that the AE may provide a more forgiving roof to the cubital tunnel syndrome than the more common fascial layer and actually be more protective from developing cubital tunnel syndrome.

Medico-Legal Traps

Failure to Diagnose Anconeus Epitrochlearis (AE) as a Cause of Cubital Tunnel Syndrome

- AE is a rare anatomical variation that can compress the ulnar nerve, leading to cubital tunnel syndrome. Failure to recognize AE as a potential cause in patients with ulnar nerve symptoms may result in delayed diagnosis and unnecessary treatments, such as therapies targeting "golfer's elbow" or idiopathic causes.
- **Thumb Rule Consideration:** Always consider AE as a differential diagnosis in patients presenting with cubital tunnel syndrome symptoms, especially if conservative treatments fail or there is an unexplained recurrence of symptoms.

Overaggressive Treatment for Golfer's Elbow

- Persistent and overaggressive treatment for "resistant golfer's elbow" without considering the possibility of AE or cubital tunnel syndrome could lead to unnecessary interventions and worsen the patient's condition. This may result in legal claims of iatrogenic harm.
- **Thumb Rule Consideration:** Avoid overaggressive treatments for medial elbow pain without investigating the possibility of ulnar nerve compression due to AE or other anatomical variations.

Delayed Surgical Intervention for Ulnar Nerve Compression

- Prolonged ulnar nerve entrapment due to AE can lead to permanent neurological deficits, including sensory loss and weakness in the hand. Delayed or inadequate surgical decompression may result in irreversible damage and legal liability for failure to provide timely care.
- **Thumb Rule Consideration:** In patients with suspected AE-related ulnar nerve compression, consider early surgical intervention to prevent permanent nerve damage, especially if symptoms progress rapidly.

Inadequate Preoperative Imaging and Misdiagnosis

- Failing to obtain detailed preoperative imaging, such as ultrasound or MRI, to confirm the presence of AE can result in misdiagnosis and inappropriate treatment. This can lead to legal challenges if a patient undergoes surgery without addressing the actual anatomical cause of their symptoms.
- **Thumb Rule Consideration:** Always obtain appropriate imaging to confirm the presence of AE in cases of cubital tunnel syndrome before proceeding with surgical decompression.

Failure to Recognize Dynamic Ulnar Neuropathy

- AE-related ulnar neuropathy may present differently from idiopathic cubital tunnel syndrome, with more rapid progression and a younger age of onset. Failure to recognize these characteristics and adjust the treatment plan accordingly can lead to suboptimal outcomes.
- **Thumb Rule Consideration:** Be aware that AE-related cubital tunnel syndrome may have dynamic features and progress more rapidly than typical cases, necessitating earlier intervention and tailored treatment.

REFERENCES

- Byun SD, Kim CH, Jeon IH. Ulnar neuropathy caused by an anconeus epitrochlearis: clinical and electrophysiological findings. J Hand Surg Eur Vol. 2011;36:607-608.
- Cheriyan T, Neuhaus V, Mudgal CS. Velocity drop in anconeus epitrochlearis-associated cubital tunnel syndrome. Am J Orthop (Belle Mead NJ). 2014;43:227-229.
- Dekelver I, Van Glabbeek F, Dijs H, et al. Bilateral ulnar nerve entrapment by the M. anconeus epitrochlearis. A case report and literature review. Clin Rheumatol. 2012;31:1139-1142.
- Erdem Bagatur A, Yalcin MB, Ozer UE. Anconeus epitrochlearis muscle causing ulnar neuropathy at the elbow: clinical and neurophysiological differential diagnosis. Orthopedics. 2016;39:e988-e991.

  Husarik DB, Saupe N, Pfirrmann CW, et al. Elbow nerves: MR findings in 60 asymptomatic subjects—normal anatomy, variants, and pitfalls. Radiology. 2009;252:148-156.
- O'Hara JJ, Stone JH. Ulnar nerve compression at the elbow caused by a prominent medial head of the triceps and an anconeus epitrochlearis muscle. J Hand Surg Br. 1996;21:133-135.

ANTERIOR CUTANEOUS NERVE ENTRAPMENT

Anterior cutaneous nerve entrapment syndrome (ACNES) is a commonly underdiagnosed and undertreated chronic state of pain. This syndrome is characterized by the entrapment of the cutaneous branches of the lower thoracoabdominal intercostal nerves at the lateral border of the rectus abdominis muscle, which causes severe, often refractory, chronic pain.

J Pain Res. 2017; 10: 145–156.

Clinical Description

Chronic abdominal wall pain might have variable etiologies, and thus it requires thorough clinical and laboratory investigations. Abdominal cutaneous nerve entrapment syndrome (ACNES) is one of the causes of chronic abdominal pain, which is mostly underdiagnosed and not appropriately treated. In this syndrome, the cutaneous branches of the lower thoracoabdominal intercostal nerves are entrapped at the lateral border of the rectus abdominis muscle, resulting in a severe, often refractory, chronic pain. The prevalence of the syndrome ranges between 15% and 30% depending on the definition and the diagnostic criteria used. In adolescents, it is reported to be diagnosed in one out of eight cases of chronic abdominal pain. In the emergency department, the prevalence of ACNES in the patients presenting with acute abdominal pain has been reported to be 2%.

Anatomically, the lower intercostal nerves (T8–T12) run between the internal oblique and transversus abdominis muscles, up to the point where they reach the rectus abdominis; here, they make a turn in their course to enter the rectus channels (commonly five at each abdominal side). Some authors have suggested that the entrapment is usually caused by this sudden turn in their course into the rectus abdominis channel, leading to ACNES. The muscle contraction at this location may cause additional nerve compression, and therefore mechanical or ischemic irritation, which results in severe pain.

The pain is usually localized with a dull and sharp component or may radiate to the ipsilateral half abdomen, following the course of the nerves. The pain, most of the times, can easily be identified by palpation at the painful site, while a positive Carnett's sign may facilitate the diagnosis. Carnett's sign, named after the scientist who described it in 1926, is when an examiner localizes the exact spot of maximal tenderness on the abdominal wall and asks the patient to raise his head and/or torso with the arms crossed over the chest. An increased or constant level of pain during this movement, with the examiner's finger in place, indicates that the cause of pain is in the abdominal wall. On the contrary, a negative Carnett's sign indicates a possible visceral cause of the pain.

Pearls & Oysters

Interventional techniques were the main therapeutic option employed in most of the studies on pain management in ACNES. These techniques include the trigger point injections (blind or ultrasound-guided), neurolytic techniques (chemical neurolysis or radiofrequency ablation), surgical techniques (anterior neurectomy and mesh reinforcement), and newer techniques such as botulinum toxin injection and neuromodulation.

Bottom Line Statement

ACNES should always be considered in the differential diagnosis of chronic abdominal pain, and specific diagnostic steps should be followed. The multimodal biopsychosocial approach should never be ignored in all cases, since interventional techniques alone may not be adequate for a successful pain management, especially in persistent refractory cases that have already undergone many treatment plan modifications. It is also wise to consider systemic drug administration following the guidelines for neuropathic pain management, since they may facilitate recovery and further improve patient's quality of life. A multimodal approach is always beneficial in such patients aiming for better long-term recovery. The best approach is yet to be defined, and further research carried out in a more systematic manner employing advanced techniques such as ultrasound-guided procedures is required on the subject.

Medico-Legal Traps

Failure to Diagnose Anterior Cutaneous Nerve Entrapment Syndrome (ACNES)

- ACNES is often underdiagnosed due to its overlapping symptoms with other causes of chronic abdominal pain, such as visceral conditions. Failure to recognize this condition can result in unnecessary diagnostic tests and treatments, such as surgeries for suspected visceral causes, leading to patient harm.
- **Thumb Rule Consideration:** Always consider ACNES in the differential diagnosis of chronic abdominal pain, especially when the pain is localized, and ensure the use of Carnett's sign to distinguish it from visceral pain.

Overlooking Carnett's Sign During Clinical Evaluation

- Carnett's sign is a key diagnostic tool for ACNES, but failure to perform or interpret it correctly can lead to misdiagnosis. Without this test, clinicians may pursue invasive investigations or treatments that do not address the true cause of the patient's pain, potentially causing legal issues due to mismanagement.

- **Thumb Rule Consideration:** Always use Carnett's sign when evaluating chronic abdominal pain to differentiate between abdominal wall and visceral pain, and document the findings clearly.

Inappropriate or Delayed Interventional Treatments

- ACNES may require interventional treatments like nerve block injections, radiofrequency ablation, or surgical neurectomy. Delaying these interventions or failing to offer them to patients with refractory pain can result in prolonged suffering and potential legal claims for neglecting effective pain management options.
- **Thumb Rule Consideration:** Consider early interventional treatments for patients with confirmed ACNES who do not respond to conservative therapy, and ensure the interventions are guided by imaging when necessary.

Mismanagement of Persistent or Refractory ACNES Cases

- ACNES can be refractory to conservative treatments, and failure to adopt a multimodal approach that includes both interventional and pharmacological management of neuropathic pain may lead to patient dissatisfaction and legal liability.
- **Thumb Rule Consideration:** For refractory ACNES cases, implement a multimodal pain management approach, including systemic medications for neuropathic pain and interventional procedures, to provide comprehensive care.

Neglecting to Follow a Multimodal Biopsychosocial Approach

- ACNES management may fail if clinicians focus solely on interventional techniques without addressing the psychological and social aspects of chronic pain. Ignoring the biopsychosocial approach can result in poor outcomes and legal repercussions for inadequate pain management.
- **Thumb Rule Consideration:** Always integrate a multimodal biopsychosocial approach when managing ACNES, addressing both physical and psychological aspects of chronic pain to improve long-term patient outcomes.

REFERENCES

- Applegate WV. Abdominal cutaneous nerve entrapment syndrome (ACNES): a commonly overlooked cause of abdominal pain. Perm J. 2002;6:20–27.
- Koop H, Koprdova S, Schurmann C. Chronic abdominal wall pain. A poorly recognized clinical problem. Dtsch Arztebl Int. 2016;113(4):51–57.
- Siawash M, de Jager-Klevit JW, Ten WT, Roumen RM, Scheltinga MR. Prevalence of anterior cutaneous nerve entrapment syndrome in a pediatric population with chronic abdominal pain. J Pediatr Gastroenterol Nutr. 2016;62(3):399–402.
- van Assen T, Brouns J, Scheltinga M, Roumen R. Incidence of abdominal pain due to the anterior cutaneous nerve entrapment syndrome in an emergency department. Scand J Trauma Resusc Emerg Med. 2015;23(19):2–6.
- Kanakarajan S, High K, Nagaraja R. Chronic abdominal wall pain and ultrasound-guided abdominal cutaneous nerve infiltration. A case series. Pain Med. 2011;12(3):382–386.
- Siawash M, Maatman R, Tjon A, Ten W, van Heurn E, Roumen R, Scheltinga M. Anterior neurectomy in children with a recalcitrant anterior cutaneous nerve entrapment syndrome is safe and successful. J Pediatr Surg. 2016 Sep 1; Epub.
- Applegate WV, Buchwalter NR. Microanatomy of the structures contributing to abdominal cutaneous nerve entrapment syndrome. J Am Board Fam Pract. 1997;10(5):329–332.
- Srinivasan R, Greenbaum DS. Chronic abdominal wall pain: a frequently overlooked problem. Practical approach to diagnosis and management. Am J Gastroenterol. 2002;97(4):824–830.
- Hooten WM, Timming R, Belgrade M, et al. Institute for Clinical Systems Improvement. Assessment and Management of Chronic Pain. Nov, 2013. Updated.
- Roderick B, Norman B. Anterior cutaneous nerve entrapment syndrome: an unusual cause of abdominal pain during pregnancy. Int J Obstet Anesth. 2016;25:96–97.
- Imajo Y, Komasawa N, Fujiwara S, Minami T. Transversus abdominal plane and rectus sheath block combination for intractable anterior cutaneous nerve entrapment syndrome after severe cholecystitis. J Clin Anesth. 2016;31:119.
- Sahoo RK, Nair A. Ultrasound guided transversus abdominis plane block for anterior cutaneous nerve entrapment syndrome. Korean J Pain. 2015;28(4):284–286.

ANTERIOR INTEROSSEOUS SYNDROME

Anterior interosseus syndrome is an isolated palsy of flexor pollicus longus, the index and long fingers of the flexor digitorum profundus, and the pronator quadratus muscles of the forearm. It manifests as pain in the forearm accompanied commonly by the weakness of the index and thumb finger pincer movement.

Aljawder A, Faqi MK, Mohamed A, Alkhalifa F. Anterior interosseous nerve syndrome diagnosis and intraoperative findings: A case report. Int J Surg Case Rep. 2016;21:44-7.

Clinical Description

The anterior interosseous nerve (AIN) is the terminal motor branch of the median nerve. It branches from the median nerve in the proximal forearm between the two heads of the pronator teres muscle to run deep along the interosseous membrane. From proximal to distal, it innervates the flexor pollicus longus (FPL), the index and long fingers of the flexor digitorum profundus (FDP), and the pronator quadratus (PQ). AIN syndrome is an isolated palsy of these three muscles. It manifests mostly as pain in the forearm accompanied frequently by a characteristic weakness of the index and thumb finger pincer movement. Many cases of AIN syndrome arise secondary to transient neuritis, although nerve compression and trauma are known etiologies as well. Different explanations have been proposed as the etiology of the disease. Controversy still exists among upper extremity surgeons about it; nevertheless, the condition is considered a neuritis in most cases.

Parsonage and Turner first described the syndrome in 1948. Leslie Gordon Kiloh and Samuel Nevin defined it as an isolated lesion of the anterior interosseous nerve in 1952. Its old name was Kiloh-Nevin syndrome. Different methods of treatment with reasonable outcomes have been reported. Both surgical and medical interventions have been addressed with different timing and variable results.

Pearls & Oysters

Complications include those of the disease process that caused the syndrome or those of the surgery intended to treat it. Anterior interosseous nerve entrapment or compression injury remains a challenging clinical diagnosis. It is difficult because it is mainly a motor nerve and the syndrome is often mistaken for a ligamentous finger injury. Differential diagnosis includes stenosing tenosynovitis, flexor tendon adherence or adhesion, flexor tendon rupture, and brachial neuritis. Brachial plexus neuritis can cause very similar syndromes.

Bottom Line Statement

Even though anterior interosseous nerve syndrome is very rare, clinical suspicion ought to arise in the presence of the radial flexor digitorum profundus and weak flexor pollicis longus muscles. The utilization of electrodiagnostic studies, coupled with MRI, is poised to assist in the diagnosis of anterior interosseous syndrome and help to specify the possible etiology.

Anterior interosseous nerve syndrome's optimal treatment has not yet been established. It is recommended that surgical interventions be offered only to those patients who do not demonstrate any clinical improvement during the first few months or to those with confirmed cases of compression neuropathy. Meticulous dissection is necessary during median nerve surgical decompression to establish sites of compression. It is critical in the identification and release of any other compressing edges or fibrous bands.

An interprofessional approach to treatment is ideal. This approach includes primary care providers who encounter the disease first and electrophysiologists who run the nerve and muscle studies. It also includes orthopedic surgeons who follow the course of treatment, pharmacists who provide the medication needed, and physical therapists who perform the rehabilitation. Other healthcare team personnel such as the nursing staff should also assist in the coordinated care of the patient. This will result in the best outcomes.

Medico-Legal Traps

Failure to Diagnose Anterior Interosseous Syndrome (AIS) Early

- AIS presents with forearm pain and motor weakness, particularly in the thumb and index finger pincer movement. Failure to recognize these symptoms and misdiagnosing it as a ligamentous injury or tendon issue can delay appropriate treatment, resulting in prolonged disability or unnecessary interventions.
- **Thumb Rule Consideration:** Always consider AIS in patients with isolated motor deficits in the forearm, particularly weakness in thumb and index finger pincer movement, and confirm with electrodiagnostic studies or MRI.

Misdiagnosis as a Tendon or Ligament Injury

- AIS can be confused with conditions such as stenosing tenosynovitis or tendon adherence, leading to inappropriate treatments like corticosteroid injections or physical therapy, which are ineffective for nerve-related issues. This can delay proper diagnosis and lead to legal repercussions for unnecessary treatments.

- **Thumb Rule Consideration:** Ensure thorough differential diagnosis by considering nerve involvement in cases of isolated motor weakness, and avoid assuming tendon or ligament pathology without proper diagnostic studies.

Inappropriate Surgical Intervention

- Surgical decompression is recommended only in cases of confirmed nerve compression or when there is no improvement after months of conservative treatment. Premature or unnecessary surgery can lead to complications, including further nerve damage or failed outcomes, increasing medico-legal risks.
- **Thumb Rule Consideration:** Reserve surgical interventions for confirmed cases of nerve compression or after a failure of conservative treatment, ensuring that the timing and necessity of surgery are fully justified.

Inadequate Use of Electrodiagnostic and Imaging Studies

- Failure to utilize electrodiagnostic studies or MRI to confirm the diagnosis of AIS and identify nerve compression can result in misdiagnosis and suboptimal treatment. This may lead to prolonged patient suffering and potential legal claims for diagnostic errors.
- **Thumb Rule Consideration:** Always use electrodiagnostic studies and MRI in patients with suspected AIS to confirm the diagnosis and identify the exact site of nerve compression or injury.

Lack of Multidisciplinary Care

- AIS treatment requires a multidisciplinary approach, including primary care, electrophysiologists, orthopedic surgeons, and physical therapists. Failure to involve the appropriate specialists in diagnosis, treatment planning, and rehabilitation can lead to incomplete care and poor outcomes, increasing legal vulnerability.
- **Thumb Rule Consideration:** Implement a multidisciplinary treatment approach for AIS, involving specialists from neurology, orthopedics, and physical therapy to ensure comprehensive care and optimal outcomes for the patient.

REFERENCES

- Tyszkiewicz T, Atroshi I. Bilateral anterior interosseous nerve syndrome with 6-year interval. SAGE Open Med Case Rep. 2018;6:2050313X18777416.
- Rodner CM, Tinsley BA, O'Malley MP. Pronator syndrome and anterior interosseous nerve syndrome. J Am Acad Orthop Surg. 2013 May;21(5):268-75.
- Ochi K, Horiuchi Y, Tazaki K, Takayama S, Matsumura T. Fascicular constrictions in patients with spontaneous palsy of the anterior interosseous nerve and the posterior interosseous nerve. J Plast Surg Hand Surg. 2012 Feb;46(1):19-24.
- Park IJ, Roh YT, Jeong C, Kim HM. Spontaneous anterior interosseous nerve syndrome: clinical analysis of eleven surgical cases. J Plast Surg Hand Surg. 2013 Dec;47(6):519-23.
- Schulte-Mattler WJ, Grimm T. [Common and not so common nerve entrapment syndromes: diagnostics, clinical aspects and therapy]. Nervenarzt. 2015 Feb;86(2):133-41.
- Feldman MI, Muhammad K, Beltran J: Preoperative diagnosis of anterior interosseous nerve syndrome resulting in complete recovery, Eur J Radiol Extra 69:e73–e76, 2009.
- Waldman SD: Anterior interosseous syndrome. In Waldman SD, editor: Pain review, Philadelphia, 2009, Saunders, pp 271–272.
- Waldman SD: Anterior interosseous syndrome. In Waldman SD, Campbell RSD, editors: Imaging of pain, Philadelphia, 2011, Saunders, pp 291–293.

ANTERIOR TALOFIBULAR PAIN SYNDROME

The Anterior Talo-Fibular Ligament (ATFL) is one of three ligaments that make up to Lateral Collateral Ligament of the ankle. The ATFL is a short ligament that widens slightly from top to bottom.

Bonnel FT, Toullec E, Mabit C, Tourné Y. Chronic ankle instability: biomechanics and pathomechanics of ligaments injury and associated lesions. Orthopaedics & traumatology: Surgery & research. 2010 Jun 1;96(4):424-32.

Clinical Description

The anterior talofibular ligament originates from the anterior edge of the lateral malleolus of the fibula and attaches to the neck of the talus, in front of the lateral malleolar facet. The function of the ATFL is to resist inversion and plantar flexion of the ankle joint. Injury to the ATFL usually occurs when the athlete's center of gravity is shifted over the lateral border of the weight-bearing leg, causing the ankle to roll inward at a high velocity. The ATFL is the weakest of the lateral collateral ligaments and therefore the first to be injured. Mechanisms of injury may include landing awkwardly on an opponent's foot, catching the outer aspect of the foot on the ground terrain, or a slide tackle that contacts the inside of the opponent's weight-bearing leg.

Ankle ligamentous sprains are the most common single type of acute sport trauma. Ankle ligament sprains were also reported to be the most common injury for college athletics in the United States. The anterior talofibular ligament is the most commonly injured ligament in the ankle.

Pearls & Oysters

A conservative approach including rest and non-steroidal anti-inflammatory drugs is the usual first-line treatment. If this fails, subtalar arthrodesis can be safely performed. For patients with an accessory anterolateral talar joint, results have been promising for a subtalar-sparing operative strategy, which may save early-onset ankle degenerative changes seen with subtalar arthrodesis, especially given the young age of patients with primary extra-articular lateral hindfoot impingement.

Bottom Line Statement

Anterior talofibular ligament injuries typically occur with an inversion injury to the ankle, either with or without plantar flexion. Approximately two-thirds of ankle sprains tend to be isolated injuries to the anterior talofibular ligament

(ATFL), the weakest ligament in the lateral collateral complex of the ankle. There is general agreement that avulsion is more common at the fibular than at the talar end of the ligament.

Anterior talofibular ligament (ATFL) injury is the most common of the ligament injuries that can occur as part of the lateral ligament complex injuries. The injuries can comprise either soft tissue tears, avulsion fractures or both.

Medico-Legal Traps

Failure to Diagnose Anterior Talofibular Ligament (ATFL) Injury

- ATFL injuries are common but can be missed or misdiagnosed as simple ankle sprains, leading to inadequate treatment and chronic instability. Delayed or improper diagnosis may result in chronic pain, instability, and further damage, potentially leading to legal claims for mismanagement.
- **Thumb Rule Consideration:** Always suspect ATFL injury in patients with ankle inversion injuries, particularly if there is persistent pain or instability, and confirm diagnosis with appropriate imaging such as MRI or ultrasound.

Inadequate Conservative Treatment

- Conservative treatments, such as rest, bracing, and physical therapy, are often the first line of management for ATFL injuries. However, failing to properly implement or monitor conservative treatment, or prematurely dismissing the need for further interventions, may result in chronic instability or long-term damage.
- **Thumb Rule Consideration:** Ensure proper and sustained conservative treatment with appropriate follow-up, and reassess if the patient continues to experience instability or pain to prevent long-term complications.

Delayed Surgical Intervention for Chronic Instability

- In cases where conservative treatments fail, delayed surgical intervention for chronic ankle instability can worsen outcomes and lead to early degenerative changes. Patients may pursue legal action if their chronic instability and pain are not adequately addressed in a timely manner.
- **Thumb Rule Consideration:** If conservative management fails and chronic instability persists, consider early surgical intervention to stabilize the ankle and prevent long-term degenerative changes.

Mismanagement of Associated Injuries

- ATFL injuries can occur with other ligament injuries or fractures, such as avulsion fractures. Failing to diagnose or manage these associated injuries can lead to poor outcomes and medico-legal issues due to incomplete or incorrect treatment.

- **Thumb Rule Consideration:** Always evaluate for associated injuries, such as avulsion fractures or additional ligament damage, when treating ATFL injuries, and ensure comprehensive management of all involved structures.

Improper Rehabilitation After Surgical or Conservative Treatment

- Whether treated conservatively or surgically, rehabilitation plays a crucial role in recovery from ATFL injuries. Inadequate or improper rehabilitation can lead to prolonged recovery, recurrent injuries, and long-term instability, increasing legal risk for poor treatment outcomes.
- **Thumb Rule Consideration:** Ensure patients receive structured rehabilitation after both conservative and surgical treatments for ATFL injuries, with tailored exercises to restore strength, stability, and range of motion in the ankle.

REFERENCES

- Dubin JC, Comeau D, McClelland RI, Dubin RA, Ferrel E. Lateral and syndesmotic ankle sprain injuries: a narrative literature review. Journal of chiropractic medicine. 2011 Sep 1;10(3):204-19.
- Fong DT, Chan YY, Mok KM, Yung PS, Chan KM. Understanding acute ankle ligamentous sprain injury in sports. BMC Sports Science, Medicine and Rehabilitation. 2009 Dec 1;1(1):14.
- Kumai T, Takakura Y, Rufai A, Milz S, Benjamin M. The functional anatomy of the human anterior talofibular ligament in relation to ankle sprains. Journal of anatomy. 2002 May;200(5):457-65.
- Clinically Relevant Technologies. Available from: http://www.youtube.com/watch?v=Z4rvAT3a7OY. [Last Accessed: 21 October 2020
- The Physio Channel. How to do the Talar Tilt Test for the ankle. Available from: https://www.youtube.com/watch?v=dp7usAmLl5c [Last Accessed: 21 October 2020]

ATYPICAL ODONTALGIA

Atypical odontalgia (AO), also termed phantom tooth pain or non-odontogenic tooth pain, is a disease characterized by continuous pain affecting the teeth or tooth sockets after extraction in the absence of any identifiable cause on clinical or radiographic examination. AO is a specific problem in the dental field, and it seems to be surprisingly complex. Antidepressants, such as amitriptyline, are reported to be effective in the treatment of AO; however, their efficacy varies depending on the case.

Marbach JJ, Raphael KG. Phantom tooth pain: a new look at an old dilemma. Pain Med. 2000;1(1):68–77.

Clinical Description

Patients with atypical odontalgia (AO) complain of medically unexplained toothache. Symptoms include pain without any pathological changes and/or stronger pain than would be expected from the clinical findings. AO is a subgroup of persistent idiopathic facial pain disorder as defined by the International Headache Society. Any dental procedures including scaling, restorative treatment, and endodontic treatment pose potential risk of AO. In many cases, the persistent nature of the pain prompts dentists to treat the teeth in the absence of any pathological findings. The treatment often exacerbates the pain instead of relieving it. Dentists usually consider a diagnosis of AO only after the failure of invasive treatment. Although it is crucial to establish diagnostic criteria for AO, the evidence-based literature to date has been insufficient to make this possible.

Several clinical management methods for AO have been reported. The pathophysiological mechanism of AO may provide useful information for effective management. Possible pathophysiological mechanisms for AO include those with neuropathic, vascular, and psychogenic origins. Since the clinical course of AO varies among patients, and each case may stem from a different origin, a universal treatment method may not be effective for all AO patients, and it may be difficult to establish an evidence base for clinical management.

Pearls & Oysters

There is insufficient evidence-based data available to establish guidelines for the diagnosis and treatment of AO thus far. Several diagnostic criteria for AO have been proposed. Common findings in the criteria are "Pain is described as a toothache" and "No radiographic or laboratory investigations demonstrate relevant abnormality." Many other findings are shown in the criteria, but may not be essential for diagnosis. The present clinical questions addressing prevalence, comorbid diseases, and the characteristics of the pain may be useful for the establishment of diagnostic criteria. Further investigations are needed to consolidate the evidence base.

Bottom Line Statement

Evidence-based data are also needed to establish guidelines for treatment and management of AO. Precise pathophysiological information about the underlying mechanisms involved in AO is needed to provide an effective strategy for treatment or management of AO. As mentioned above, the three main hypotheses about the pathophysiology of AO relate to whether the condition has a psychogenic, vascular or neuropathic derivation. Diagnostic criteria of defined neuropathic pain and a treatment algorithm for neuropathic pain based on evidence-based research are available. These criteria and the algorithm could be applied to AO patients whose pain can be attributed to neuropathic factors. Recently, Patient-Oriented Evidence that Matters (POEM) is emerging as a more significant approach than evidence-based data for use in clinical practice. Given that in psychosomatic diseases, doctor-centered interventions, and close observation of the doctor-patient relationship are of particular importance, clinicians may need to treat AO patients using the POEM approach.

Medico-Legal Traps

Failure to Diagnose Atypical Odontalgia (AO) Early

- Atypical odontalgia is often misdiagnosed as a typical dental issue, leading to unnecessary dental procedures such as extractions or root canals. These invasive treatments can exacerbate the condition, causing the patient more pain and increasing legal risk for misdiagnosis and unnecessary interventions.
- **Thumb Rule Consideration:** Always consider AO in patients with unexplained tooth pain, particularly when there are no radiographic or clinical findings, and avoid invasive treatments without clear pathological evidence.

Invasive Treatment Without Proper Diagnostic Workup

- Dentists may rush to perform dental procedures in response to persistent pain, even in the absence of diagnostic evidence. This can worsen the patient's condition and lead to claims of medical negligence for unnecessary interventions.
- **Thumb Rule Consideration:** Before performing any invasive dental

procedures, ensure thorough diagnostic workup, including imaging and patient history, to rule out non-odontogenic causes like AO.

Mismanagement of Neuropathic Pain

- AO is often neuropathic in origin, and failure to manage it with appropriate treatments, such as neuropathic pain medications, can result in prolonged patient suffering and dissatisfaction, leading to potential legal consequences for inadequate pain management.
- **Thumb Rule Consideration:** When AO is suspected, consider neuropathic pain management strategies, such as prescribing antidepressants like amitriptyline, and avoid relying solely on traditional dental treatments.

Lack of Clear Communication with the Patient

- Failing to explain the complex nature of AO and setting unrealistic expectations for traditional dental treatments can lead to patient frustration and legal claims. Miscommunication can make patients believe their pain is being dismissed or mistreated.
- **Thumb Rule Consideration:** Clearly communicate with patients about the nature of AO, its chronic and complex nature, and the limitations of traditional dental treatments, setting appropriate expectations for pain management.

Delayed Referral to Specialists

- Dentists may hesitate to refer patients with AO to pain specialists, neurologists, or psychiatrists, delaying appropriate treatment. This can lead to prolonged pain and potential legal consequences for not providing timely care.
- **Thumb Rule Consideration:** Refer patients with persistent, unexplained dental pain to pain specialists or neurologists early on, especially if initial dental treatments fail, to ensure proper management of neuropathic pain.

REFERENCES

- Headache Classification Committee of the International Headache Society, "Classification and diagnostic criteria for headache disorders, cranial neuralgias and facial pain," Cephalalgia, vol. 8, 7, pp. 1–96, 1988.
- J. J. Marbach, "Is phantom tooth pain a deafferentation (neuropathic) syndrome? Part I: evidence derived from pathophysiology and treatment," Oral Surgery Oral Medicine and Oral Pathology, vol. 75, no. 1, pp. 95–105, 1993.
- R. A. Pertes, D. R. Bailey, and A. S. Milone, "Atypical odontalgia—a nondental toothache," Journal of the New Jersey Dental Association, vol. 66, no. 1, pp. 29–33, 1995.
- R. L. Campbell, K. W. Parks, and R. N. Dodds, "Chronic facial pain associated with endodontic therapy," Oral Surgery Oral Medicine and Oral Pathology, vol. 69, no. 3, pp. 287–290, 1990.
- C. Feinmann and T. Newton-John, "Psychiatric and psychological management considerations associated

with nerve damage and neuropathic trigeminal pain," Journal of Orofacial Pain, vol. 18, no. 4, pp. 360–365, 2004.

- G. A. Kaspo, "Atypical odontalgia in the dental office," The Journal of the Michigan Dental Association, vol. 77, no. 5, pp. 34–36, 1995.
- T. List, G. Leijon, M. Helkimo, A. Öster, and P. Svensson, "Effect of local anesthesia on atypical odontalgia—a randomized controlled trial," Pain, vol. 122, no. 3, pp. 306–314, 2006.
- J. J. Marbach, "Is phantom tooth pain a deafferentation (neuropathic) syndrome? Part I: evidence derived from pathophysiology and treatment," Oral Surgery Oral Medicine and Oral Pathology, vol.75, no.1, pp. 95–105, 1993.

AVASCULAR NECROSIS OF THE HIP

Osteonecrosis of the hip, commonly known as avascular necrosis (AVN) of the hip, is the death of the femoral head as a result of vascular disruption. AVN is more common in males than in females. It typically presents as the insidious onset of pain around the hip.

Bergman J, Nordström A, Nordström P. Epidemiology of osteonecrosis among older adults in Sweden. Osteoporos Int. 2019 May;30(5):965-973.

Clinical Description

Osteonecrosis of the hip, commonly known as avascular necrosis (AVN) of the hip, is the death of the femoral head as a result of the vascular disruption. AVN of the hip results in pain around the hip which is insidious in onset. The cause is generally multifactorial and more commonly seen in males compared to females. Furthermore, the age of presentation from symptomatic AVN of the hip is younger than that of osteoarthritis. The treatment of AVN of the hip is controversial, and as such, there are many different treatment options for AVN. The ideal treatment option depends on the severity and stage of the disease.

AVN of the femoral head results from disruption of the vascular supply to the bone. Potential causes of AVN of the femoral head include causes that are clearly known such as when direct trauma has occurred, and in instances where the inciting event is unknown and only can be associated with risk factors that predispose to the disease process.

Pearls & Oysters

Mnemonic to help remember the most common causes of AVN

ASEPTIC

A – Alcohol/AIDS

S – Steroids, sickle cell disease, SLE

E – Erlenmeyer flask (Gaucher disease)

P – Pancreatitis

T – Trauma

I – Idiopathic, infection

C – Caisson's disease

Bottom Line Statement

Hip osteonecrosis is associated with very high morbidity if the diagnosis is missed. Thus, the condition is best managed by an interprofessional team that includes a radiologist, orthopedic surgeon, rheumatologist, internist, nurse practitioner and a pharmacist. There is no one single test that can make the diagnosis of this disorder and hence, communication and discussion with other healthcare workers is vital. The offending drug must be discontinued right away. The patients are managed medically and surgically but a complete recovery is not always guaranteed. Some patients are left with a permanent gait alteration and this can significantly affect the quality of life.

Medico-Legal Traps

Failure to Diagnose Avascular Necrosis (AVN) Early

- AVN often presents with insidious hip pain, which can be mistaken for more common conditions like osteoarthritis or muscle strain. Delayed diagnosis may lead to disease progression, hip joint collapse, and increased morbidity, making the patient susceptible to unnecessary pain and dysfunction.
- **Thumb Rule Consideration:** Always consider AVN in patients with unexplained hip pain, especially those with risk factors such as steroid use or alcohol consumption, and promptly order imaging studies such as MRI to confirm the diagnosis.

Mismanagement of Risk Factors

- AVN is linked to several modifiable risk factors, including steroid use, alcohol abuse, and conditions like sickle cell disease. Failure to manage or mitigate these risks, such as by continuing corticosteroid treatment when contraindicated, can exacerbate the condition and lead to medico-legal consequences.
- **Thumb Rule Consideration:** Always assess and address risk factors in patients at risk for AVN, particularly in those receiving long-term corticosteroids or with underlying conditions like sickle cell disease, and adjust treatments accordingly.

Delayed Referral to Orthopedic Specialists

- Inadequate referral to orthopedic specialists for patients with suspected or confirmed AVN can lead to delayed surgical interventions, worsening joint damage, and poor functional outcomes. Prolonged delays may result in the need for more invasive procedures, such as total hip replacement.
- **Thumb Rule Consideration:** Refer patients with confirmed or suspected

AVN to an orthopedic specialist early to ensure timely intervention and to discuss both non-surgical and surgical treatment options, depending on the stage of the disease.

Inappropriate or Delayed Surgical Intervention

- AVN may require surgical treatment depending on the stage of the disease. Delaying necessary surgery or opting for inappropriate conservative management in advanced cases can lead to irreversible damage and poor outcomes. This can result in legal liability for not providing timely or adequate care.
- **Thumb Rule Consideration:** Ensure that surgical interventions, such as core decompression or hip replacement, are considered promptly for patients with advanced AVN who do not respond to conservative treatment.

Inadequate Postoperative Rehabilitation

- Recovery from AVN-related surgery, such as hip replacement, requires structured rehabilitation. Failure to provide appropriate postoperative care, including physical therapy, can lead to suboptimal recovery, gait abnormalities, and potential long-term disability, increasing the risk of litigation.
- **Thumb Rule Consideration:** Always provide structured rehabilitation plans post-surgery and ensure regular follow-up to monitor recovery and address any gait abnormalities or complications.

REFERENCES

- Pascarella R, Fantasia R, Sangiovanni P, Maresca A, Massetti D, Politano R, Cerbasi S. Traumatic hip fracture-dislocation: A middle-term follow up study and a proposal of new classification system of hip joint associated injury. Injury. 2019 Aug;50 Suppl 4:S11-S20.
- Belmahi N, Boujraf S, Larwanou MM, El Ouahabi H. Avascular necrosis of the femoral head: An exceptional complication of cushing's disease. Ann Afr Med. 2018 Oct-Dec;17(4):225-227.
- Duan Y, Xi Y, Cun X, Yang Y, Li B, Zhou J, Tang X, Li Z. [Treatment of avascular necrosis of femoral head in patients with human immunodeficiency virus infection by cementless total hip arthroplasty]. Zhongguo Xiu Fu Chong Jian Wai Ke Za Zhi. 2018 Dec 15;32(12):1507-1511.
- Suksathien Y, Sueajui J. Mid-term results of short stem total hip arthroplasty in patients with osteonecrosis of the femoral head. Hip Int. 2019 Nov;29(6):603-608.
- Goyal T. Early results of surgery for femoroacetabular impingement in patients with osteonecrosis of femoral head. SICOT J. 2018;4:47.
- Wang C, Meng H, Wang Y, Zhao B, Zhao C, Sun W, Zhu Y, Han B, Yuan X, Liu R, Wang X, Wang A, Guo Q, Peng J, Lu S. Analysis of early stage osteonecrosis of the human femoral head and the mechanism of femoral head collapse. Int J Biol Sci. 2018;14(2):156-164.
- Kawano K, Motomura G, Ikemura S, Kubo Y, Fukushi J, Hamai S, Fujii M, Nakashima Y. Long-term hip survival and factors influencing patient-reported outcomes after transtrochanteric anterior rotational osteotomy for osteonecrosis of the femoral head: A minimum 10-year follow-up case series. Mod Rheumatol. 2020 Jan;30(1):184-190.

AVASCULAR NECROSIS OF THE SCAPHOID

Idiopathic avascular necrosis (AVN) of the scaphoid was first described by Georg Preiser in 1910. It is a rare condition that can cause pain and sometimes swelling around the anatomical snuffbox, which may be associated with loss of strength and reduced range of motion in the wrist.

Arch Bone Jt Surg. 2020 Jan; 8(1): 94–98.

Clinical Description

Post-traumatic avascular necrosis (AVN) of the scaphoid is a common complication probably due to the precarious blood supply. The rate of incidence is about 13% to 40% and almost all are seen in the proximal fragmen. Careful review of the literature revealed six cases of distal AVN in three studie. The diagnosis of AVN of the scaphoid is made by combining the MRI findings with direct observation of the punctuate bleeding during the operation. However, the diagnosis of AVN is suspicious in these cases, as MRI investigation had been performed in one case [5] and preoperative bleeding was observed in the other.

Pearls & Oysters

As the disease progresses, the scaphoid collapses to the extent that the distal pole becomes deformed and arthr!itic, mimicking the appearance of avascular necrosis. The prognosis would appear to depend on the stage of the disease, and treatment should be planned accordingly.

It appears that the aetiology may be related to interference in the extrinsic blood supply to the proximal pole of the scaphoid in susceptible patients, and it appears that positive ulnar variance may be significant.

Bottom Line Statement

Post-traumatic AVN of the scaphoid occurs as a result of impairment of the vascular supply to the involved bone fragment. Several studies had demonstrated a strikingly poor blood supply to the proximal pole, particularly in comparison with the abundant supply to the distal two-thirds of the scaphoid. Review of the literature revealed six cases in three reports. There may be several explanations for this condition. According to Espinosa et al., AVN in the distal fragment occurs if the volar vessel is damaged and the fracture line is distal to the line of entry of the dorsal vessels. Another explanation maybe the anomalous different vascularization of the distal pole.

Medico-Legal Traps

Failure to Diagnose Avascular Necrosis (AVN) of the Scaphoid Early

- AVN of the scaphoid is often misdiagnosed as a simple wrist sprain or fracture due to its rarity and vague symptoms. Delayed or missed diagnosis can lead to the collapse of the scaphoid bone and subsequent arthritis, resulting in long-term disability. This can lead to legal claims for negligence or misdiagnosis.
- **Thumb Rule Consideration:** Always consider AVN of the scaphoid in patients with persistent wrist pain, especially after trauma, and confirm the diagnosis with MRI if symptoms persist despite conservative treatment.

Inadequate Imaging and Diagnostic Workup

- Failure to utilize advanced imaging, such as MRI, to detect early signs of AVN can result in a missed or delayed diagnosis, leading to disease progression. Relying solely on X-rays may overlook early AVN, particularly in the proximal pole of the scaphoid.
- **Thumb Rule Consideration:** Use MRI as the imaging modality of choice for diagnosing suspected AVN of the scaphoid, especially in patients with ongoing wrist pain and no clear radiographic abnormalities on X-ray.

Inappropriate or Delayed Surgical Intervention

- AVN of the scaphoid often requires timely surgical intervention, such as bone grafting or revascularization, to restore blood supply and prevent bone collapse. Delaying surgery or opting for inappropriate conservative treatments in advanced stages can lead to irreversible joint damage and future legal challenges.
- **Thumb Rule Consideration:** Consider early surgical intervention for patients with confirmed AVN of the scaphoid, especially if the proximal pole is affected, to prevent bone collapse and arthritic changes.

Failure to Monitor Post-Traumatic Scaphoid Fractures for AVN

- Scaphoid fractures, especially of the proximal pole, are at high risk of developing AVN due to poor blood supply. Failure to monitor patients with scaphoid fractures for signs of AVN through follow-up imaging can lead to missed diagnoses and worsening of the condition.
- **Thumb Rule Consideration:** Closely monitor scaphoid fractures, particularly of the proximal pole, with follow-up imaging (MRI or CT) to detect any signs of AVN, especially if healing is delayed.

Inadequate Postoperative Rehabilitation

- Proper rehabilitation is crucial after surgical intervention for AVN of the scaphoid. Failure to provide structured rehabilitation can result in poor recovery, reduced wrist function, and long-term disability, increasing the risk of legal repercussions for suboptimal outcomes.
- **Thumb Rule Consideration:** Ensure patients receive appropriate postoperative rehabilitation following surgery for AVN of the scaphoid to restore wrist function and prevent long-term complications.

REFERENCES

- Botte MJ, Pacelli LL, Gelberman RH. Vascularity and osteonecrosis of the wrist. Orthop Clin North Am. 2004;35:405–21.
- Amadio PC, Taleisnik J. Fractures of the carpal bones. In: Green DP, Hotchkiss RN, editors. Green's operative hand surgery. 3rd edition. New York, NY: Churchill Livingstone; 1993. pp. 799–801. p.
- Freedman DM, Botte MJ, Gelberman RH. Vascularity of the carpus. Clin Orthop Relat Res. 2001;383:47–59.
- Espinosa GA, Michael AS, Wilbur AC, McKusick MA, et al. Osteonecrosis of the distal pole of the carpal navicular following fracture. Mil Med. 1986;151:663–5.
- Garg B, Gupta H, Kotwal PP. Nontraumatic osteonecrosis of the distal pole of the scaphoid. Indian J Orthop. 2011;45:185–7.
- Sherman SB, Greenspan A, Norman A. Osteonecrosis of the distal pole of the carpal scaphoid following fracture-a rare complication. Skeletal Radiol. 1983;9:189–91.

BOXER'S KNUCKLE

Boxing is a popular sport throughout the world and injuries to the dorsum of the hand are fairly common in this sport. Whether recreational or professional, the spectrum of injury varies. The characteristic injury is the 'boxer's knuckle', which involves disruption of the extensor hood mechanism with dorsal capsule rupture. This injury can be severely disabling with devastating effects for the athlete. The spectrum of injuries further extends to simple contusions, lacerations, extensor tendon ruptures or subluxation and MC/ CMC fractures.

Ann R Coll Surg Engl. 2011 Jul; 93(5): e55–e56.

Clinical Description

Sagittal band rupture is often referred to as a "Boxer's knuckle". This lesion, which is common in boxers, occurs often after clenched-fist trauma and mostly at the third MCP. Clinical findings consist of pain, swelling, incomplete joint extension, and subluxation of the extensor tendon. Usually, the mechanism of injury is severe blunt trauma with forceful flexion of joints resulting in stretching of the extensor mechanism. The injury could be closed or open. The mechanism of open injuries can involve avulsion, crushing or impact with a sharp object. A thorough history and clinical examination is crucial to identifying the extent of the injury as sinister injuries can be easily overlooked, especially capsular tears, which could result in synovitis, and fistulas between joint cavity and subcutaneous tissue. Sagittal bands are transversely located ligaments, centralizing the extensor tendon. Due to ulnar deviation predisposition of the MCP joint and anatomic weakness, the radial band ruptures more often than ulnar sagittal bands. Abnormal signal intensity or echogenicity of the thickened and possible discontinuity of the sagittal band with edema of the dorsal soft tissues suggest the diagnosis on MRI and ultrasound. Dynamic ultrasound (US) can confirm the extensor tendon subluxation during MCP joint flexion, which is an advantage compared to static MRI. Conservative treatment can be considered in acute cases, while surgical repair of the sagittal bands is standard of care in severe acute and chronic ruptures.

Pearls & Oysters

Treatment of extensor mechanism injuries depends on the severity of the injury and structures involved. Simple lacerations to the skin and extensor tendons can be repaired primarily. However, management of deeper structures such as sagittal bands, tendon dislocation and capsular tears remains controversial. Some authors advocate surgical treatment while others prefer a non-operative course. Usually, extensor mechanism disruption is treated with surgery. For capsular tears, Arai et al suggested surgical repair but in another study complete functional recovery was seen in athletes without repair. Meticulous postoperative care is needed for complex injuries with appropriate splinting and follow-up. Whatever the course, the prime goal is to return the hand to its previous functional state.

Bottom Line Statement

Boxer's knuckle must be distinguished from stress fracture, arthritis, and other occult pathological conditions of the wrist and hand. Traumatic injuries of the metacarpophalangeal joints are a common occurrence in professional and recreational sports such as boxing and martial arts, especially the fourth and fifth metacarpals. Injury usually results from a forceful impact with a clenched fist. The spectrum of injuries varies from simple skin laceration to extensor mechanism disruption, dorsal capsule rupture, metacarpal fractures and carpometacarpal joint injuries. These injuries are well documented in boxers as well as in patients who had been involved in fights and assaults. Coexistent arthritis bursitis and tendinitis may contribute to the patient's pain, necessitating additional treatment with more localized injection of local anesthetic and steroid.

Medico-Legal Traps

Failure to Diagnose Boxer's Knuckle Early

- Boxer's knuckle, involving sagittal band rupture and extensor mechanism disruption, may be misdiagnosed as a simple hand contusion or sprain, leading to improper treatment. This can result in long-term joint dysfunction and chronic pain, exposing the clinician to potential legal action for delayed diagnosis.
- **Thumb Rule Consideration:** Always consider Boxer's knuckle in patients presenting with hand pain, swelling, and limited extension after trauma, especially in boxers or individuals involved in fist-related activities, and confirm with dynamic ultrasound or MRI to assess extensor tendon subluxation.

Inadequate Assessment of Capsular Tears and Extensor Mechanism Injuries

- Capsular tears and deeper extensor mechanism injuries can be easily missed if a thorough clinical examination is not performed. Neglecting these injuries can lead to chronic synovitis, fistulas, and persistent hand dysfunction, leading to medico-legal consequences for incomplete assessment.

- **Thumb Rule Consideration:** Perform a comprehensive clinical examination and utilize imaging (e.g., dynamic ultrasound or MRI) to fully assess capsular integrity and extensor tendon involvement in patients with suspected Boxer's knuckle.

Inappropriate or Delayed Surgical Intervention

- Surgical repair is often necessary for severe extensor mechanism disruptions and chronic sagittal band ruptures. Delayed or inappropriate conservative treatment in severe cases can lead to irreversible joint damage and decreased hand function, prompting legal claims for inadequate care.
- **Thumb Rule Consideration:** Recommend surgical intervention for severe sagittal band ruptures or chronic cases of Boxer's knuckle to restore joint stability and hand function, especially when conservative measures fail or the injury is severe.

Misdiagnosis of Boxer's Knuckle as Arthritis or Tendinitis

- Misdiagnosing Boxer's knuckle as arthritis, tendinitis, or stress fractures may result in inappropriate treatments like steroid injections or physical therapy, which can aggravate the underlying condition. This can result in worsening symptoms and potential legal action for mismanagement.
- **Thumb Rule Consideration:** Differentiate Boxer's knuckle from conditions like arthritis or tendinitis by focusing on the mechanism of injury and performing targeted imaging, such as dynamic ultrasound, to visualize sagittal band rupture and extensor tendon dislocation.

Inadequate Postoperative Rehabilitation

- After surgical repair of Boxer's knuckle, proper rehabilitation and splinting are crucial for recovery. Failing to provide structured postoperative care can result in poor outcomes, delayed recovery, and permanent loss of hand function, increasing legal risks for inadequate follow-up care.
- **Thumb Rule Consideration:** Ensure comprehensive postoperative rehabilitation and splinting for patients recovering from surgical repair of Boxer's knuckle, with regular follow-up to monitor recovery and prevent complications.

REFERENCES

- Cockenpot E, Lefebvre G, Demondion X, Chantelot C, Cotten A. Imaging of sports-related hand and wrist injuries: Sports imaging series. Radiology. 2016. Jun; 279(3): 674–92.
- Bents RT, Metz JP, Topper SM. Traumatic extensor tendon dislocation in a boxer: a case study. Med Sci

Sports Exerc 2003; 35: 1,645–1,647.

- Gladden JR. Boxer's knuckle; a preliminary report. Am J Surg 1957; 93: 388–397.
- Hame SL, Melone CP Jr. Boxer's knuckle in the professional athlete. Am J Sports Med 2000; 28: 879–882.
- Posner MA, Ambrose L. Boxer's knuckle – dorsal capsular rupture of the metacarpophalangeal joint of a finger. J Hand Surg Am 1989; 14: 229–236.
- Arai K, Toh S, Nakahara K et al.. Treatment of soft tissue injuries to the dorsum of the metacarpophalangeal joint (Boxer's knuckle). J Hand Surg Br 2002; 27: 90–95.
- Waldman SD: Painful conditions of the wrist and hand. Physical diagnosis of pain: an atlas of signs and symptoms, ed 2, Philadelphia, 2010, Saunders, pp 153–154.

BREASTSTROKER'S KNEE

Swimmers Knee is the second most common injury related to swimming, with Swimmers Shoulder being the most common. Sometimes called Breaststroke Knee or Breaststrokers Knee, it is a painful condition affecting the inner side of the knee, and is most common with the swim stroke of breaststroke. The leg action of breaststroke is a wide circular, sweeping motion of the legs. The powerful inward movement causes a lateral stress on the knee such that as the medial collateral ligament, that runs along the inner side of the knee joint can be strained and stretched with overuse, or if the knee is already injured or unstable.

Am J Sports Med. 1987 Jan-Feb;15(1):63-71.

Clinical Description

Breaststroker's Knee is a combination of a strain to the medial collateral ligament (MCL) and compression on the lateral knee, seen largely in response to the kick performed in breaststroke. The breaststroke kick is a high valgus load produced during sudden flexion-extension, adduction and external rotation of the knee against the hydrodynamic environment, resulting in stress to the medial compartment.

As a result, it is not uncommon for swimmers to present with ligament sprains on the MCL, irritation of the medial plica and bursal irritation at the muscular insertions of the adductor and hamstring muscles. Furthermore, strain injuries can be present in the adductor muscles (adductor magnus and brevis, especially). Breaststroker's Knee is largely due to the overuse of the knee in the breaststroke kick. This is especially true if the technique used isn't correct, or after intense or prolonged sessions of kicking training.

Pearls & Oysters

The most common cause of swimmer's knee is poor technique in inexperienced swimmers. The main problem is the performance of the 'whip-kick' movement during breaststroke.

The breaststroke kick is a high valgus load produced during sudden flexion-extension, adduction and external rotation of the knee against the hydrodynamic environment resulting in stress to the medial compartment. Hence a strain occurs to the medial collateral ligament and compression on the lateral knee. Inexperienced swimmers with poor technique may put too much pressure on this ligament but swimmer's knee can also occur in experienced swimmers as a result of overuse.

Bottom Line Statement

The breaststroke is one of the most complicated swim strokes to learn and requires a completely different technique than the other three swim styles.

One of the differences between this style and the others lies in the distribution of forward propulsion. In breaststroke 70% of propulsion comes from your legs with the rest of the power coming from breaststroke arm pull, meaning there is more strain put on the legs and knees than in any of the other swim strokes.

The most popular breaststroke swimming technique is the so-called whip kick motion. This technique involves bending the legs toward the thighs and thighs toward the hips at an angle of approximately 120 degrees with feet almost at the surface of the water and the knees quite close together.

The legs play a key role throughout the entire stroke particularly the position of knees. That is why the knees are a breaststroker's weak point.

Medico-Legal Traps

Failure to Diagnose Breaststroker's Knee Early

- Breaststroker's Knee, a strain of the medial collateral ligament (MCL), is often underdiagnosed or misdiagnosed as a general knee strain or overuse injury. Delayed diagnosis can worsen the condition, leading to prolonged recovery or chronic pain, which may result in medico-legal consequences for improper management.
- **Thumb Rule Consideration:** Always consider Breaststroker's Knee in swimmers, especially those who perform the breaststroke regularly, and promptly assess the MCL and medial knee structures to prevent worsening of the condition.

Inadequate Assessment of Swimming Technique

- Poor swimming technique, especially improper execution of the whip kick in breaststroke, is a common cause of Breaststroker's Knee. Failing to assess and correct a swimmer's technique may lead to recurring injuries and possible legal claims for negligence in addressing the root cause of the condition.
- **Thumb Rule Consideration:** Always evaluate the swimmer's technique, particularly the whip kick movement, and recommend corrective coaching or physical therapy to prevent further injury.

Neglecting Conservative Management Options

- Conservative treatments, such as rest, physical therapy, and technique modification, are often the first line of defense for Breaststroker's Knee. Failing to implement or monitor conservative treatments may result in the progression of the injury, leading to the need for surgical intervention and potential legal action for inadequate care.
- **Thumb Rule Consideration:** Ensure conservative management, including rest, physical therapy, and technique adjustments, is thoroughly explored and monitored before considering more invasive interventions for Breaststroker's Knee.

Delayed Referral to Specialists

- In cases where conservative management fails, timely referral to a sports medicine specialist or orthopedic surgeon is essential. Delaying this referral can lead to prolonged symptoms, joint instability, and further complications, increasing the risk of medico-legal claims for delayed care.
- **Thumb Rule Consideration:** Refer swimmers with persistent or worsening symptoms of Breaststroker's Knee to a specialist early, especially if conservative treatment does not yield improvement within a reasonable timeframe.

Inadequate Post-Recovery Rehabilitation

- After treatment or recovery from Breaststroker's Knee, structured rehabilitation is crucial to restore strength and prevent re-injury. Failing to provide or recommend proper rehabilitation may lead to long-term knee instability, chronic pain, and legal repercussions for inadequate follow-up care.
- **Thumb Rule Consideration:** Always provide or recommend a structured rehabilitation program post-recovery to restore knee function and reduce the risk of recurrence in swimmers.

REFERENCES

- Beall DP, Googe JD, Moss JT, et al: Magnetic resonance imaging of the collateral ligaments and the anatomic quadrants of the knee, Radiol Clin North Am 45:983–1002, 2007.
- Jones L, Bismil Q, Alyas F, Connell D, Bell J: Persistent symptoms following nonoperative management in low grade MCL injury of the knee: the role of the deep MCL, Knee 16:64–68, 2009.
- Kastelein M, Wagemakers HPA, Luijsterburg PAJ, et al: Assessing medial collateral ligament knee lesions in general practice, Am J Med 121:982–988, 2008.
- Kennedy JC, Hawkins R, Krissoff WB: Orthopaedic manifestations of swimming, Am J Sports Med 6:309–322, 1978.
- Malone WJ, Verde F, Weiss D, Fanelli GC: MR imaging of knee instability, MRI Clin North Am 17:6102–6724, 2009.
- Stulberg SD, Shulman K, Stuart S, et al: Breaststroker's knee: pathology, etiology, and treatment, Am J Sports Med 8:164–171, 1980.

BUNIONETTE PAIN

Also called Tailor's bunions, a bunionette is similar to a bunion, but occurs on the outside of the foot. It is a raised portion of skin that often becomes irritated and sore. Bunionettes cause pain on the outside portion of the foot where it is raised. The pain or discomfort usually occurs when shoes that rub that area are worn. If the rubbing breaks the skin, an infection can result.

DAVIES H. Metatarsus quintus valgus. Br Med J. 1949 Apr 16. 1 (4606):664.

Clinical Description

The term tailor's bunion (a synonym for bunionette) initially described an acquired lesion that caused chronic pain and swelling over the lateral aspect of the fifth metatarsal (MT) head. These lesions often were present on tailors, whose traditional cross-legged sitting posture on benches resulted in pressure being placed on the lateral side of the foot, leading to the development of painful bunionettes. Davies described the lesion in the English literature in 1949.

A bunionette is defined as a painful prominence on the lateral aspect of the fifth MT head. Although it is not as common as a medial bunion, it is a cause of chronic pain and shoe-fitting problems in individuals whose feet are characterized by a widened forefoot or in those who have a lateral splaying or prominence over the fifth MT.

Treatment often can be nonoperative. Surgery for a bunionette is performed when symptoms of an unacceptable degree are not relieved by conservative treatments, such as shaving the callus or wearing wider shoes, silicon pads, softer shoe coverings, or sandals. Surgical procedures are determined by the pathoanatomy. No single, universally acceptable procedure exists for all patients.

Presenting symptoms of a bunionette (tailor's bunion) usually include painful keratoses over the lateral aspect of the metatarsal (MT) head, but they also may be present on the plantar and dorsal aspects. Medial deviation of the fifth phalanx with some rotation is frequently seen. Determining whether the patient is truly having pain or whether he or she just finds the foot cosmetically unacceptable is important. Assessing whether the deformity is fixed or correctable also is important.

Pearls & Oysters

Surgery for a bunionette (tailor's bunion) is performed when symptoms of an unacceptable degree are not relieved by conservative treatments, such as shaving the callus or wearing wider shoes, silicon pads, softer shoe coverings, or sandals. The use of minimal-incision surgery in the management of this condition has grown; various percutaneous approaches appear promising, and some authors have reported results comparable to those of open surgery. Future developments may include different osteotomies.

Recurrence can occur from poor procedure selection or performance or from progression of underlying pathophysiology (eg, arthropathy). Nonunion is a significant risk with proximal MT osteotomy, though it can occur with midshaft osteotomies.

Some of these contraindications apply to specific reconstructive procedures. For example, severe refractory deformities, inflammatory conditions, and infected neuropathic arthritic or failed surgical procedures may necessitate treatment with ablative rather than reconstructive procedures.

Bottom Line Statement

The bony prominence on the lateral side of the fifth metatarsal head often is called atailor's bunion, referring to the position in which tailors would sit on the floor with their legs crossed, forcing the lateral border of the foot against the floor. It often is seen in splay foot combined with hallux valgus, or the head of the fifth metatarsal may be congenitally or traumatically enlarged. Also, the shaft may be angulated laterally, making the fifth metatarsal head more prominent. Standard weight-bearing views of the foot, including dorsoplantar, lateral, and oblique, should be obtained for measurement of the 4-5 intermetatarsal angle (4-5 IMA). This angle is formed by two lines that bisect the fourth and fifth metatarsals. The normal 4-5 IMA is less than 6.5 to 8 degrees; the average 4-5 IMA is 6.5 degrees in normal feet and 9.6 degrees in feet with a symptomatic bunionette. Bunionettes also are classified based on these weight-bearing radiographs: type I, enlargement of the fifth metatarsal head or alateral exostosis; type II, abnormal lateral bend to the distal fifth metatarsal with a normal 4-5 IMA; and type III, an increased 4-5 IMA (>8 degrees) that results in a widened forefoot. Type III is the most common deformity. Other angles that may be useful are the lateral deviation angle, which is formed by a line from the center of the metatarsal head and neck to the metatarsal base and a line along the medial cortex of the fifth metatarsal (normal, 2.6 degrees; with bunionette, 8 degrees), and the fifth metatarsophalangeal angle, which usually is more than 14 degrees in symptomatic patients. Shimobayashi et al. analyzed the radiographic morphologic characteristics of the entire foot in patients with symptomatic bunionette deformity and found that the third, fourth, and fifth metatarsal heads were more displaced laterally in patients with deformity than those without deformity. In addition, all intermetatarsal angles were larger in patients with deformity compared with normal feet. They suggest assessing the entire foot for width and splaying of all metatarsals, not just the fifth, which may represent only one cause of the deformity.

Medico-Legal Traps

Failure to Diagnose Bunionette (Tailor's Bunion) Early

- Bunionettes may present as simple lateral foot pain, and clinicians may overlook the deformity, dismissing it as a minor irritation. Delayed diagnosis can lead to worsening deformity and pain, which may result in legal claims for negligence in identifying the condition.
- **Thumb Rule Consideration:** Always assess for a bunionette in patients complaining of lateral foot pain, especially those with a history of wearing tight or narrow shoes, and confirm with weight-bearing radiographs if necessary.

Inadequate Conservative Management

- Conservative management, such as recommending wider shoes or using silicone pads, is often the first-line treatment. Failure to adequately advise or monitor these interventions may lead to persistent symptoms and patient dissatisfaction, resulting in potential legal claims for inadequate care.
- **Thumb Rule Consideration:** Ensure comprehensive conservative treatment, including footwear modifications and protective padding, and follow up regularly to monitor patient progress before considering surgical options.

Inappropriate or Premature Surgical Intervention

- Surgery for bunionettes should be reserved for cases where conservative treatments fail. Premature or inappropriate surgical intervention, especially without proper evaluation of the foot's anatomy and metatarsal angles, can lead to complications like nonunion, poor healing, or recurrence of the deformity.
- **Thumb Rule Consideration:** Reserve surgical intervention for cases where conservative management fails, and ensure thorough preoperative assessment, including measurement of metatarsal angles, to guide appropriate procedure selection.

Misdiagnosis of Cosmetic Concerns as Pain

- Patients with bunionettes may present for cosmetic reasons rather than functional pain. Failure to differentiate between cosmetic dissatisfaction and actual symptomatic deformity may result in unnecessary treatments, potentially leading to medico-legal disputes over inappropriate care.

- **Thumb Rule Consideration:** Carefully evaluate whether the patient's concern is cosmetic or functional, and tailor treatment recommendations accordingly, being cautious about recommending surgery for cosmetic reasons alone.

Inadequate Postoperative Care and Rehabilitation

- After surgical correction of a bunionette, improper postoperative care or rehabilitation may result in complications such as nonunion, recurrence, or joint stiffness. Failure to ensure adequate follow-up can lead to poor outcomes and increased legal risk.
- **Thumb Rule Consideration:** Provide comprehensive postoperative care, including appropriate splinting, rehabilitation, and regular follow-up visits, to ensure proper healing and minimize the risk of recurrence or complications.

REFERENCES

- Ceccarini P, Rinonapoli G, Nardi A, Bisaccia M, Di Giacomo LM, Caraffa A. Bunionette. Foot Ankle Spec. 2017 Apr. 10 (2):157-161.
- Ajis A, Koti M, Maffulli N. Tailor's bunion: a review. J Foot Ankle Surg. 2005 May-Jun. 44 (3):236-45.
- Cooper PS. Disorders and deformities of the lesser toes. Myerson MS, ed. Foot and Ankle Disorders. Philadelphia: Saunders; 2000. Vol 1: 335-340.
- Shi GG, Humayun A, Whalen JL, Kitaoka HB. Management of Bunionette Deformity. J Am Acad Orthop Surg. 2018 Oct 1. 26 (19):e396-e404.
- Coughlin MJ. Etiology and treatment of the bunionette deformity. Instr Course Lect. 1990. 39:37-48. [
- Necas L, Hrubina M, Skotak M, Melisik M, Lisy P, Cibula Z. Bunionette deformity corrected with "shortening" scarf osteotomy of the fifth metatarsal: mid-term results of a 34-cases. Foot Ankle Surg. 2020 Jul. 26 (5):541-546.
- Cohen BE, Nicholson CW. Bunionette deformity. J Am Acad Orthop Surg. 2007 May. 15 (5):300-7.
- Shimobayashi M, Tanaka Y, Taniguchi A, Kurokawa H, Tomiwa K, Higashiyama I. Radiographic Morphologic Characteristics of Bunionette Deformity. Foot Ankle Int. 2016 Mar. 37 (3):320-6.
- Laffenêtre O, Millet-Barbé B, Darcel V, Lucas Y Hernandez J, Chauveaux D. Percutaneous bunionette correction: results of a 49-case retrospective study at a mean 34 months' follow-up. Orthop Traumatol Surg Res. 2015 Apr. 101 (2):179-84.
- Morawe GA, Schmieschek MHT. Minimally invasive bunionette correction. Oper Orthop Traumatol. 2018 Jun. 30 (3):184-194.
- Teoh KH, Hariharan K. Minimally Invasive Distal Metatarsal Metaphyseal Osteotomy (DMMO) of the Fifth Metatarsal for Bunionette Correction. Foot Ankle Int. 2018 Apr. 39 (4):450-457.
- Michels F, Guillo S. Bunionette: Is There a Minimally Invasive Solution?. Foot Ankle Clin. 2020 Sep. 25 (3):425-439.
- Kay DB, Sabetta JA. Fifth Metatarsal Bunionette Correction Using a Stable Intramedullary Device. Foot Ankle Orthop. 2022 Jan. 7 (1):24730114211S00273.

BURNING MOUTH SYNDROME

Burning mouth syndrome (BMS) is a chronic debilitating oral condition characterised by a burning sensation of the oral mucosa in an otherwise apparently normal person. Its aetiology and pathogenesis are obscure, but both psychogenic factors and peripheral and central neuropathies appear to be implicated. There is no cure for BMS, and treatment with either local or systemic medications focuses on the relief of symptoms and on improving quality of life. In recalcitrant cases, psychological/psychiatric intervention may be helpful. In order to improve treatment outcomes, a better understanding of the pathogenesis of this syndrome might provide a basis for the development of more effective management strategies.

Clark GT: Persistent orodental pain, atypical odontalgia, and phantom tooth pain: when are they neuropathic disorders? J Calif Dent Assoc 34:599–609, 2006.

Clinical Description

The International Association for the Study of Pain (IASP) has described burning mouth syndrome as a chronic condition characterised by a burning sensation of the oral mucosa for which no cause can be found. The anterior part of the tongue is most commonly affected, followed by the labial mucosa and occasionally the palate. The burning pain is often accompanied by tingling or numbness and the sensation of dryness of the mouth. Reduced taste intensity and a bitter or a metallic taste are experienced by about two-thirds of those with BMS. Despite all these symptoms, the oral mucosa and the salivary flow rate are normal.

The burning sensation of BMS is moderate to severe in intensity, is usually bilaterally symmetrical, and is present every day for most of the day. It is minimal or even absent early in the morning and during mealtimes and it seldom interferes with sleep. In most cases, BMS starts spontaneously and continues for several years. Only about 3% of cases resolve over a 5-year observation period and even with treatment only about 30% of affected persons report any improvement.

Pearls & Oysters

The main complications surrounding the treatment of burning mouth syndrome are those associated with its misdiagnosis. Chemical dependence, depression, and multiple failed therapeutic procedures are the rule rather than the exception. A diagnosis of a psychiatric basis for the patient's pain should be made only after all somatic causes of burning mouth syndrome have carefully been ruled out.

Bottom Line Statement

The pathogenesis of BMS is complex involving psychogenic factors and dysregulated peripheral and central pain pathways. Genetic factors determining the function of neural pain pathways may play an important role in individual susceptibility to BMS, and while there is no standard treatment protocol for its management, both drugs and psychological services may be required. Once causes of burning mouth and tongue that have clinically identifiable pathological processes have been ruled out, a rational treatment plan addressing the often multifactorial nature of the patient's pain can be initiated. A supportive therapeutic environment is crucial if symptom reduction is to be achieved.

Medico-Legal Traps

Failure to Diagnose Burning Mouth Syndrome (BMS) Early

- BMS is often underdiagnosed or misdiagnosed as other oral conditions due to its vague and complex symptoms. Delayed diagnosis can lead to prolonged patient suffering, unnecessary treatments, and legal claims for mismanagement.
- **Thumb Rule Consideration:** Always consider BMS in patients with chronic, unexplained oral burning sensations, especially when no clinical abnormalities are found on examination, and rule out other somatic causes early.

Misdiagnosis as a Local Oral Condition

- BMS may be mistaken for local conditions such as candidiasis, oral lichen planus, or allergies. Treating patients for these unrelated conditions without recognizing the neuropathic or psychogenic nature of BMS can lead to worsening symptoms and legal consequences for incorrect treatment.
- **Thumb Rule Consideration:** After ruling out common oral conditions, consider BMS as a differential diagnosis and avoid unnecessary local treatments if no clinical evidence supports a local pathology.

Inadequate Management of Psychogenic Factors

- Psychological or psychiatric factors play a significant role in BMS, yet failing to address these aspects of the condition can result in ineffective treatment. Patients may become chemically dependent on medications or develop depression, leading to potential legal issues for inadequate holistic care.

- **Thumb Rule Consideration:** Integrate psychological and psychiatric evaluations early in the treatment plan for BMS, and consider a multidisciplinary approach that includes both medical and mental health care.

Overuse of Medications Without Improvement

- Due to the lack of a cure for BMS, patients may be prescribed multiple medications, such as antidepressants or anticonvulsants, with little symptom relief. Overprescription without proper monitoring can lead to medication dependence or side effects, increasing medico-legal risks.
- **Thumb Rule Consideration:** Carefully monitor medication use in BMS patients, ensuring regular follow-ups to assess efficacy, and avoid long-term prescriptions without demonstrable improvement.

Failure to Set Realistic Expectations

- Given the chronic nature of BMS and the limited success rates of current treatments, failing to set realistic expectations with patients regarding the potential outcomes can lead to dissatisfaction and claims of inadequate care.
- **Thumb Rule Consideration:** Clearly communicate the challenges of treating BMS, set realistic expectations for symptom management rather than cure, and provide ongoing support to improve the patient's quality of life.

REFERENCES

- https://www.iasp-pain.org/files/Content/ContentFolders/Global Year Against Pain2/20132014 OrofacialPain/FactSheets/Burning_Mouth_Syndrome_2016.pdf.
- L. L. Patton, M. A. Siegel, R. Benoliel, and A. de Laat, "Management of burning mouth syndrome: systematic review and management recommendations," Oral Surgery, Oral Medicine, Oral Pathology, Oral Radiology, and Endodontology, vol. 103, suppl. 39, pp. S39.e1–S39.e13, 2007.
- J. A. G. Buchanan and J. M. Zakrzewska, "Burning mouth syndrome," BMJ Clinical Evidence, vol. 2010, 2010.
- G. E. Gurvits and A. Tan, "Burning mouth syndrome," World Journal of Gastroenterology, vol. 19, no. 5, pp. 665–672, 2013.
- M. Grushka, J. Epstein, and A. Mott, "An open-label, dose escalation pilot study of the effect of clonazepam in burning mouth syndrome," Oral Surgery, Oral Medicine, Oral Pathology, Oral Radiology, and Endodontology, vol. 86, no. 5, pp. 557–561, 1998.
- H. Forssell, S. Jääskeläinen, T. List, P. Svensson, and L. Baad-Hansen, "An update on pathophysiological mechanisms related to idiopathic oro-facial pain conditions with implications for management," Journal of Oral Rehabilitation, vol. 42, no. 4, pp. 300–322, 2015.
- A. Scala, L. Checchi, M. Montevecchi, I. Marini, and M. A. Giamberardino, "Update on burning mouth syndrome: Overview and patient management," Critical Reviews in Oral Biology and Medicine, vol. 14, no. 4, pp. 275–291, 2003.
- J. G. Speciali and J. Stuginski-Barbosa, "Burning mouth syndrome," Current Pain and Headache Reports, vol. 12, no. 4, pp. 279–284, 2008.

CERVICOTHORACIC INTERSPINOUS BURSITIS

The interspinous ligaments of the lower cervical and upper thoracic spine and their associated muscles are susceptible to the development of acute and chronic pain symptoms following overuse. Bursitis is thought to be responsible for this pain. Frequently, the patient presents with midline pain after prolonged activity requiring hyperextension of the neck, such as painting a ceiling, or following prolonged use of a computer monitor with too high a focal point.

https://aneskey.com/cervicothoracic-interspinous-bursitis/

Clinical Description

Cervicothoracic Interspinous Bursitis is a painful condition of the upper back and neck. A bursa is a fluid-filled sac that is present in many areas of the body. After injury or overuse, these bursa can become inflamed and cause pain. The pain of cervicothoracic interspinous bursitis is dull and aching. It is usually confined to the midline area without much radiation outward. It is worse with activity and relieved with rest. Thrusting the neck forward will also tend to decrease the pain. This condition is usually precipitated after extending the neck for prolonged periods. The neurological exam is normal with the exception of localized pain in the area. X-rays, MRIs and CT scans are useful to look for underlying anatomic problems that should be excluded such as disease of the spinal chord.• Electromyography and Nerve Conduction Studies are useful to exclude diseases of the muscle and nerves. Blood work is used to look for auto-immune and collagen vascular diseases. The treatment of cervicothoracic interspinous bursitis begins with conservative modalities such as heat, ice, rest and physical therapy. Non-steroidal anti-inflammatory medications will decrease the pain and inflammation. Injection into the area of a local anesthetic and a corticosteroid is also useful for treatment.

Pearls & Oysters

The diagnosis of cervicothoracic bursitis is typically made based on the patient's symptoms and physical examination. These may include pain and tenderness in the cervicothoracic region, decreased range of motion, and muscle spasm. Other conditions, such as syringomyelia, tumors, ankylosing spondylitis, and fibromyalgia, may present with similar symptoms and may need to be ruled out as a possible cause of the patient's symptoms.

Imaging tests, such as X-rays, MRI, or CT scans, may also be helpful in making a diagnosis of cervicothoracic bursitis. These tests can help to identify any abnormalities in the spine or surrounding structures that may be contributing to the patient's symptoms.

Treatment for cervicothoracic bursitis may include non-steroidal anti-inflammatory drugs (NSAIDs) to reduce inflammation, physical therapy to help improve range of motion and strengthen the muscles in the affected area, and, in some cases, injections of corticosteroids to reduce inflammation. In severe cases, surgery may be necessary to remove the inflamed bursa.

Failure to recognize inadvertent epidural, subdural, or dural puncture can result in significant motor and sensory block with the potential for associated loss of consciousness, hypotension, and apnea.

If subdural placement is unrecognized, and the previously mentioned doses of local anesthetics are administered, the signs and symptoms are similar to those of subarachnoid injection, although the resulting motor and sensory block may be spotty.

Bottom Line Statement

The pain with cervicothoracic interspinous bursitis is localized to the interspinous region between C7 and T1 and does not radiate. It is constant, dull, and aching. The patient may attempt to relieve the constant ache by assuming a posture of dorsal kyphosis with a thrusting forward of the neck. In contrast to the pain of cervical strain, the pain of cervicothoracic interspinous bursitis often lessens with activity and worsens with rest. Pain syndromes that may mimic cervicothoracic bursitis include cervical strain, cervical fibromyositis, inflammatory arthritis, and disorders of the cervical spinal cord, roots, plexus, and nerves. Congenital abnormalities such as Arnold-Chiari malformation and Klippel-Feil syndrome may also manifest similarly to cervicothoracic bursitis. Correction of the functional abnormalities responsible for the development of cervicothoracic interspinous bursitis is mandatory if long-lasting relief is to be achieved.

Medico-Legal Traps

Failure to Diagnose Cervicothoracic Interspinous Bursitis Early

- Cervicothoracic interspinous bursitis can be misdiagnosed as more common conditions such as cervical strain, fibromyalgia, or inflammatory arthritis. Failure to correctly diagnose this condition may lead to unnecessary treatments and prolonged patient suffering, increasing the risk of legal claims for mismanagement.

- **Thumb Rule Consideration:** Always consider cervicothoracic interspinous bursitis in patients with midline neck and upper back pain, particularly after hyperextension activities, and rule out other conditions through imaging and physical examination.

Inadequate Exclusion of Differential Diagnoses

- Conditions such as syringomyelia, tumors, and ankylosing spondylitis can present similarly to cervicothoracic interspinous bursitis. Failing to properly exclude these serious conditions may result in missed diagnoses, potentially leading to legal action for inadequate diagnostic workup.
- **Thumb Rule Consideration:** Always perform a thorough diagnostic workup, including imaging (X-ray, MRI, or CT) and blood tests, to rule out other serious conditions that could mimic cervicothoracic interspinous bursitis before initiating treatment.

Improper Use of Corticosteroid Injections

- Corticosteroid injections are a common treatment for cervicothoracic bursitis, but improper administration, such as inadvertent epidural or subdural puncture, can result in significant complications including motor and sensory block, hypotension, or even loss of consciousness. These errors can lead to serious medico-legal consequences.
- **Thumb Rule Consideration:** Ensure that corticosteroid injections are administered with precision, using imaging guidance when necessary, to avoid complications such as inadvertent epidural or subdural puncture.

Delayed or Inadequate Conservative Treatment

- Initial conservative treatments like NSAIDs, physical therapy, and lifestyle modifications are crucial for managing cervicothoracic interspinous bursitis. Failure to adequately implement or monitor these treatments can lead to worsening symptoms, necessitating more invasive procedures and increasing legal exposure.
- **Thumb Rule Consideration:** Prioritize early and consistent conservative management with NSAIDs, physical therapy, and ergonomic adjustments, and monitor patient progress to adjust treatment as needed.

Failure to Address Underlying Functional Abnormalities

- Recurrence of cervicothoracic interspinous bursitis is common if the underlying functional abnormalities (e.g., poor posture, improper ergonomics) that caused the condition are not corrected. Neglecting these factors can lead to chronic pain and potential legal claims for ineffective treatment.

- **Thumb Rule Consideration:** Correct underlying functional abnormalities, such as poor posture or ergonomic issues, to prevent recurrence and ensure long-term relief from cervicothoracic interspinous bursitis.

REFERENCES

- Hull JJ, Tomaski SM: Osteomyelitis of the cervical spine: case report and literature review, Otolaryngol Head Neck Surg 113:193, 1995.
- Perka C, Schneider SV, Buttgereit F, Matziolis G: Development of cervical interspinous bursitis after prolonged sports trauma: a case report, Joint Bone Spine73:118–120, 2006.
- Reckelhoff KE, Green MN, Kettner NW: Cervical spine osteochondroma: rare presentation of a common lesion, J Manipulative Physiol Ther 33:711–715, 2010.
- Waldman SD: Cervicothoracic interspinous bursitis. In Waldman SD, editor: Pain review, Philadelphia, 2009, Saunders, pp 238–239.

CHARLIN'S SYNDROME

Although rare, a painful neuroma of the nerve stump, results in devastating symptoms of headache including upper facial and ocular pain, severe ipsilateral rhinorrhea and mucosal congestion, conjunctival injection. These symptoms and signs are called Charlin `s syndrome.

(Becker M, Kohler R, Vargas MI, Viallon M, Delavelle J. Pathology of the trigeminal nerve. Neuroimaging Clin N Am. 2008;18:283–307.)

Clinical Description

Charlin's syndrome is a very rare pathological condition, resulting from neuralgia of the nasociliary nerve. It is also called nasal nerve syndrome, nasociliaris nerve syndrome, and nasociliary syndrome. Some authors have referred to it as nasociliary neuralgia. In this syndrome, touching the outer aspect of one nostril causes a lancinating pain, which mainly radiates to the eyebrow, orbit, or into the nose or jaw, and is also accompanied by lacrimation, conjunctival infection, nasal congestion, sneezing, and redness of the skin on the forehead. However, the pathogenesis of this uncommon cause of head and face pain is thought to be dysfunction of the nasociliary ganglion in a manner analogous to the dysfunction of the sphenopalatine ganglion thought to be the source of cluster headache. The pain of Charlin's syndrome has a rapid onset to peak, with attacks lasting 45 to 60 minutes. In some patients, these attacks can be triggered by sensory stimulation of the affected areas. Although in many ways similar to cluster headache (e.g., retroorbital location of pain, profuse unilateral rhinorrhea, rapid onset to peak, and short duration of attacks), many dissimilarities also exist. In contrast to cluster headache, alcohol consumption does not appear to trigger attacks of Charlin's syndrome and the seasonal and chronobiological patterns so characteristic of cluster headache do not seem to be a factor. Patients suffering from Charlin's syndrome uniformly respond to daily nasociliary nerve blocks with local anesthetic, as described subsequently.

Pearls & Oysters

Patients suffering from Charlin's syndrome present with the complaint of severe paroxysms of ocular or retro-orbital pain that radiates into the ipsilateral forehead, nose, and maxillary region. The pain is associated with voluminous ipsilateral rhinorrhea and congestion of the nasal mucosa and significant inflammation of the affected eye (from Waldman SD: Atlas of uncommon pain syndromes. 3rd ed., Elsevier 2013).

Failure to diagnose Charlin's syndrome correctly may put the patient at risk if an intracranial pathological condition or demyelinating disease, which may mimic the clinical presentation of Charlin's syndrome, is overlooked. MRI is indicated in all patients thought to have Charlin's syndrome. Failure to diagnose glaucoma or temporal arteritis, which also may cause intermittent ocular pain, may result in permanent loss of sight.

Bottom Line Statement

Nasociliary nerve block via the medial orbital approach is especially useful in the diagnosis and palliation of pain secondary to Charlin's syndrome. Given the uncommon nature of this headache syndrome and its overlap with the symptoms of cluster headache and other neurological problems, including cavernous sinus thrombosis and intracranial and retroorbital tumors, Charlin's syndrome must remain a diagnosis of exclusion. All patients suspected to have Charlin's syndrome require MRI of the brain with and without gadolinium contrast material and thorough ophthalmological and neurological evaluation. Nasociliary nerve block via the medial orbital approach should be performed only by clinicians familiar with the regional anatomy.

Medico-Legal Traps

Failure to Diagnose Charlin's Syndrome Early

- Charlin's syndrome is often misdiagnosed due to its rare occurrence and overlapping symptoms with other conditions like cluster headaches, sinusitis, or neuralgias. Delayed or missed diagnosis can lead to unnecessary treatments and prolonged patient suffering, potentially leading to medico-legal consequences for mismanagement.
- **Thumb Rule Consideration:** Always consider Charlin's syndrome in patients presenting with severe ocular or retro-orbital pain and rhinorrhea, and confirm the diagnosis by ruling out more common conditions such as cluster headaches or sinusitis.

Overlooking Differential Diagnoses of Ocular Pain

- Charlin's syndrome can mimic conditions such as glaucoma, temporal arteritis, or intracranial pathologies like tumors. Failure to exclude these serious differential diagnoses can result in missed diagnoses of life-threatening conditions or permanent vision loss, leading to legal repercussions for inadequate diagnostic workup.
- **Thumb Rule Consideration:** Always rule out more serious conditions like glaucoma, temporal arteritis, or intracranial masses through comprehensive evaluation, including MRI and ophthalmological

examination, before diagnosing Charlin's syndrome.

Inappropriate or Delayed Imaging

- Given the rarity of Charlin's syndrome, it is crucial to use MRI with gadolinium contrast to exclude intracranial pathology. Failing to perform appropriate imaging can result in missed diagnoses of tumors or vascular anomalies, which could worsen the patient's prognosis and lead to legal action.
- **Thumb Rule Consideration:** Always perform MRI with and without gadolinium contrast in patients suspected of having Charlin's syndrome to rule out intracranial pathology and ensure an accurate diagnosis.

Improper Administration of Nasociliary Nerve Blocks

- Nasociliary nerve blocks are an effective treatment for Charlin's syndrome but must be performed by clinicians with expertise in the regional anatomy. Improper administration can lead to complications, including orbital damage or incomplete relief of symptoms, increasing the risk of legal claims for procedural errors.
- **Thumb Rule Consideration:** Ensure that nasociliary nerve blocks are administered only by clinicians familiar with the anatomy and technique, and monitor for potential complications during and after the procedure.

Failure to Manage Patient Expectations

- Charlin's syndrome can be challenging to manage due to its chronic and severe nature. Failure to set realistic expectations for treatment outcomes, especially regarding the frequency and effectiveness of nerve blocks, may lead to patient dissatisfaction and legal claims for inadequate care.
- **Thumb Rule Consideration:** Clearly communicate with patients about the chronic nature of Charlin's syndrome, the limitations of current treatments, and the importance of ongoing management to set realistic expectations for pain relief.

REFERENCES

- Charlin C. Le Syndrome du Nerf Nasal. Ann Ocul 1931;168:86.
- Roy FH. Ocular Syndromes and Systemic Diseases. 4th Ed. Coralville, Iowa: FEP international; 2008. p. 233.
- Syndromes and eponimes in Otolaryngology. Romanian J Rhinol 2011;1:223.
- Farri A, Enrico A, Farri F. Headaches of otolaryngological interest: Current status while awaiting revision of classification. Practical considerations and expectations. Acta Otorhinolaryngol Ital 2012;32:77-86.
- Becker M, Kohler R, Vargas MI, Viallon M, Delavelle J: Pathology of the trigeminal nerve, Neuroimaging Clin N Am 18:283–307, 2008.
- Craven J: Anatomy of the cranial nerves, Anaesth Intensive Care Med 11:529–534, 2010.
- Lewis DW, Gozzo YF, Avner MT: The "other" primary headaches in children and adolescents [review], Pediatr Neurol 33:303–313, 2005.

CHEIRALGIA PARESTHETICA

Cheiralgia paresthetica is a compression neuropathy of the superficial radial nerve. It manifests as sensory disturbances, such as paresthesias, to the dorsal and radial aspect of the wrist and hand. Treatment of this condition is straightforward for most patients with conservative measures directed at removing the offending agent.

Tosun N, Tuncay I, Akpinar F. Entrapment of the sensory branch of the radial nerve (Wartenberg's syndrome): an unusual cause. Tohoku J Exp Med. 2001 Mar;193(3):251-4.

Clinical Description

The radial nerve is susceptible to compression at many different locations throughout its course. Cheiralgia paresthetica is compression of the superficial branch of the radial nerve in the forearm. This condition was first described by Dr. Wartenberg in 1932 when he introduced the term cheiralgia paresthetica and reported five clinical cases. It is also commonly known as Wartenburg syndrome and superficial radial nerve palsy. The superficial radial nerve is purely sensory and does not have any motor component. The condition presents with symptoms such as pain and burning located on the dorsal and radial side of the hand. Often it is aggravated by activities such as pronation, pinching, and gripping.

The radial nerve derives from the posterior cord of the brachial plexus and consists of fibers from the nerve roots at C5, C6, C7, C8, and sometimes T1. It descends between the long head of the triceps and axillary artery and enters the posterior compartment of the arm via the triangular interval. It continues to descend along the medial proximal upper arm between the long and medial head of the triceps until it reaches the spiral groove. The nerve passes distally and laterally around the posterior humerus, where it penetrates the lateral intermuscular septum and gains access to the anterior compartment of the brachium. The nerve enters the anterior compartment distal to the deltoid insertion at approximately 11 cm proximal to the elbow. It continues anteriorly to the lateral epicondyle between the brachialis and brachioradialis at the elbow to enter the forearm.

Roughly 3 to 5 cm proximal to the supinator, the radial nerve separates into the posterior interosseous nerve and the superficial branch of the radial nerve. The posterior interosseous nerve proceeds deep to the supinator. The superficial branch of the radial nerve continues superficially to the supinator and deep to the ulnar margin of the brachioradialis in the anterolateral aspect of the forearm to where it briefly runs alongside the radial artery. At roughly 9 cm proximal to the radial styloid process, it then pierces the deep fascia between the middle and distal third of the forearm, to emerge between the brachioradialis and extensor carpi radialis longus to eventually become subcutaneous. The superficial branch of the radial nerve then ramifies again at approximately 4.9 cm proximal to the styloid process into dorsomedial and dorsolateral branches. These branches travel alongside the cephalic vein and proceed across the first dorsal compartment of the wrist and its tendons, the abductor pollicis longus and the extensor pollicis brevis. The dorsolateral branch supplies the dorsolateral thumb proximal to the interphalangeal joint. The dorsomedial branch supplies the dorsomedial thumb proximal to the interphalangeal joint, dorsoradial half of the hand and dorsal aspect of the index, long, and radial half of ring fingers proximal to the distal interphalangeal joint.

Pearls & Oysters

Complications include but are not limited to unsuccessful surgical decompression, persistent symptoms, worsening of symptoms, iatrogenic nerve injury or injury to surrounding structures, and wound problems.

Cheiralgia paresthetica can be treated well with straightforward nonoperative interventions. The key to treatment is an accurate diagnosis and identification of the cause of the compression. Once the cause is determined, patients should be educated on techniques to remove the compression and to avoid activities that will aggravate the symptoms. These conservative measures will lead to symptom resolution in the majority of patients.

Bottom Line Statement

Cheiralgia paresthetica is a relatively common disorder that is underdiagnosed. The diagnosis is often confused with other wrist disorders. Successful management of cheiralgia paresthetica encompasses an interprofessional team approach. Clinicians, including the primary care provider and nurse practitioner who first see the patient, must be familiar with this disease and its presentation to diagnose it correctly. Having a high index of suspicion will lead to prompt diagnosis and initiation of treatment. Radiologists and neurologists can further verify the disease and identify the location of compression through imaging and electrodiagnostic tests.

Treatment initially consists of multifactoral conservative management with the removal of compression and avoidance of provocative activities. Brace therapy may be an initial approach with input from orthotists. NSAIDs and other nerve medications may also be options; the pharmacist should verify appropriate agent selection, dosing, perform medication reconciliation, and counsel the patient regarding optimal use of NSAID to avoid complications such as gastric upset, reporting any issues to the nurse or physician. If patients fail to improve with conservative management, a surgeon can remove anatomic nerve compression through a variety of techniques. Postoperatively, the patient will benefit from physical therapy and occupational therapy focusing on early range of motion, nerve gliding exercises, and avoiding activities that exacerbate the condition. Specialty-trained nurses can monitor progress and provide patient education at follow-up visits and also watch for adverse medication effects, and let the treating physician know if there are any concerns. Open discussion and communication with the patient and between all of the health care providers on the interprofessional healthcare team is key to the successful treatment of this disease.

Medico-Legal Traps

Failure to Diagnose Cheiralgia Paresthetica Early

- Cheiralgia paresthetica is often misdiagnosed as other wrist conditions such as carpal tunnel syndrome or de Quervain's tenosynovitis. This delay in diagnosis can result in prolonged symptoms, inappropriate treatments, and potential legal claims for mismanagement.
- **Thumb Rule Consideration:** Always consider cheiralgia paresthetica in patients presenting with isolated sensory disturbances on the dorsal-radial aspect of the hand, and confirm the diagnosis through clinical examination and electrodiagnostic studies.

Inadequate Assessment of Compression Causes

- Failing to identify and address the source of radial nerve compression, such as wearing tight wristbands or repetitive motions, can result in persistent symptoms and recurrence. Neglecting to modify these risk factors may lead to worsening of the condition and legal action for incomplete treatment.
- **Thumb Rule Consideration:** Always thoroughly evaluate and educate patients on potential compression causes, such as tight accessories or repetitive activities, and ensure they modify these behaviors to prevent recurrence.

Overuse of Surgical Interventions

- While surgery may be necessary for refractory cases, premature or unnecessary surgical decompression can lead to complications such as iatrogenic nerve injury, persistent symptoms, or poor surgical outcomes, increasing the risk of medico-legal claims.

- **Thumb Rule Consideration:** Reserve surgical decompression for cases where conservative treatment fails, and ensure a thorough evaluation, including imaging and nerve studies, before recommending surgery.

Inadequate Conservative Treatment

- Cheiralgia paresthetica typically responds well to non-operative treatments such as NSAIDs, splinting, and activity modification. Failing to implement or inadequately monitor conservative management can result in prolonged symptoms and patient dissatisfaction, leading to potential legal issues.
- **Thumb Rule Consideration:** Prioritize conservative treatment measures, including rest, NSAIDs, splinting, and behavior modification, and regularly follow up with patients to monitor symptom resolution.

Failure to Provide Proper Postoperative Rehabilitation

- After surgical intervention, failing to ensure proper postoperative care, including physical therapy and nerve gliding exercises, can delay recovery and lead to persistent symptoms or recurrent nerve compression, resulting in potential legal claims for poor postoperative management.
- **Thumb Rule Consideration:** Provide comprehensive postoperative care, including physical therapy, nerve gliding exercises, and patient education on avoiding provocative activities, to optimize recovery and prevent recurrence.

REFERENCES

- Tosun N, Tuncay I, Akpinar F. Entrapment of the sensory branch of the radial nerve (Wartenberg's syndrome): an unusual cause. Tohoku J Exp Med. 2001 Mar;193(3):251-4.
- Braidwood AS. Superficial radial neuropathy. J Bone Joint Surg Br. 1975 Aug;57(3):380-3.
- Doughty CT, Bowley MP. Entrapment Neuropathies of the Upper Extremity. Med Clin North Am. 2019 Mar;103(2):357-370.
- Knutsen EJ, Calfee RP. Uncommon upper extremity compression neuropathies. Hand Clin. 2013 Aug;29(3):443-53.
- Popinchalk SP, Schaffer AA. Physical examination of upper extremity compressive neuropathies. Orthop Clin North Am. 2012 Oct;43(4):417-30.
- Jacobson JA, Fessell DP, Lobo Lda G, Yang LJ. Entrapment neuropathies I: upper limb (carpal tunnel excluded). Semin Musculoskelet Radiol. 2010 Nov;14(5):473-86.
- Latef TJ, Bilal M, Vetter M, Iwanaga J, Oskouian RJ, Tubbs RS. Injury of the Radial Nerve in the Arm: A Review. Cureus. 2018 Feb 16;10(2):e2199.
- Chodoroff G, Honet JC. Cheiralgia paresthetica and linear atrophy as a complication of local steroid injection. Arch Phys Med Rehabil. 1985 Sep;66(9):637-9.
- Patel A, Pierce P, Chiu DTW. A fascial band implicated in Wartenberg syndrome. Plast Reconstr Surg. 2014 Mar;133(3):440e-442e.
- Waldman SD: Cheiralgia paresthetica. In Waldman SD, editor: Pain review, Philadelphia, 2009, Saunders, pp 275–276

CHRONIC PAROXYSMAL HEMICRANIA (CPH)

Chronic paroxysmal hemicrania (CPH) is a primary headache syndrome characterized by recurrent unilateral episodes of headache associated with cranial autonomic symptoms. Headaches are sharp and stabbing in nature and occur greater than five times per day, up to forty times per day in some cases.

Headache Classification Committee of the International Headache Society (IHS) The International Classification of Headache Disorders, 3rd edition. Cephalalgia. 2018 Jan;38(1):1-211.

Clinical Description

Paroxysmal hemicrania is a rare form of headache that usually begins in adulthood. Patients experience severe throbbing, claw-like, or boring pain usually on one side of the face; in, around, or behind the eye; and occasionally reaching to the back of the neck. This pain may be accompanied by red and tearing eyes, a drooping or swollen eyelid on the affected side of the face, and nasal congestion. Patients may also feel dull pain, soreness, or tenderness between attacks. Attacks of paroxysmal hemicrania typically occur from 5 to 40 times per day and last 2 to 30 minutes. The disorder has two forms: chronic, in which patients experience attacks on a daily basis for a year or more, and episodic, in which the headaches may remit for months or years. Certain movements of the head or neck or external pressure to the neck may trigger these headaches in some patients. The disorder is more common in women than in men.

Many patients experience complete to near-complete relief of symptoms following physician-supervised medical treatment. Paroxysmal hemicrania may last indefinitely but has been known to go into remission or stop spontaneously. CPH is in a family of headache syndromes called the trigeminal autonomic cephalgias (TACs). TACs are characterized by unilateral trigeminal nerve distribution pain that occurs in tandem with ipsilateral cranial nerve autonomic symptoms. The TACs include paroxysmal hemicrania, cluster headache, hemicrania continua, short-lasting unilateral neuralgiform headache attacks with conjunctival injection and tearing (SUNCT).

The etiology of chronic paroxysmal hemicrania (CPH) is unknown.

Pearls & Oysters

Chronic paroxysmal hemicrania (CPH) is a significant headache syndrome for medical providers to be aware of because it can cause significant disability if left untreated, and it generally responds very well to treatment with indomethacin. Taking a thorough history, including headache frequency and duration, as well as the presence of associated cranial autonomic symptoms, is the key to diagnosing CPH. Cranial imaging and laboratory workup can help to rule out alternative diagnoses.

Failure to diagnose chronic paroxysmal hemicrania correctly may put the patient at risk if intracranial pathological conditions or demyelinating disease that may mimic the clinical presentation of chronic paroxysmal hemicrania is overlooked. MRI is indicated in all patients thought to have chronic paroxysmal hemicrania. Failure to diagnose glaucoma, which may cause intermittent ocular pain, may result in permanent loss of sight.

Bottom Line Statement

Chronic paroxysmal hemicrania is classified as a trigeminal autonomic cephalgia. The trigeminal autonomic cephalgias are a group of distinct headache syndromes that share a number of common and often overlapping clinical characteristics. The diagnosis of chronic paroxysmal hemicrania is made by obtaining a thorough, targeted headache history. Between attacks, patients with chronic paroxysmal hemicrania should have a normal neurological examination. If the neurological examination is abnormal between attacks, the diagnosis of chronic paroxysmal hemicrania should be discarded and a careful search for the cause of the patient's neurological findings should be undertaken.

Medico-Legal Traps

Failure to Diagnose Chronic Paroxysmal Hemicrania (CPH) Early

- CPH can be mistaken for other headache disorders such as migraines or cluster headaches. Delayed diagnosis may result in unnecessary treatments and prolonged patient suffering, as CPH typically responds well to indomethacin, unlike other headaches.
- **Thumb Rule Consideration:** Always consider CPH in patients with frequent unilateral headaches (5 to 40 times per day) and cranial autonomic symptoms, and confirm diagnosis with a positive indomethacin trial.

Misdiagnosis of Ocular Pain as Glaucoma

- Ocular pain associated with CPH can mimic conditions such as glaucoma.

Failure to differentiate between the two can lead to inappropriate ophthalmologic treatments and potential vision loss, increasing the risk of medico-legal claims.

- **Thumb Rule Consideration:** Perform thorough cranial imaging and clinical evaluation in patients presenting with ocular pain to rule out glaucoma and other ocular pathologies before diagnosing CPH.

Inadequate Use of Imaging to Rule Out Serious Conditions

- Serious conditions such as intracranial pathologies or demyelinating diseases may present similarly to CPH. Failing to perform MRI or other imaging studies to rule out these causes can result in missed diagnoses and potential legal consequences for neglecting thorough diagnostic workup.
- **Thumb Rule Consideration:** Always obtain an MRI in patients with suspected CPH to rule out intracranial pathologies and demyelinating diseases, ensuring a safe and accurate diagnosis.

Overlooking the Importance of Indomethacin for Diagnosis

- Indomethacin is the treatment of choice for CPH, and failure to use it in the diagnostic process can result in unnecessary or ineffective treatments. Mismanagement of medication can lead to prolonged patient discomfort and dissatisfaction.
- **Thumb Rule Consideration:** Use indomethacin as a diagnostic tool for CPH; a positive response confirms the diagnosis, while failure to respond should prompt consideration of alternative diagnoses.

Inadequate Follow-Up and Monitoring

- CPH may persist for long periods, and failing to provide adequate follow-up to adjust treatment or monitor for remission can lead to recurrence or exacerbation of symptoms, resulting in legal claims for inadequate care.
- **Thumb Rule Consideration:** Ensure regular follow-up for CPH patients to monitor symptom progression, treatment response, and adjust medications as needed to prevent relapse or complications.

REFERENCES

- Cittadini E, Matharu MS, Goadsby PJ. Paroxysmal hemicrania: a prospective clinical study of 31 cases. Brain. 2008 Apr;131(Pt 4):1142-55.
- Boes CJ, Dodick DW. Refining the clinical spectrum of chronic paroxysmal hemicrania: a review of 74 patients. Headache. 2002 Sep;42(8):699-708.
- Antonaci F, Sjaastad O. Chronic paroxysmal hemicrania (CPH): a review of the clinical manifestations. Headache. 1989 Nov;29(10):648-56.
- Benitez-Rosario MA, McDarby G, Doyle R, Fabby C: Chronic cluster-like headache secondary to prolactinoma: uncommon cephalalgia in association with brain tumors, J Pain Symptom Manage 37:271–276, 2009.

- Benoliel R, Sharav Y: Paroxysmal hemicrania: case studies and review of the literature, Oral Surg Oral Med Oral Pathol Oral Radiol Endodontol 85:285–292, 1998.
- Camarda C, Camarda R, Monastero R: Chronic paroxysmal hemicrania and hemicrania continua responding to topiramate: two case reports, Clin Neurol Neurosurg 110:88–91, 2008.

CLITORAL PRIAPISM

Clitoral priapism is a rare condition that is associated with an extended duration of clitoral erection due to local engorgement of clitoral tissue resulting in pain. Although the pathophysiology is not completely understood, it has been associated with specific classes of medications, diseases that alter clitoral blood flow or others associated with small to large vessel disease.

Thompson JW, Jr, Ware MR, Blashfield RK. Psychotropic medication and priapism: a comprehensive review. J Clin Psychiatry. 1990;51:430–433.

Clinical Description

Clitoral priapism is a rare cause of clitoral pain. It is thought to be a result of alterations in local hemodynamics leading to incomplete venous or lymphatic drainage of the clitoral tissue, resulting in edema and tissue swelling with concomitant pain. Due to the increasing number of medications being prescribed that can cause priapism as well as the resultant deficiency in blood flow to the clitoral region, it is paramount for the emergency physician (EP) to diagnose and treat appropriately. The prolonged erection is not associated with sexual stimulation, can last from minutes to days, and is frequently uncomfortable. Embarrassment can preclude patients from describing the exact nature of their symptoms, emphasizing the importance of a complete physical exam that includes an evaluation of the clitoris.

Clitoral priapism has been associated with medications producing alpha blockade, inhibition of serotonin reuptake, and non-SSRI antidepressants. It has also been associated with transitional cell carcinoma obstructing venous and lymphatic clitoral outflow.Since cases are rare, there is inadequate evidence to determine the incidence of this condition or the likelihood of a particular cause. However, it has been shown that discontinuing the offending agent can result in a therapeutic resolution within 24–72 hours.Other treatment modalities include imipramine, non-steroidal anti-inflammatory medications (NSAIDs), ice packs, opiates, and, rarely, intracavernous injection of adrenaline

Pearls & Oysters

No specific treatment regimen has been proven to be effective in managing clitoral priapism. However, cause-specific treatment frequently reverses the condition and has responded well, in case reports, to the usage of NSAIDS, cooling pads, and opiates, although their effectiveness is inconclusive.When the etiology in unknown, the course of treatment becomes more confused and uncertain. While several case reports have discussed the use of imipramine as the initial drug of choice, its effect is poorly understood.More likely, the patient's condition resolved because the offending agent was removed. Intracavernous administration of alpha agonists similar to the treatment of penile priapism has also been reported with success.Therefore, the accepted management involves removal of the offending agent, replacement with an agent from another therapeutic class, and coordinated treatment with imipramine for symptomatic episodes.

Bottom Line Statement

Priapism is defined as a persistent and painful erection of penile or clitoral tissue with a duration of more than six hours and is not associated with sexual arousal. Clitoral priapism is an infrequent cause of clitoral or vulvar pain and can result in unnecessary and extensive laboratory and radiographic testing if not diagnosed appropriately through the history and clinical examination. Although only infrequently associated with etiologies that can cause long-term morbidity, the episodes themselves can be incapacitating and can require multiple hospital or clinic visits for pain control, according to sporadic case reports in the literature. Often a vague history is obtained as a function of embarrassment and frequently the episode has abated by the time the clinician evaluates the patient, making it difficult to diagnose. The details of specific clitoral swelling followed by pain with concomitant erection of the clitoral tissue can be suggestive of the diagnosis. Often, patients will describe an episode of perceived vulvar or labial swelling or pain that leads to clitoral swelling, erection, and extensive pain. Others will describe symptoms of dysuria, anorgasmia, intestinal complaints, and even cramping pain in the pelvic or lower abdominal region within the episode of clitoral priapism. A search for antecedent or proximate causes should ensue, and would likely include a complete recent medication and illicit drug history, a complete physical and gynecological examination, relevant urine and pregnancy studies, and adjunct testing depending upon the physical exam and history findings.

The mechanism of clitoral priapism is theorized to be similar to the pathophysiology of male priapism, which involves altered circulation of the corpora cavernosa and increased clitoral intracavernous pressure resulting in erection of the glans. Decreasing venous outflow results in increased blood volume and pressure in the corpora. Although in men an increase in arterial inflow is an additional mechanism for producing priapism, this does not appear to be a relevant etiology in women.

Corporeal venous outflow obstruction is likely a result of the following causes:

1) alpha sympathomimetic blockade resulting in extended relaxation of corporal smooth muscle,

2) physical obstruction or sinus compression, and

3) venous drainage occlusion.

Medico-Legal Traps

Failure to Diagnose Clitoral Priapism Early

- Clitoral priapism is often misdiagnosed or overlooked due to its rarity and the patient's reluctance to describe symptoms. Delayed diagnosis can lead to unnecessary tests and prolonged discomfort, increasing the risk of medico-legal claims for delayed treatment or mismanagement.
- **Thumb Rule Consideration:** Always consider clitoral priapism in patients presenting with unexplained vulvar or clitoral pain, especially if there is a history of medication use that affects blood flow, and conduct a thorough physical exam including the clitoris.

Overlooking Medication as a Cause

- Clitoral priapism can be associated with specific medications, such as those affecting alpha blockade or serotonin reuptake. Failure to review the patient's medication history and recognize drug-induced priapism can lead to persistence of symptoms and potential legal repercussions for inadequate assessment.
- **Thumb Rule Consideration:** Always review a complete medication history, including psychotropic and non-SSRI antidepressants, in patients with suspected clitoral priapism, and consider discontinuing the offending agent as a first-line treatment.

Inadequate Pain Management

- Clitoral priapism can cause significant pain, and inadequate pain control may lead to multiple hospital visits and patient dissatisfaction. Failing to manage pain effectively can result in legal claims for suboptimal treatment.
- **Thumb Rule Consideration:** Provide prompt and adequate pain relief using NSAIDs, opiates, or other appropriate modalities such as ice packs, while treating the underlying cause of the priapism.

Failure to Explore Underlying Causes

- Although medication is a common cause, clitoral priapism can also result from conditions affecting venous or lymphatic drainage. Failure to investigate other potential causes, such as tumors or systemic diseases, can lead to missed diagnoses and legal liability for inadequate workup.
- **Thumb Rule Consideration:** If medication is not the cause, conduct a thorough evaluation, including imaging and lab tests, to rule out other causes of venous or lymphatic outflow obstruction, such as tumors or vascular disease.

Improper Use of Invasive Interventions

- Invasive treatments like intracavernous injection of alpha agonists should be reserved for severe cases. Premature or improper use of such treatments can lead to complications, increasing the risk of legal consequences for inappropriate interventions.
- **Thumb Rule Consideration:** Reserve invasive treatments, such as alpha agonist injections, for cases where conservative measures fail, and ensure they are administered by a clinician experienced in the technique to avoid complications.

REFERENCES

- Medina CA. Clitoral priapism: a rare condition presenting as a cause of vulvar pain. Obstet Gynecol. 2002;100:1089–1091.
- Klein DF. Repeated observations of yawning, clitoral engorgement, and orgasm associated with fluoxetine administration. J Clin Psychopharmacol. 1989;9:384.
- Slavin RE, et al. Locally aggressive granular cell tumor causing priapism of the crus of the clitoris. A light and ultrastructural study, with observations concerning the pathogenesis of fibrosis of the corpus cavernosum in priapism. Am J Surg Pathol. 1986;10:497–507.
- DiGiorgi S, Schnatz PF, Mandavilli S, Greene JF, Curry SL. Transitional cell carcinoma presenting as clitoral priapism. Gynecol Oncol. 2004;93:540–542.
- Berk M, Acton M. Citalopram-associated clitoral priapism: a case series. Int Clin Psychopharmacol. 1997;12:121–122.
- Pohl J, Pott B, Kleinhans G. Priapism: a three-phase concept of management according to etiology and prognosis. Br J Urol. 1986;58:113–118.
- Gordon SA, Stage KH, Tansey KE, Lotan Y. Conservative management of priapism in acute spinal cord injury. Urology. 2005;65:1195–1197.
- Yamamoto K. Priapism successfully treated with indomethacin: report of a case. Hinyokika Kiyo. 1970;16:283–286.
- Brodie-Meijer CC, Diemont WL, Buijs PJ. Nefazodone-induced clitoral priapism. Int Clin Psychopharmacol. 1999;14:257–258.
- Teixeira CE, Faro R, Moreno RA, et al. Nonadrenergic, noncholinergic relaxation of human isolated corpus cavernosum induced by scorpion venom. Urology. 2001;57:816–820.

CLIVAL CHORDOMA SYNDROME

Chordomas are rare tumors that can develop anywhere along the craniospinal axis. These tumors present challenges with respect to diagnosis and treatment due to a high rate of recurrence, even after multiple surgeries, and the propensity to involve any region within the craniospinal axis. New developments in radiation therapy have improved recurrence-free survival in patients with chordomas. Different regimens of chemotherapy and molecularly-targeted therapies, as adjuvants to surgery, have been described in individual case reports and case series.

McMaster ML, Goldstein AM, Bromley CM, et al. Chordoma: Incidence and survival patterns in the United States, 1973–1995. Cancer Causes Control. 2001;12(1):1–11.

Clinical Description

Clival chordoma is a rare type of neoplasm that arises from embryological remnants of the notochord along the spinal axis. These tumors are usually benign, although aggressive clival chordomas have been reported. They make up approximately one third of all central nervous system chordomas and tend to grow slowly, producing symptoms through the compression of adjacent brainstem and cranial nerves. Despite this, the long-term outcome for patients diagnosed with clival chordoma is generally poor due to the location of the tumors and their tendency to recur regardless of the treatment method chosen. Clival chordomas can occur at any age and are slightly more common in men. Early diagnosis is important to prevent acute neurological disasters, but the slow growth of these tumors results in an average time of 2 years from the onset of symptoms to diagnosis.

Pearls & Oysters

The slow-growing nature of clival chordomas can lead to delayed diagnosis, which can complicate the treatment of these tumors. Additionally, the clinical presentation of clival chordoma can be confusing because many of the clinical syndromes that mimic its signs and symptoms are also difficult to diagnose. This can make it challenging to accurately identify and treat clival chordoma.

Treatment options for clival chordoma may include surgery, radiation therapy, and chemotherapy, depending on the specific characteristics of the tumor and the overall health of the patient. Surgery is often the first line of treatment for clival chordoma, with the goal of removing as much of the tumor as possible. However, these tumors can be difficult to completely remove due to their location in the spine, and they may recur after surgery. In some cases, radiation therapy or chemotherapy may be used to slow the growth of the tumor or to help reduce the risk of recurrence.

Overall, the management of clival chordoma can be complex and requires the expertise of a multidisciplinary team of healthcare professionals. It is important for patients with clival chordoma to work closely with their healthcare team to develop a treatment plan that is tailored to their individual needs.

Bottom Line Statement

Clival chordoma is a rare type of neoplasm, or abnormal growth of tissue, that arises from embryological remnants of the notochord along the spinal axis. These tumors are usually benign, although aggressive clival chordomas have been reported. Clival chordomas tend to grow slowly and produce symptoms through the compression of adjacent brainstem and cranial nerves. Despite this, the long-term outlook for patients with clival chordoma is generally poor due to the location of these tumors and their tendency to recur regardless of the treatment method chosen. Clival chordomas can occur at any age and are slightly more common in men. Early diagnosis is important to prevent acute neurological problems, but the slow growth of these tumors can result in a delay in diagnosis. Treatment options for clival chordoma may include surgery, radiation therapy, and chemotherapy, depending on the specific characteristics of the tumor and the overall health of the patient. It is important for patients with clival chordoma to work closely with their healthcare team to develop a treatment plan that is tailored to their individual needs.

Medico-Legal Traps

Failure to Diagnose Clival Chordoma Early

- Clival chordomas are slow-growing and often mimic other neurological conditions, which can lead to delayed diagnosis. Missing early signs of the tumor can result in severe neurological deficits or a more complicated treatment process, increasing the risk of medico-legal claims for diagnostic delays.
- **Thumb Rule Consideration:** Always consider clival chordoma in patients presenting with progressive neurological symptoms and brainstem compression signs, and prioritize MRI imaging to detect the tumor early.

Inadequate Surgical Resection

- Complete surgical resection is difficult due to the tumor's location near vital structures, but incomplete resection can lead to recurrence. Failure to plan or perform surgery with appropriate expertise can result in residual tumor tissue and complications, leading to potential legal action for inadequate care.

- **Thumb Rule Consideration:** Ensure that surgical resection of clival chordoma is performed by an experienced neurosurgical team, and combine it with adjunct therapies like radiation to reduce the likelihood of recurrence.

Delayed Use of Radiation Therapy

- Postoperative radiation therapy is essential for improving long-term survival and reducing recurrence in clival chordoma patients. Delayed or inadequate use of radiation can lead to tumor recurrence and worsening patient outcomes, resulting in legal claims for improper treatment planning.
- **Thumb Rule Consideration:** Implement radiation therapy early in the postoperative period for clival chordoma patients to ensure the best chance of recurrence-free survival.

Failure to Implement Multidisciplinary Care

- Clival chordoma requires a multidisciplinary approach, including neurosurgeons, oncologists, radiologists, and rehabilitation specialists. Failure to coordinate care across disciplines can lead to suboptimal outcomes and increased medico-legal risks for incomplete management.
- **Thumb Rule Consideration:** Involve a multidisciplinary team in the treatment of clival chordoma, ensuring that all aspects of the patient's care—surgery, radiation, and follow-up—are managed cohesively.

Inadequate Follow-up and Monitoring

- Clival chordomas have a high risk of recurrence, even after aggressive treatment. Failure to provide adequate follow-up with regular imaging and clinical evaluations can result in missed recurrences, leading to avoidable complications and legal claims for inadequate long-term care.
- **Thumb Rule Consideration:** Ensure patients with clival chordoma receive long-term follow-up with regular MRI scans and clinical evaluations to monitor for recurrence and address any new symptoms promptly.

REFERENCES

- Stacchiotti S, Sommer J, Chordoma Global Consensus Group. Building a global consensus approach to chordoma: a position paper from the medical and patient community. Lancet Oncology. 2015 Feb;16(2):e71-83. doi: 10.1016/S1470-2045(14)71190-8.
- Stacchiotti S, Gronchi A, Fossati P, et al. Best practices for the management of local-regional recurrent chordoma: a position paper by the Chordoma Global Consensus Group. Ann Oncol. 2017 Jun 1;28(6):1230-

1242. doi: 10.1093/annonc/mdx054.

- Walcott BP, Nahed BV, Mohyeldin A, Coumans JV, Kahle KT, Ferreira MJ. Chordoma: current concepts, management, and future directions. Lancet Oncology. 2012 Feb;13(2):e69-76. doi: 10.1016/S1470-2045(11)70337-0.
- Diaz RJ, Cusimano MD. The biological basis for the modern treatment of chordoma. J Neurooncol. 2011 Sep;104(2):411-22. doi: 10.1007/s11060-011-0559-8. Epub 2011 Mar 8.
- Sciubba DM, Cheng JJ, Petteys RJ, Weber KL, Frassica DA, Gokaslan ZL. Chordoma of the sacrum and vertebral bodies. J Am Acad Orthop Surg. 2009 Nov;17(11):708-17.

CORONARY LIGAMENT STRAIN

Preservation of the meniscus whenever possible is essential in maintaining knee stability and preventing premature osteoarthritis. Peripheral meniscal tears are the most amenable to surgical repair. This study evaluates the peripheral attachments of the medial meniscus and focuses on a specific tear limited to the meniscotibial ligament (coronary ligament). The diagnosis is made arthrographically when the medial meniscus floats above the tibial plateau without separating completely from the capsule. The lateral meniscus is rarely involved in this type of injury.

Skeletal Radiol. 1984;11(3):191-6. doi: 10.1007/BF00349493.

Clinical Description

The coronary ligaments, also known as the meniscotibial ligaments, are part of the fibrous capsule of the knee joint. They are made up of the medial coronary ligament and the lateral coronary ligament. They connect the inferior edges of the menisci to the of the tibial plateau. The coronary ligaments support rotational stability of the knee and prevent anterior tibial translation.

Coronary ligament injuries can lead to other knee joint pathology and negatively alter the biomechanics of the knee. Lesions to the coronary ligaments can increase rotational instability. They can also cause increased strain on the anterior cruciate ligament or menisci . This leads to risk of meniscal extrusion or other injury to these structures. Research suggests coronary ligament injuries are under diagnosed and untreated, as they present similar to meniscus pathologies.

Pearls & Oysters

Perhaps even more important to manual practitioners are incidences of injury to these ligaments from non-traumatic factors. Such injuries can often develop slowly over time through constant pounding from some of the previously mentioned sports (in addition to distance running, especially if performed over inconsistent terrains). Clinically I have found these injuries to be very common and often mis-diagnosed for example as Iliotibial band syndrome at the lateral attachment to the knee. Chronic injury to the ligaments will result in connective tissue fibrosis/contraction, which then, in addition to causing pain, can limit proper translation of the menisci; this can theoretically lead to injury to the menisci, or the stabilizing ligaments of the knee due to altered biomechanics.

Bottom Line Statement

Named after the Latin word corona, meaning crown (referring to their crown-like shape), the coronary ligaments are two in number and are termed medial and lateral coronary ligaments. These often forgotten, but clinically important ligaments are in truth part of the fibrous capsule of the knee joint.

Injury to these structures is very common, however more commonly overlooked. Activities that particularly stress them involve rotation/torsion of the tibia on the femur as often occurs during sports such as dancing, martial arts, racquet sports, football, and soccer; particularly if the athlete has poor foot and/or knee alignment. Another pre-disposing factor is laxity in either the cruciate and/or collateral ligaments.

Injury to the coronary ligaments commonly stems from traumatic injury. For example, they are frequently ruptured in medial collateral ligament disruption and lateral collateral ligament complex tears; although injury to the structures can occur independently. Typically, the precipitating incident is a sudden and forceful medial or lateral twist of the knee occurring on a planted foot. The resultant pain is often sharp with sudden movements and may or may not be accompanied by mild swelling depending on the degree of the injury. In most cases flexion and extension ROM will remain full with discomfort at end range although with higher grades, effusion may restrict full end ranges.

As the coronary ligaments are not clearly described in most anatomy texts, many manual therapists are unaware of their significance. Injury to these structures are often confused with damage to other structures in the knee. For example, acute, traumatic injury is often misdiagnosed as meniscal tears, or collateral ligament sprains. Confounding the incidence of incorrect diagnoses is the misinterpretation of a widely utilized orthopedic test, namely 'joint line tenderness.' This test is performed by simply applying pressure to the medial or lateral joint line. Pain with pressure is often considered a positive test for meniscal tears/damage...however more often this represents injury to the collateral ligaments. This misinterpretation occurs, as coronary ligament damage can be present with meniscal injury, however from my clinical experience sole injury to the coronary ligaments is most often the case.

Medico-Legal Traps

Failure to Diagnose Coronary Ligament Strain Early

- Coronary ligament injuries are often overlooked or misdiagnosed as more common knee injuries like meniscal tears or Iliotibial Band Syndrome (ITBS). This delay in diagnosis can result in improper treatment, prolonged pain, and worsening of the injury, increasing the risk of medico-legal claims for mismanagement.

- **Thumb Rule Consideration:** Always consider coronary ligament strain in patients with knee pain, especially those involved in sports requiring rotational knee movements, and use targeted imaging to differentiate it from meniscal or collateral ligament injuries.

Misinterpretation of Joint Line Tenderness Test

- The joint line tenderness test is commonly used to diagnose meniscal injuries, but it can be falsely positive in cases of coronary ligament injury. Misinterpreting this test can lead to incorrect treatment plans focused on meniscal repair or other knee structures, which may result in poor outcomes and legal liability.
- **Thumb Rule Consideration:** Be cautious when using the joint line tenderness test, as coronary ligament injuries can present similarly to meniscal injuries. Ensure further diagnostic imaging is used to confirm the diagnosis before proceeding with treatment.

Inadequate Treatment of Non-Traumatic Coronary Ligament Injuries

- Non-traumatic, overuse injuries to the coronary ligaments, especially in activities like running or martial arts, are often misdiagnosed or untreated. Failing to address the underlying biomechanical causes can lead to chronic pain, fibrosis, and further knee instability, exposing clinicians to medico-legal risks for poor management.
- **Thumb Rule Consideration:** Assess patients for chronic or overuse injuries to the coronary ligaments, particularly in athletes, and focus on addressing biomechanical issues such as foot and knee alignment alongside treatment.

Overlooking the Role of Coronary Ligament in Knee Stability

- Coronary ligaments play a key role in rotational stability of the knee, and injury to them can increase strain on other knee structures, such as the anterior cruciate ligament (ACL) or menisci. Failure to recognize and treat coronary ligament injury can lead to secondary injuries and legal claims for incomplete diagnosis and treatment.
- **Thumb Rule Consideration:** Always consider the potential impact of coronary ligament strain on knee biomechanics, especially in patients with rotational instability, and include rehabilitation strategies aimed at preventing further knee damage.

Failure to Provide Adequate Post-Injury Rehabilitation

- Coronary ligament injuries require proper rehabilitation, including strengthening and stabilization exercises, to prevent long-term instability or chronic pain. Failing to implement a structured rehabilitation plan can lead to recurrent injury, worsening of symptoms, and potential legal claims for inadequate care.
- **Thumb Rule Consideration:** Ensure patients receive a comprehensive rehabilitation program after coronary ligament injury, focusing on knee stability, rotational control, and addressing any contributing biomechanical factors to prevent recurrence or further injury.

REFERENCES

- Guy S, Ferreira A, Carrozzo A, Delaloye JR, Cavaignac E, Vieira TD, Sonnery-Cottet B. Isolated Meniscotibial Ligament Rupture: The Medial Meniscus "Belt Lesion". Arthrosc Tech. 2022 Jan 13;11(2):e133-e138.
- Feger J, Knipe H, Knipe H, et al. Meniscotibial ligaments. Available from: https://radiopaedia.org/articles/meniscotibial-ligaments(Accessed on 21 Nov 2022)
- Smith PA, Humpherys JL, Stannard JP, Cook JL. Impact of Medial Meniscotibial Ligament Disruption Compared to Peripheral Medial Meniscal Tear on Knee Biomechanics. J Knee Surg. 2021 Jun;34(7):784-792
- A. Peltier, T. Lording, L. Maubisson, R. Ballis, P. Neyret, S. Lustig. The role of the meniscotibial ligament in posteromedial rotational knee stability Knee Surg Sports Traumatol Arthrosc 2015 23:2967–2973
- Krych AJ, Bernard CD, Leland DP, Camp CL, Johnson AC, Finnoff JT, Stuart MJ. Isolated meniscus extrusion associated with meniscotibial ligament abnormality. Knee Surg Sports Traumatol Arthrosc. 2020 Nov;28(11):3599-3605.
- Smith PA, Humpherys JL, Stannard JP, Cook JL. Impact of Medial Meniscotibial Ligament Disruption Compared to Peripheral Medial Meniscal Tear on Knee Biomechanics. J Knee Surg. 2021 Jun;34(7):784-792.
- Mariani PP, Torre G, Battaglia MJ. The post-traumatic meniscal extrusion, sign of meniscotibial ligament injury. A case series. Orthop Traumatol Surg Res. 2022 May;108(3):103226.
- Otten MHC. Pain in the Coronary Ligaments of the Knee: How Regenerative Therapies Can Help. Available from: https://cellaxys.com/pain-in-the-coronary-ligaments-of-the-knee-how-regenerative-therapies-can-help/ (Accessed 22/11/2022).
- Paletta GA Jr, Crane DM, Konicek J, Piepenbrink M, Higgins LD, Milner JD, Wijdicks CA. Surgical Treatment of Meniscal Extrusion: A Biomechanical Study on the Role of the Medial Meniscotibial Ligaments With Early Clinical Validation. Orthop J Sports Med. 2020 Jul 29;8(7):2325967120936672.

COUGH HEADACHE

Cough headache is a well described, but rare headache. Headaches are characteristically triggered by a rapid increase in intra-abdominal pressure which occurs with coughing, sneezing or straining.

Tinel J. La Céphalée à l'effort. Syndrome de distension douloureuse des veines intracrâniennes. Méd (Paris) 1932;14:113–8.

Clinical Description

Primary cough headache which has a lifetime prevalence of 1%, is a sudden-onset bilateral or unilateral headache lasting seconds to 2 hours without associated symptoms provoked by coughing, sudden postural movements, weightlifting, laughing, and defecating and usually occurring in people over the age of 40 years.

Cough headache is a term used to describe headaches triggered by coughing and other activities associated with a Valsalva maneuver, such as laughing, straining at stool, lifting, and bending the head toward the ground.

Clinicians have identified the following two types of cough headache:

- Benign
- Symptomatic

Secondary pathology should be excluded including Chiari type 1 malformation, posterior fossa lesions, unruptured cerebral aneurysms, spontaneous intracranial hypotension, and subdural hematoma by obtaining an MRI of the brain with and without contrast, and MRA (magnetic resonance angiogram) of the brain.

Initially, both types of cough headache were thought to be related to sexual and exertional headaches, but they are now considered distinct clinical entities. A strong male predilection is seen for benign cough headache and no gender predilection for symptomatic cough headache.

Pearls & Oysters

Failure to diagnose cough headache correctly may put the patient at risk if intracranial pathology or demyelinating disease (which may mimic the clinical presentation of cough headache) is overlooked. MRI and MRA are indicated in all patients thought to have cough headache. Failure to diagnose glaucoma, which also may cause intermittent ocular pain, may result in permanent loss of sight.

Bottom Line Statement

Any patient presenting with headaches associated with exertion or Valsalva maneuver should be taken very seriously. Although statistically most of these headaches ultimately are proved to be of benign cause, a few patients have potentially life-threatening disease. The diagnosis of cough headache is made by obtaining a thorough, targeted headache history and performing a careful physical examination.

The clinician must separate patients suffering from benign cough headache from patients suffering from symptomatic cough headache. Patients with benign cough headache should have a normal neurological examination. If the neurological examination is abnormal, the diagnosis of benign cough headache should be discarded and a careful search for the cause of the patient's neurological findings should be undertaken.

Medico-Legal Traps

Failure to Differentiate Between Benign and Symptomatic Cough Headache

- Cough headaches can be either benign or symptomatic of a more serious underlying condition such as Chiari malformation or intracranial pathology. Failing to distinguish between these can result in a missed diagnosis of a potentially life-threatening condition, leading to medico-legal consequences for negligence.
- **Thumb Rule Consideration:** Always differentiate between benign and symptomatic cough headaches by obtaining detailed imaging, including MRI and MRA, to rule out structural or vascular abnormalities in patients presenting with cough-induced headaches.

Failure to Perform Adequate Imaging

- Symptomatic cough headaches can be linked to serious conditions like posterior fossa lesions or unruptured cerebral aneurysms. Failing to order comprehensive imaging (MRI and MRA) may lead to missed diagnoses and severe outcomes such as brainstem compression or hemorrhage, exposing clinicians to legal liability for incomplete workup.
- **Thumb Rule Consideration:** Always perform MRI and MRA of the brain in patients with cough headaches to exclude serious underlying pathology, especially if the patient has abnormal neurological findings.

Misdiagnosis of Cough Headache as a Benign Condition

- Cough headaches may be misdiagnosed as benign without proper investigation, leading to potential harm if the headache is symptomatic of a serious condition. Misdiagnosis can result in delayed or missed treatment for intracranial pathologies, increasing the risk of legal action.
- **Thumb Rule Consideration:** Do not assume a cough headache is benign without ruling out symptomatic causes, particularly in patients over 40 or those with additional neurological symptoms.

Inadequate Patient History and Examination

- Cough headache diagnosis relies heavily on a detailed history and thorough physical examination. Failing to gather comprehensive information on the frequency, duration, and triggers of the headache can lead to incorrect diagnosis and treatment, raising legal risks for incomplete assessment.
- **Thumb Rule Consideration:** Obtain a thorough headache history focused on triggers like coughing, sneezing, and exertion, and perform a complete neurological exam to guide appropriate diagnostic testing.

Failure to Rule Out Ocular Conditions Such as Glaucoma

- Cough headache can mimic ocular conditions like glaucoma, which can present with intermittent ocular pain. Failing to consider and rule out glaucoma in patients presenting with headache and ocular symptoms could lead to permanent vision loss and potential medico-legal liability.
- **Thumb Rule Consideration:** Always consider and rule out ocular conditions such as glaucoma in patients presenting with ocular pain associated with a cough headache, especially if there are visual disturbances or increased intraocular pressure.

REFERENCES

- Berciano J, Poca M-A, García A, Sahuquillo J: Paroxysmal cervicobrachial coughinduced pain in a patient with syringomyelia extending into spinal cord posterior gray horns, J Neurol 54:678–681, 2007.
- Pareja JA, Álvarez M: The usual treatment of trigeminal autonomic cephalalgias. Headache 53(9):1401-1414, 2013.
- Cutrer FM, DeLange J: Cough, exercise, and sex headaches. Neurol Clin 32:433-450, 2014.
- Chen YY, Lirng JF, Fuh JL, et al: Primary cough headache is associated with posterior fossa crowdedness: a morphometric MRI study, Cephalalgia 24:694–699, 2004.
- Pascual J: Primary cough headache, Curr Pain Headache Rep 9:272–276, 2005.
- Pascual J, Rubén Martín A, Oterino A: Headaches precipitated by cough, prolonged exercise or sexual activity: a prospective etiological and clinical study, J Headache Pain 9:259–266, 2008.
- Waldman SD: Arnold Chiari malformation type I. In Waldman SD, Campbell RS, editors: Imaging of pain, Philadelphia, 2011, Saunders, pp 27–28.

CUBITAL BURSITIS

The bicipitoradial bursa lies at the insertion of the biceps tendon on the radial tuberosity. It is an unusual site for chronic bursitis and most often results from repetitive mechanical trauma or overuse. Other causes include tuberculosis, immunological complications of rheumatological disease and synovial chondromatosis. Accurate diagnosis requires imaging studies and sometimes histological study.

Journal of Orthopaedics, Trauma and Rehabilitation Volume 18, Issue 1, June 2014, Pages 7-11

Clinical Description

Cubital bursitis is a condition that causes inflammation and swelling of the cubital bursa, a small fluid-filled sac located in the anterior aspect of the elbow. This condition is becoming more common due to the increasing number of people using exercise equipment. Cubital bursitis can be caused by acute trauma to the elbow, such as a direct injury or repetitive movements such as biceps strengthening exercises or throwing sports. It can also be caused by conditions such as gout or rheumatoid arthritis. If the inflammation of the cubital bursa becomes chronic, calcification of the bursa may occur. Symptoms of cubital bursitis include elbow pain, swelling, and tenderness in the affected area. Treatment may include rest, ice, physical therapy, and medications to reduce inflammation. In severe cases, surgery may be necessary to remove the bursa. It is important to seek medical attention if you experience persistent elbow pain or other symptoms of cubital bursitis.

Elbow pain can be caused by a variety of conditions, including arthritis of the elbow joint, tennis elbow, golfer's elbow, and olecranon bursitis. Arthritis of the elbow joint can cause pain similar to that seen in cubital bursitis, but the point tenderness seen in cubital bursitis is absent in arthritis of the elbow. Tennis elbow and golfer's elbow are characterized by pain and tenderness over the lateral and medial epicondyles, rather than at the midline as seen with cubital bursitis. Acute gout affecting the elbow may present as a diffuse, inflammatory condition that may be difficult to distinguish from infection of the joint, rather than as a localized musculoskeletal pain syndrome. It is important to seek medical attention if you experience persistent elbow pain or other symptoms, as these conditions can be managed with appropriate treatment.

Pearls & Oysters

Misdiagnosis is the major complication associated with the diagnosis of cubital bursitis. If a clinician fails to recognize an acute inflammatory or infectious arthritis of the elbow, this can result in permanent damage to the joint and chronic pain and functional disability. Injection of the cubital bursa at the elbow is generally a safe procedure, but there is a risk of inadvertent intravascular injection or persistent paresthesia due to needle trauma to the median nerve. To decrease the risk of these complications, a 25- or 37-gauge needle may be used, although this may increase the risk of hematoma. Applying manual pressure to the area of the block immediately after injection and using cold packs for 20-minute periods after the procedure can also help to reduce postprocedure pain and bleeding. It is important to follow the instructions of your healthcare provider and to report any adverse reactions or complications to your provider as soon as possible.

Bottom Line Statement

Bursae are small, fluid-filled sacs that are found around joints and help to reduce friction and allow muscles and tendons to move smoothly over each other. They are lined with a synovial membrane and contain synovial fluid, which is produced by the blood vessels in the synovial membrane. When a bursa becomes inflamed, there is an increase in the production of synovial fluid, which can cause swelling of the bursal sac. Overuse or misuse of a joint can lead to inflammation, enlargement, and, rarely, infection of the bursae. Coexisting conditions such as tendinitis and epicondylitis may also contribute to elbow pain and may require additional treatment with local anesthetic and depot steroid injections. These injections can be a safe procedure if care is taken to avoid the median nerve and use sterile technique to prevent infection. The use of physical modalities, such as heat and gentle range-of-motion exercises, can be helpful several days after the injection, while avoiding vigorous exercises that may exacerbate symptoms. Simple analgesics and nonsteroidal anti-inflammatory drugs (NSAIDs) may also be used in conjunction with this injection technique for elbow pain.

Medico-Legal Traps

Failure to Differentiate Cubital Bursitis from Other Elbow Conditions

- Cubital bursitis can mimic conditions such as arthritis, tennis elbow, and olecranon bursitis. Misdiagnosing cubital bursitis as one of these other conditions may lead to improper treatment, worsening the condition, and increasing the risk of medico-legal claims for diagnostic errors.

- **Thumb Rule Consideration:** Always perform a thorough physical exam and use imaging studies to differentiate cubital bursitis from other elbow pathologies, such as arthritis or epicondylitis, to ensure appropriate treatment.

Inadequate Diagnostic Workup to Rule Out Infection or Gout

- Cubital bursitis can be caused by gout, infections, or inflammatory conditions like rheumatoid arthritis. Failing to investigate and rule out these underlying causes can lead to persistent symptoms or worsening of the condition, increasing legal exposure for inadequate diagnostic workup.
- **Thumb Rule Consideration:** Always perform diagnostic tests, including blood work or joint aspiration, to rule out infection, gout, or inflammatory arthritis in patients presenting with symptoms of cubital bursitis.

Complications from Injections into the Cubital Bursa

- Injection therapy can be a safe and effective treatment for cubital bursitis, but improper technique can lead to complications such as nerve injury or intravascular injection. Mismanagement of these complications may result in legal claims for procedural errors.
- **Thumb Rule Consideration:** Use proper injection techniques with small-gauge needles to minimize risks, and take care to avoid nerve trauma or intravascular injection when administering treatment for cubital bursitis.

Failure to Address Underlying Causes or Contributing Factors

- Cubital bursitis may develop due to overuse or repetitive trauma, and failing to address these contributing factors can result in recurrent bursitis or further joint damage. This may lead to claims for inadequate or incomplete treatment.
- **Thumb Rule Consideration:** Always assess and address underlying causes such as repetitive movements or improper exercise techniques, and incorporate activity modification or ergonomic changes into the treatment plan to prevent recurrence.

Inadequate Post-Injection Care and Monitoring

- Post-injection care, including monitoring for complications like infection or hematoma, is critical. Failure to provide proper follow-up or manage adverse effects promptly can result in patient harm and legal liability for inadequate care.

- **Thumb Rule Consideration:** Provide clear post-injection instructions, including monitoring for signs of infection or nerve damage, and ensure timely follow-up to assess the effectiveness of the treatment and any complications.

REFERENCES

- A.Y. Skaf, R.D. Boutin, R.W. Dantas, et al. Bicipitoradial bursitis: MR imaging findings in eight patients and anatomic data from contrast material opacification of bursae followed by routine radiography and MR imaging in cadavers Radiology, 212 (1999), pp. 111-116.
- D.R. Wenzke MR imaging of the elbow in the injured athlete Radiol Clin N Am, 51 (2013), pp. 195-213.
- S. Kannangara, D. Munidasa, J. Kross, et al. Scintigraphy of cubital bursitis Clin Nucl Med, 27 (2002), pp. 348-350.
- N.D. Karanjia, P.J. Stiles Cubital bursitis J Bone Joint Surg Br, 70 (1988), pp. 832-833.
- F. Draghi, B. Gregoli, C. Sileo Sonography of the bicipitoradial bursa: a short pictorial essay J Ultrasound, 15 (2012), pp. 39-41.
- K. Matsumoto, S. Hukuda, M. Fujita, et al. Cubital bursitis caused by localized synovial chondromatosis of the elbow. A case report J Bone Joint Surg, 78A (1996), pp. 275-277.
- Skaf AY, Boutin RD, Dantas RW et al. Bicipitoradial bursitis: MR imaging findings in eight patients and anatomic data from contrast material opacification of bur- sae followed by routine radiography and MR imaging in cadavers. Radiology. 1999 Jul;212(1):111-6.
- Karanja ND, Stiles PJ. Cubital bursitis. J Bone Joint Surg Br. 1988 Nov;70(5):832-3.
- Matsumoto K, Hukuda S, Fujita M, Kakimoto A, Tachibana S. Cubital bursitis caused by localized synovial chondromatosis of the elbow : A case report. J Bone Joint Surg Am. 1996 Feb;78(2):275-7.
- Yamamoto T, Mizuno K, Soejima T, Fujii M. Bicipital radial bursitis - CT and MR appearance. Comput Med Imaging Graph. 2001 Nov-Dec;25(6):531-3
- Liessi G, Cesari S, Spaliviero B, Dell?Antonio C, Avventi P. The US, CT and MR findings of cubital bursitis : A report of five cases. Skeletal Radiol. 1996 Jul;25(5):471-5.
- Kannangara S, Munidasa D, Kross J, Van der Wall H. Scintigraphy of cubital bursitis. Clin Nucl Med. 2002 May;27(5):348-50.

CUBITAL TUNNEL SYNDROME

Cubital tunnel syndrome is neuropathy of the ulnar nerve causing symptoms of numbness and shooting pain along the medial aspect of the forearm, also including the medial half of the fourth digit and the fifth digit. It is caused by compression of the ulnar nerve at the elbow region. Ulnar nerve neuropathy is the second most common compression neuropathy of the arm, following carpal tunnel syndrome.

Filippou G, Mondelli M, Greco G, Bertoldi I, Frediani B, Galeazzi M, Giannini F. Ulnar neuropathy at the elbow: how frequent is the idiopathic form? An ultrasonographic study in a cohort of patients. Clin Exp Rheumatol. 2010 Jan-Feb;28(1):63-7.

Clinical Description

Cubital tunnel syndrome (CBTS) is a peripheral nerve compression syndrome. It is an irritation or injury of the ulnar nerve in the cubital tunnel at the elbow. This is also termed ulnar nerve entrapment and is the second most common compression neuropathy in the upper extremity after carpal tunnel syndrome. It represents a source of considerable discomfort and disability for the patient and may, in extreme, cases lead to a loss of function of the hand. Cubital tunnel syndrome is also often misdiagnosed.

Peripheral nerve compression syndromes are characterised by chronic irritation and pressure lesions on the sites where nerves have to pass through narrow anatomic spaces and fibro-osseous structures. The main clinical manifestation of this type of compression are paresthesia, sensory impairment and paresis.

Cubital tunnel syndrome can also be caused by traction, pressure or ischemia of the ulnar nerve which passes through the cubital tunnel at the medial side of the elbow.[5] Pain or paraesthesia in the fourth and fifth finger and pain in the medial aspect of the elbow, which may extend proximally or distally, is caused by compression of the ulnar nerve. There is only limited evidence that proves the effectiveness of nonsurgical and surgical interventions to treat cubital tunnel syndrome.

Pearls & Oysters

Cubital tunnel syndrome is a condition that occurs when the ulnar nerve, which runs from the neck down the arm to the hand, becomes compressed or entrapped as it passes through the cubital tunnel at the elbow. This can lead to pain, numbness, and tingling in the hand and fingers, as well as weakness in the hand and wrist.

Golfer's elbow, also known as medial epicondylitis, is a condition that causes pain and inflammation on the inside of the elbow. It is often caused by overuse or repetitive stress on the muscles and tendons of the elbow and is common in athletes, particularly golfers.

Cubital tunnel syndrome can be misdiagnosed as golfer's elbow because the symptoms of these two conditions can be similar. However, there are some key differences between the two conditions. In cubital tunnel syndrome, the maximal tenderness to palpation is typically found 1 inch below the medial epicondyle, while in golfer's elbow, the maximal tenderness is typically found directly over the medial epicondyle. Additionally, cubital tunnel syndrome may be accompanied by weakness in the hand and wrist, while golfer's elbow typically does not cause these symptoms.

It is important for a healthcare provider to accurately diagnose cubital tunnel syndrome, as the treatment for this condition differs from the treatment for golfer's elbow. Treatment for cubital tunnel syndrome may include non-surgical options such as splinting, physical therapy, and corticosteroid injections, as well as surgical options such as decompression surgery to relieve the pressure on the ulnar nerve.

Bottom Line Statement

Despite the significant amount of literature devoted to the diagnosis and treatment of cubital tunnel syndrome, optimal treatment often requires two very simple components of treatment - time and rest. While surgical intervention can greatly ease symptoms, successful lifelong management of cubital tunnel syndrome also demands education and a dedicated effort at activity modification. Hopefully, with better environmental work conditions and early detection, can the expenses involved, the time spent in rehabilitation and most importantly the pain and disability patients experience decrease with the help of the patient, employers and the medical management team.

Medico-Legal Traps

Failure to Differentiate Cubital Tunnel Syndrome from Golfer's Elbow

- Cubital tunnel syndrome and golfer's elbow share similar symptoms such as pain in the medial elbow, leading to frequent misdiagnosis. Treating cubital tunnel syndrome as golfer's elbow can result in prolonged symptoms, further nerve damage, and medico-legal risks for inadequate diagnosis and treatment.

- **Thumb Rule Consideration:** Always differentiate between cubital tunnel syndrome and golfer's elbow by assessing the location of tenderness (1 inch below the medial epicondyle for cubital tunnel syndrome) and by testing for sensory and motor deficits.

Inadequate Diagnostic Workup

- Cubital tunnel syndrome is often misdiagnosed due to a failure to perform adequate nerve conduction studies or imaging. Missing an early diagnosis can lead to permanent nerve damage and claims for medical negligence.
- **Thumb Rule Consideration:** Always confirm cubital tunnel syndrome through clinical examination combined with nerve conduction studies or ultrasound imaging to assess the extent of nerve compression.

Delayed Surgical Intervention

- While nonsurgical treatments such as splinting and physical therapy are recommended first, delaying necessary surgical decompression when nonsurgical measures fail can lead to irreversible nerve damage. Patients may pursue legal claims for failure to provide timely and appropriate care.
- **Thumb Rule Consideration:** If conservative management does not improve symptoms within a reasonable timeframe (e.g., 3-6 months), consider early referral for surgical evaluation to prevent permanent ulnar nerve damage.

Inadequate Patient Education and Activity Modification

- Cubital tunnel syndrome can be aggravated by repetitive activities and improper ergonomics. Failure to educate patients on activity modification, ergonomic adjustments, and protective measures can lead to recurrence or worsening of symptoms, raising legal concerns over incomplete treatment.
- **Thumb Rule Consideration:** Always provide comprehensive patient education on activity modification, ergonomic strategies, and the importance of rest to prevent worsening of cubital tunnel syndrome and improve long-term outcomes.

Failure to Follow Up After Treatment

- Both surgical and nonsurgical treatments require careful follow-up to monitor progress and address any persistent or worsening symptoms. Failing to provide adequate follow-up care can lead to complications, unsatisfactory outcomes, and potential legal action for neglectful care.
- **Thumb Rule Consideration:** Ensure regular follow-up after treatment

for cubital tunnel syndrome to assess symptom improvement, nerve function, and the need for further intervention.

REFERENCES

- Aalmer BA, Hughes TB. Cubital Tunnel Syndrome. J Hand Surg. 2010; 35(1): 153–163.
- Han HH, Kang HW, Lee JL, Jung S. Fascia Wrapping Technique: A Modified Method for the Treatment of Cubital Tunnel Syndrome. The Scientific World Journal. 2014; Article ID 482702, 6 pages. doi:10.1155/2014/482702
- Cutts S. Cubital tunnel syndrome. Postgrad Med J. 2007; 83(975): 28–31.
- Assmus H, Antoniadis G, Bischoff C. Carpal and cubital tunnel and other, rarer nerve compression syndromes. Dtsch Arztebl Int. 2015;112(1-2):14-25; quiz 26.
- Lund AT, Amadio PC. Treatment of cubital tunnel syndrome: perspectives for the therapist. J Hand Ther. 2006;19(2):170-8.
- Rinkel WD, Schreuders TA, Koes BW, Huisstede BM. Current evidence for effectiveness of interventions for cubital tunnel syndrome, radial tunnel syndrome, instability, or bursitis of the elbow: a systematic review. Clin J Pain. 2013;29(12):1087-96.
- Feindel W, Stratford J. Cubital tunnel compression in tardy ulnar nerve palsy. Can Med Assoc J. 1958;78:351.
- Osborne GV. The surgical treatment of tardy ulnar neuritis. J Bone Joint Surg Br. 1957;39B:782.
- Tetro AM, Pichora DR. Cubital tunnel syndrome and the painful upper extremity. Hand Clin. 1996;12(4):665-677.
- Wheeless CR. Cubital tunnel syndrome. http://www.wheelessonline.com/ortho/cubital_tunnel_syndrome. Updated June 5, 2010. Accessed November 1, 2010.

DEVIL'S GRIP

Devil's grip is an uncommon cause of chest pain. Also known as Bornholm disease and Pleurodynia, the grip of the phantom, dry pleurisy, and Sylvest's disease, devil's grip is caused by acute infection with coxsackievirus. This virus is transmitted via the fecal–oral route and is highly contagious, owing to a long period of viral shedding of 6 weeks. In some patients, their immune system limits the infection to a mild fever or flulike illness called summer fever. In others, a full-fledged infection with resultant pleurodynia and cough develops.

Steven D. Waldman MD, JD, in Atlas of Uncommon Pain Syndromes (Third Edition), 2014.

Clinical Description

Pleurodynia (formerly called Bornholm disease) is a form of viral myalgia defined by the sudden occurrence of lancinating chest pain or abdominal pain, commonly associated with fever, malaise, and headaches. Pleurodynia should be considered in all cases of acute and subacute chest pain that present in the ER or in internal medicine, cardiology, or cardiothoracic surgery outpatient clinics. The onset of chest pain is acute. During attacks, the pain is severe, intense, and excruciating, lasting seconds to a minute. Pain is paroxysmal, occurring in attacks separated by minutes to hours. Severe attacks can result in difficulty breathing. The thoracic pain is usually over the lower ribs and is unilateral, but it can also occur over the front, back, or substernal area. Between attacks, patients usually have a constant, dull, pleuritic chest pain. A very important quality of the pain is its direct relationship to sneezing, coughing, laughing and deep breathing, which can cause the patient to look tachypneic and even diaphoretic. The pain typically lasts 1 to 4 days, although pain lasting as long as 45 days has been reported.

Symptoms can easily be mistaken for acute coronary syndrome in adults. Lower back pain can mimic acute purulent spondylitis and discitis. Children are more likely to have involvement of the upper abdominal wall; presentation in infants may mimic intussusception, whereas older children and adolescents may present with suspected appendicitis or perforated peptic ulcer. Bruehl et al reported a case of pleurodynia in an adolescent who had been previously misdiagnosed with costochondritis and acute anxiety.

Other conditions to consider in the diagnosis of pleurodynia include bronchiolitis obliterans organizing pneumonia, drug-induced myalgias, intercostal neuralgia, tumors of the pleural space, soft tissue sarcoma, viral or idiopathic pleurisy, postthoracotomy pain syndrome, and sickle cell crisis.

Pearls & Oysters

Common hygiene measures aid in the prevention of the oral-fecal transmission of coxsackievirus B. Encourage proper hygiene measures in the patient's household to avoid intrafamilial spread of the virus.

An outbreak of pleurodynia among high school football players was traced to contaminated water; therefore, avoid direct oral contact with common drinking or ice containers in favor of individual water containers and ice packs.

Coxsackievirus B is a small RNA virus that lacks a lipoprotein envelope and, hence, may be resistant to physical and chemical inactivation, including 70% alcohol or 1% quaternary ammonium compounds. Sodium hypochlorite at a concentration of 3120 ppm, at a contact time of 5 minutes, was sufficient to completely inactivate different Enterovirus strains. Good sterilization techniques that include ethylene oxide have been shown to inactivate the virus on electrophysiologic catheters.

Bottom Line Statement

Devil's grip is an uncommon cause of chest pain that is frequently misdiagnosed. Correct diagnosis is necessary to treat this painful condition properly and to avoid overlooking serious intrathoracic or intra-abdominal pathology. Intercostal nerve block is a simple technique that can produce dramatic relief for patients with devil's grip. As mentioned, the proximity of the intercostal nerve to the pleural space makes careful attention to technique mandatory.

Medico-Legal Traps

Misdiagnosis as Acute Coronary Syndrome or Other Thoracic Conditions

- Devil's grip, or pleurodynia, is often mistaken for serious conditions like acute coronary syndrome or pleuritis due to its severe chest pain presentation. Misdiagnosis can lead to unnecessary cardiac testing, delays in appropriate care, and potential legal claims for diagnostic errors.
- **Thumb Rule Consideration:** Always consider pleurodynia in cases of acute chest pain, especially when it is related to coughing, sneezing, or deep breathing, and confirm with clinical history and viral studies before proceeding with invasive diagnostic procedures.

Failure to Consider Viral Etiology and Mode of Transmission

- Coxsackievirus B, which causes pleurodynia, is highly contagious. Failing to recognize the viral cause or to educate patients on hygiene measures can lead to further transmission within families or communities, increasing liability for preventable outbreaks.
- **Thumb Rule Consideration:** Educate patients and their families on hygiene measures to prevent the spread of coxsackievirus, especially in communal settings, and encourage proper handwashing and sterilization practices.

Overlooking Differential Diagnosis in Children and Adolescents

- Pleurodynia can present with varied symptoms in children, mimicking conditions like appendicitis or intussusception. Failing to consider pleurodynia can result in unnecessary surgeries or delayed treatment, raising the risk of medico-legal claims for mismanagement.
- **Thumb Rule Consideration:** Consider pleurodynia in pediatric patients presenting with acute abdominal or chest pain, and use imaging or clinical history to differentiate from surgical emergencies like appendicitis or intussusception.

Inappropriate Treatment or Delayed Pain Relief

- Failure to provide adequate pain relief in patients with devil's grip can lead to prolonged suffering. Mismanagement of pain, especially in severe cases, can result in dissatisfaction or legal claims for inadequate care.
- **Thumb Rule Consideration:** Use appropriate pain management strategies, including NSAIDs or intercostal nerve blocks, to provide rapid and effective relief for patients with devil's grip, while monitoring for signs of complications.

Failure to Use Proper Disinfection and Sterilization Techniques

- Coxsackievirus B is resistant to some common disinfectants. Failure to properly sterilize equipment or patient areas may contribute to viral spread, potentially resulting in preventable infections and legal claims for inadequate infection control.
- **Thumb Rule Consideration:** Ensure proper sterilization techniques, such as using sodium hypochlorite or ethylene oxide, are employed in medical settings to inactivate the virus, particularly in high-risk environments like hospitals and sports teams.

REFERENCES

- ABell EJ, Grist NR. ECHO viruses, carditis, and acute pleurodynia. Am Heart J. 1971 Jul. 82(1):133-5.
- Kenzaka T, Hida Y, Matsumoto M, Akita H. A case of epidemic myalgia with symptoms resembling acute purulent spondylitis and discitis. BMC Musculoskelet Disord. 2016 Aug 4. 17:323.
- Tariq N, Kyriakopoulos C. Group B coxsackie virus. StatPearls [Internet]. 2020 Jan.
- Mizuta K, Yamakawa T, Kurokawa K, et al. Epidemic myalgia and myositis associated with human parechovirus type 3 infections occur not only in adults but also in children: findings in Yamagata, Japan, 2014. Epidemiol Infect. 2016 Apr. 144(6):1286-90.
- Leendertse M, van Vugt M, Benschop KS, et al. Pleurodynia caused by an echovirus 1 brought back from the tropics. J Clin Virol. 2013 Oct. 58(2):490-3. [Full Text].
- Moore M, Kaplan MH, McPhee J, Bregman DJ, Klein SW. Epidemiologic, clinical, and laboratory features of Coxsackie B1-B5 infections in the United States, 1970-79. Public Health Rep. 1984 Sep-Oct. 99(5):515-22.
- Romero JR. Reverse-transcription polymerase chain reaction detection of the enteroviruses. Arch Pathol Lab Med. 1999 Dec. 123(12):1161-9.
- Nolte FS. Case studies in cost effectiveness of molecular diagnostics for infectious diseases: pulmonary tuberculosis, enteroviral meningitis, and BK virus nephropathy. Clin Infect Dis. 2006 Dec 1. 43(11):1463-7.
- Noordhoek GT, Weel JF, Poelstra E, Hooghiemstra M, Brandenburg AH. Clinical validation of a new real-time PCR assay for detection of enteroviruses and parechoviruses, and implications for diagnostic procedures. J Clin Virol. 2008 Feb. 41(2):75-80.
- Patel DD, Kapoor A, Ayyagari A, Dhole TN. Development of a simple restriction fragment length polymorphism assay for subtyping of coxsackie B viruses. J Virol Methods. 2004 Sep 15. 120(2):167-72.
- Druce JD, Russell JS, Birch CJ, Vickery K, Harper RW, Smolich JJ. Cleaning and sterilization protocol for reused cardiac electrophysiology catheters inactivates hepatitis and coxsackie viruses. Infect Control Hosp Epidemiol. 2005 Aug. 26(8):720-5.
- McEvoy GK. Nonsteroidal anti-inflammatory agents. AHFS Drug information. Bethesda, Md: American Society of Health-System Pharmacists; 2000.
- Yang L, He D, Tang M, et al. Development of an enzyme-linked immunosorbent spot assay to measure serum-neutralizing antibodies against coxsackievirus B3. Clin Vaccine Immunol. 2014 Mar. 21(3):312-20.

DIFFUSE IDIOPATHIC SKELETAL HYPEROSTOSIS

Diffuse idiopathic skeletal hyperostosis (DISH) is a systemic condition characterized by characteristic ossification patterns that can occur in the spine and peripheral entheses. DISH most commonly affects the spine and often presents as back pain and stiffness. Resnick et al. originally coined the term DISH in 1975 and is now the most commonly used term to describe this condition in the literature. The term is both inclusive and descriptive of the disorder. The ossifications are classically described in the spine as flowing ossifications along the anterolateral aspect in at least three successive vertebral levels or four contiguous vertebrae. Although less common, peripheral enthesopathy can occur at the shoulder, elbow, knee, or calcaneus. DISH in the spine most commonly occurs on the right side of the thoracic spinal segment.

Mader R, Verlaan JJ, Buskila D. Diffuse idiopathic skeletal hyperostosis: clinical features and pathogenic mechanisms. Nat Rev Rheumatol. 2013 Dec;9(12):741-50.

Clinical Description

Diffuse idiopathic skeletal hyperostosis (DISH) is a systemic condition characterized by characteristic ossification patterns that can occur in the spine and peripheral entheses. DISH most commonly affects the spine and often presents as back pain and stiffness. Resnick et al. originally coined the term DISH in 1975 and is now the most commonly used term to describe this condition in the literature. The term is both inclusive and descriptive of the disorder. Forestier and Rotes-Querol initially described the underlying pathology in specimens and a series of 200 patients in 1950, who called it "senile ankylosing hyperostosis."

The ossifications are classically described in the spine as flowing ossifications along the anterolateral aspect in at least three successive vertebral levels or four contiguous vertebrae. Although less common, peripheral enthesopathy can occur at the shoulder, elbow, knee, or calcaneus. DISH in the spine most commonly occurs on the right side of the thoracic spinal segment.

While the etiology remains poorly defined, various risk factors have been identified in the literature, including gout, hyperlipidemia, and diabetes. HLA-B8 is common in both DISH and diabetes mellitus. As such, high rates of diabetes mellitus, hyperuricemia, and hyperlipidemia have been present in patients with DISH. Unlike other seronegative spondyloarthropathies, no apparent relationship has been identified between DISH and HLA-B27.

Pearls & Oysters

Patients with DISH who sustain spine fractures are at increased risk of instability due to ligamentous calcification and increased deforming forces secondary to vertebral ankylosis. Increased length of instrumentation is often necessary to accommodate the lever arms acting on the fracture site. Meyer demonstrated that surgical treatment of cervical fractures in elderly patients with DISH correlates with a 15% rate of mortality compared to 67% after conservative treatment, highlighting the importance of prompt diagnosis, evaluation, and treatment after trauma in patients with DISH.

Heterotopic ossification (HO) is a frequent complication following total hip arthroplasty (THA) in patients with DISH (30 to 56%). In contrast, patients without DISH in the cited series only had a 10 to 22% rate of HO. Fahrer et al. reported low rates of pain and functional limitations and recommended no prophylaxis against HO in patients with DISH after undergoing THA.

Bottom Line Statement

While semantics exist regarding the absolute and consensus agreement of DISH diagnostic criteria, there remain several critical components to the workup and management of these patients when presenting even in the setting of minor traumas. Emergency medical services (EMS) providers, nurses, advanced practitioners, clinicians, and surgeons require efficient and coordinated care to obtain comprehensive histories, examinations (including mandatory neurovascular examinations), and to have a low threshold to obtain appropriate imaging to ensure underlying fractures do not go undetected. Clinical deterioration warrants urgent evaluation and management modalities.

Medico-Legal Traps

Failure to Diagnose Diffuse Idiopathic Skeletal Hyperostosis (DISH) Early

- DISH can present with subtle symptoms like back pain and stiffness, which can be mistaken for other common spinal conditions. Delayed diagnosis or misdiagnosis can lead to worsened spinal deformities, missed fractures, and increased risk of instability, creating potential legal exposure for inadequate care.
- **Thumb Rule Consideration:** Always consider DISH in patients with back pain and stiffness, especially those with known risk factors like diabetes, hyperlipidemia, and gout, and confirm diagnosis with imaging showing characteristic ossifications.

Inadequate Imaging and Failure to Detect Fractures

- Patients with DISH are at increased risk for spinal fractures, especially after minor trauma, due to ligamentous calcification and vertebral ankylosis. Failure to obtain appropriate imaging, such as X-rays or CT scans, can result in missed or undiagnosed fractures, leading to spinal instability and legal consequences.
- **Thumb Rule Consideration:** Always perform thorough imaging, including CT or MRI, in patients with suspected DISH following trauma, even if the trauma appears minor, to detect any underlying fractures or spinal instability.

Mismanagement of Post-Trauma Instability

- DISH patients who sustain spinal fractures may require more extensive surgical stabilization due to their increased risk of instability. Failure to properly stabilize the spine in these cases can lead to neurological deficits or worsening deformities, exposing healthcare providers to legal claims for improper surgical management.
- **Thumb Rule Consideration:** When treating spinal fractures in DISH patients, ensure that longer instrumentation and more extensive stabilization are considered to accommodate for increased lever forces on the ankylosed spine.

Overlooking Heterotopic Ossification After Surgery

- Patients with DISH have a higher risk of heterotopic ossification (HO) after surgical procedures like total hip arthroplasty (THA). Failing to recognize or prevent HO can lead to decreased range of motion and functional limitations, potentially resulting in medico-legal claims for postoperative complications.
- **Thumb Rule Consideration:** Monitor for heterotopic ossification in patients with DISH undergoing THA, and consider prophylactic measures if necessary, depending on patient history and surgical outcomes.

Failure to Implement Multidisciplinary Management

- DISH can affect multiple areas of the body, including the spine and peripheral joints. Failing to coordinate care between specialties, such as orthopedics, neurology, and rheumatology, can lead to incomplete treatment plans and further complications, increasing the risk of legal claims for inadequate patient management.
- **Thumb Rule Consideration:** Ensure a multidisciplinary approach to managing patients with DISH, involving specialists in spine, joint care, and metabolic conditions like diabetes, to optimize outcomes and reduce the

risk of complications.

REFERENCES

- Belanger TA, Rowe DE. Diffuse idiopathic skeletal hyperostosis: musculoskeletal manifestations. J Am Acad Orthop Surg. 2001 Jul-Aug;9(4):258-67.
- Resnick D, Shaul SR, Robins JM. Diffuse idiopathic skeletal hyperostosis (DISH): Forestier's disease with extraspinal manifestations. Radiology. 1975 Jun;115(3):513-24.
- FORESTIER J, ROTES-QUEROL J. Senile ankylosing hyperostosis of the spine. Ann Rheum Dis. 1950 Dec;9(4):321-30.
- Vezyroglou G, Mitropoulos A, Antoniadis C. A metabolic syndrome in diffuse idiopathic skeletal hyperostosis. A controlled study. J Rheumatol. 1996 Apr;23(4):672-6.
- Mader R, Novofastovski I, Schwartz N, Rosner E. Serum adiponectin levels in patients with diffuse idiopathic skeletal hyperostosis (DISH). Clin Rheumatol. 2018 Oct;37(10):2839-2845.
- Mader R, Novofestovski I, Adawi M, Lavi I. Metabolic syndrome and cardiovascular risk in patients with diffuse idiopathic skeletal hyperostosis. Semin Arthritis Rheum. 2009 Apr;38(5):361-5.
- Paley D, Schwartz M, Cooper P, Harris WR, Levine AM. Fractures of the spine in diffuse idiopathic skeletal hyperostosis. Clin Orthop Relat Res. 1991 Jun;(267):22-32.
- Nascimento FA, Gatto LA, Lages RO, Neto HM, Demartini Z, Koppe GL. Diffuse idiopathic skeletal hyperostosis: A review. Surg Neurol Int. 2014;5(Suppl 3):S122-5.
- Guillemin F, Mainard D, Rolland H, Delagoutte JP. Antivitamin K prevents heterotopic ossification after hip arthroplasty in diffuse idiopathic skeletal hyperostosis. A retrospective study in 67 patients. Acta Orthop Scand. 1995 Apr;66(2):123-6.
- Fahrer H, Koch P, Ballmer P, Enzler P, Gerber N. Ectopic ossification following total hip arthroplasty: is diffuse idiopathic skeletal hyperostosis a risk factor? Br J Rheumatol. 1988 Jun;27(3):187-90.

DRIVER'S ELBOW

Driver's elbow is an entrapment neuropathy resulting from external compression of the ulnar nerve that clinically mimics cubital tunnel syndrome. It is often is misdiagnosed as golfer's elbow, which accounts for the many patients with "golfer's elbow" who fail to respond to conservative measures. Driver's elbow can be distinguished from golfer's elbow in that in driver's elbow, the maximal tenderness to palpation is over the ulnar nerve 1 inch below the medial epicondyle, whereas with golfer's elbow, the maximal tenderness to palpation is directly over the medial epicondyle.

Palmer BA, Hughes TB: Cubital tunnel syndrome, J Hand Surg 35:153–163, 2010.

Clinical Description

The ulnar nerve is susceptible to compression when a driver or passenger rests his or her elbow on the lower sill of the vehicle window while the shoulder is abducted and the elbow flexed. When the elbow is flexed, the proximal edge of the arcuate ligament becomes taut and the total volume of the cubital tunnel is decreased, resulting in increased intratunnel pressure further compromising the ulnar nerve. Vibration transmitted from the car body to the elbow also may further contribute to compromise of the ulnar nerve. This entrapment neuropathy presents as pain and associated paresthesias in the lateral forearm that radiate to the wrist and ring and little finger. Untreated, progressive motor deficit and, ultimately, flexion contracture of the affected fingers can result.

Pearls & Oysters

The major complications associated with the diagnosis and treatment of patients with driver's elbow fall into two categories:

(1) iatrogenically induced complications resulting from persistent and overaggressive treatment of "resistant golfer's elbow" and

(2) the potential for permanent neurological deficits as a result of prolonged untreated entrapment of the ulnar nerve.

Failure of the clinician to recognize acute inflammatory or infectious arthritis of the elbow may result in permanent damage to the joint, chronic pain, or functional disability.

Bottom Line Statement

Ulnar nerve entrapment at the elbow is often misdiagnosed as golfer's elbow, and this fact accounts for the many patients whose "golfer's elbow" fails to respond to conservative measures. Driver's elbow can be distinguished from golfer's elbow in that in driver's elbow, the maximal tenderness to palpation is over the ulnar nerve 1 inch below the medial epicondyle, whereas with golfer's elbow, the maximal tenderness to palpation is directly over the medial epicondyle. If cubital tunnel syndrome is suspected, injection of the ulnar nerve at the elbow with local anesthetic and steroid gives almost instantaneous relief.

Medico-Legal Traps

Misdiagnosis of Driver's Elbow as Golfer's Elbow

- Driver's elbow is often mistaken for golfer's elbow due to similar symptoms, leading to prolonged ineffective treatment. Failing to differentiate these conditions can result in unresolved pain and permanent neurological damage, raising legal risks for diagnostic errors.
- **Thumb Rule Consideration:** Always assess the location of tenderness—driver's elbow has maximal tenderness over the ulnar nerve 1 inch below the medial epicondyle, while golfer's elbow is tender directly over the medial epicondyle—to ensure accurate diagnosis and avoid unnecessary treatments.

Failure to Recognize Ulnar Nerve Entrapment Early

- Delayed diagnosis of ulnar nerve entrapment can lead to progressive motor deficits, sensory loss, and even flexion contractures of the fingers. Missing early signs of entrapment increases the risk of medico-legal claims for failing to prevent permanent damage.
- **Thumb Rule Consideration:** Consider ulnar nerve entrapment in any patient with pain and paresthesias radiating to the wrist, ring, and little fingers, and promptly order diagnostic tests (e.g., nerve conduction studies) if symptoms persist.

Overaggressive Treatment for Misdiagnosed Golfer's Elbow

- Persistently treating "golfer's elbow" with aggressive therapies when the true diagnosis is driver's elbow or cubital tunnel syndrome can result in iatrogenic harm and further nerve damage. This increases legal exposure for unnecessary interventions.
- **Thumb Rule Consideration:** When conservative treatments fail for suspected golfer's elbow, reconsider the diagnosis and assess for ulnar

nerve involvement before proceeding with invasive procedures.

Inadequate Patient Education on Activity Modification

- Not informing patients about proper ergonomic adjustments, such as avoiding resting their elbow on hard surfaces during driving, can lead to recurrence of driver's elbow or worsening symptoms. This oversight may expose healthcare providers to legal claims for inadequate preventive care.
- **Thumb Rule Consideration:** Educate patients with driver's elbow on activity modification, including avoiding prolonged elbow flexion and resting the elbow on hard surfaces, to prevent recurrence and long-term nerve damage.

Neglecting to Rule Out Infectious or Inflammatory Arthritis

- Failure to consider and exclude inflammatory or infectious arthritis when diagnosing elbow pain can lead to mismanagement of serious underlying conditions, resulting in joint damage and legal liability for neglecting comprehensive care.
- **Thumb Rule Consideration:** Always perform a thorough clinical assessment, including blood tests and imaging, to rule out inflammatory or infectious causes of elbow pain when diagnosing driver's elbow, particularly in cases of unexplained swelling or persistent pain.

REFERENCES

- Abdel-Salam A, Eyres KS, Cleary J: Drivers' elbow: a cause of ulnar neuropathy, J Hand Surg 16:436–437, 1991.
- Palmer BA, Hughes TB: Cubital tunnel syndrome, J Hand Surg 35:153–163, 2010.
- Szabo RM, Kwak C: Natural history and conservative management of cubital tunnel syndrome, Hand Clin 23:311–318, 2007.
- Waldman SD: Golfer's elbow. In Waldman SD, editor: Pain review, Philadelphia, 2009, Saunders, pp 267–268.
- Waldman SD: The ulnar nerve. In Waldman SD, editor: Pain review, Philadelphia, 2009, Saunders, pp 76.
- Waldman SD: Ulnar nerve entrapment at the elbow. In Waldman SD, editor: Pain review, Philadelphia, 2009, Saunders, pp 270–271.

EAGLE SYNDROME

Eagle syndrome is characterized by recurrent pain in the middle part of the throat (oropharynx) and face. Classic Eagle syndrome is typically seen in patients after throat trauma or tonsillectomy. Other symptoms may include difficulty swallowing, feeling of something stuck in the throat, tinnitus, and neck or facial pain. A second form of Eagle syndrome unrelated to tonsillectomy causes compression of the vessel that carries blood to the brain, neck, and face (carotid artery). This form can cause headache and dizziness.

Waldman SD (6 June 2013). Atlas of Uncommon Pain Syndromes. Elsevier Health Sciences. pp. 35–36.

Clinical Description

Eagle's syndrome, defined by Eagle in 1949, is characterised by morphological abnormality/ossification of the styloid process. The average length of the styloid process is 20-30 mm in the adult Caucasians and 15.4-18.8 mm in the Asian population. An elongated styloid process is defined by being at least 30 mm long. The clinical picture is composed of recurrent throat and neck pain, radiating into the ear and dysphagia. Symptoms can be bilateral or, more frequently, unilateral. The incidence is 4-8 per 10,000 people.

The aetiology is not well defined and a number of theories have been suggested, such as congenital elongation due to the persistence of an embryonic cartilaginous outgrowth, calcification of the stylohyoid ligament and formation of bone tissue at the insertion of the ligament. This clinical picture might also be seen in patients after tonsillectomy. Clinical presentation is varied and establishing a causative relationship between the styloid process/stylohyoid ligament and symptoms can be challenging. Classically, the pain develops following tonsillectomy, presumably due to distortion of the local anatomy following surgery; however, it is frequently found in patients who have not had regional surgery.

Pearls & Oysters

Eagle syndrome is a rare condition that occurs when the styloid process, a small bony structure on the side of the skull, becomes elongated or misaligned. This can cause a variety of symptoms, including pain in the throat, ear, and face, difficulty swallowing, and pain when moving the head or neck.

Glossopharyngeal neuralgia is a condition that causes sudden, severe pain in the throat, tongue, and ear. The pain of glossopharyngeal neuralgia is often described as shock-like and may be triggered by activities such as swallowing or speaking. In contrast, the pain associated with Eagle syndrome is typically a sharp, shooting pain that is triggered by movement of the head or neck.

It is important for healthcare providers to distinguish between these two conditions because the treatment for each condition is different. Eagle syndrome is typically treated with medications to control pain and inflammation, as well as physical therapy or surgery to correct the misalignment of the styloid process. Glossopharyngeal neuralgia may be treated with medications to control pain and prevent further attacks, as well as surgery to remove the cause of the pain, such as a blood vessel that is compressing the glossopharyngeal nerve.

Because tumors in the neck and throat region may cause symptoms similar to those of Eagle syndrome, it is important for healthcare providers to evaluate patients with pain in this region for the presence of cancer. Eagle syndrome should be considered a diagnosis of exclusion after other potential causes have been ruled out.

Bottom Line Statement

Eagle's syndrome should always be suspected when idiopathic unilateral pain occurs, especially in adult women and when the pain is not responsive to painkillers. In addition, the exacerbation of the pain by swallowing, yawning and crying, as in our patient, should help in diagnosis. Patients often seek assistance by many clinicians, which is related to the non-specificity of symptoms, with poor success. Multidisciplinary approach, early indication to radiological investigation, especially MDCT of the styloid process is advisable in such cases. The elongation of the styloid process is a relatively common condition, although not all the affected patients complain of symptoms. When occurring, the diagnostic workup may be critical, since throat and neck pain, mild dysphagia and foreign body sensation in the pharynx are misleading symptoms. Otolaryngologists, neurologists and dental surgeons should be aware of the existence and incidence of this clinical entity, which is associated with a critical decay in the quality of life.

Medico-Legal Traps for Eagle Syndrome

Misdiagnosis as Glossopharyngeal Neuralgia or Other Throat Conditions

- Eagle syndrome shares similar symptoms with other conditions like glossopharyngeal neuralgia and neck or throat tumors. Misdiagnosing Eagle syndrome can lead to incorrect treatment approaches such as unnecessary medications or surgeries. This can expose the physician to legal claims for failure to accurately diagnose the condition.

- **Thumb Rule Consideration:** Always differentiate Eagle syndrome from glossopharyngeal neuralgia and other throat conditions through careful assessment, including imaging such as a CT scan of the styloid process to confirm elongation and rule out malignancy.

Overlooking Symptoms Following Tonsillectomy

- Eagle syndrome can arise or worsen after tonsillectomy due to anatomical changes. Failing to recognize post-tonsillectomy Eagle syndrome can lead to prolonged patient suffering, misdiagnosis, and unsuccessful treatment plans, increasing legal risks.
- **Thumb Rule Consideration:** In any patient with throat and neck pain post-tonsillectomy, consider Eagle syndrome as a possible diagnosis, especially if pain worsens with swallowing, yawning, or neck movement.

Delayed or Inadequate Imaging Studies

- Inadequate or delayed imaging can result in missed diagnosis of an elongated styloid process, leaving Eagle syndrome untreated. This can lead to ongoing pain, reduced quality of life, and potential legal repercussions for delayed care.
- **Thumb Rule Consideration:** Promptly order detailed imaging, such as MDCT, to evaluate the styloid process in patients with persistent, idiopathic throat, neck, or facial pain, particularly when routine treatments fail.

Failure to Consider Surgical Treatment When Indicated

- Some patients with severe Eagle syndrome require surgical intervention (styloidectomy) to alleviate their symptoms. Failure to discuss or offer surgery when conservative treatments fail could result in accusations of medical negligence.
- **Thumb Rule Consideration:** Offer surgical options, such as styloidectomy, when patients with Eagle syndrome do not respond to medication or physical therapy, ensuring they are aware of all treatment modalities.

Neglecting Multidisciplinary Collaboration

- Eagle syndrome requires a multidisciplinary approach involving otolaryngologists, neurologists, and dental surgeons for proper diagnosis and treatment. Lack of coordination between specialties can lead to inadequate care, resulting in medico-legal risks.

- **Thumb Rule Consideration:** Engage a multidisciplinary team, including ENT specialists and neurologists, for comprehensive evaluation and management of Eagle syndrome, especially in complex or unresponsive cases.

REFERENCES

- Murtagh RD, Caracciolo JT, Fernandez G. CT findings associated with Eagle syndrome. AJNR Am J Neuroradiol. 2001;22 (7): 1401-2. Pubmed citation
- Lorman JG, Biggs JR. The Eagle syndrome. AJR Am J Roentgenol. 1983;140 (5): 881-2. doi:10.2214/ajr.140.5.881 - Pubmed citation
- Chuang WC, Short JH, McKinney AM et-al. Reversible left hemispheric ischemia secondary to carotid compression in Eagle syndrome: surgical and CT angiographic correlation. AJNR Am J Neuroradiol. 2007;28 (1): 143-5. Pubmed citation
- Eagle WW. Elongated styloid processes: report of two cases. Arch Otolaryngol 1937;47:584–87
- Faivre A, Abdelfettah Z, Rodriguez S et-al. Neurological picture. Bilateral internal carotid artery dissection due to elongated styloid processes and shaking dancing. J. Neurol. Neurosurg. Psychiatr. 2009;80 (10): 1154-5.
- Blythe JN, Matthews NS, Connor S: Eagle's syndrome after fracture of the elongated styloid process, Br J Oral Maxillofac Surg 47:233–235, 2009.
- Callahan B, Kang J, Dudekula A, Eusterman V, Rabb CH: New Eagle's syndrome variant complicating management of intracranial pressure after traumatic brain injury, Injury Extra 41:41–44, 2010.
- Johnson GM, Rosdy NM, Horton SJ: Manual therapy assessment findings in patients diagnosed with Eagle's syndrome: a case series, Man Ther 16:199–202, 2011.

EPIDURAL ABSCESS

An epidural abscess is an infection within the epidural space anywhere in the brain or spinal cord. Epidural abscesses occur as a result of infections involving the spinal or cranial epidural space. Intracranial epidural abscesses (IEA) are complications of cranial surgery or trauma; they may also develop as complications of otorhinolaryngological infections or other neck and thoracic procedures.

Chow F. Brain and Spinal Epidural Abscess. Continuum (Minneap Minn). 2018 Oct;24(5, Neuroinfectious Disease):1327-1348.

Clinical Description

An epidural abscess is an infection within the epidural space anywhere in the brain or spinal cord.

Dura mater forms the inner lining of the bony skull, and under normal conditions, there is no space between the skull and the dura. Intracranial pressure (ICP) elevation related to infections, inflammation, or tumors opens up the epidural space and separates bone from the tissue. This newly formed epidural space may contain blood, pus, or an abscess. Below the foramen magnum, the epidural space extends the length of the spine.

It has 2 compartments:

(1) a true space posterior and lateral to the spinal cord containing a cushioning layer of fat embedded with penetrating arteries and an extensive venous plexus, and

(2) a potential anterior space where the dura adheres to the posterior surface of the vertebral body.

Epidural abscesses occur as a result of infections involving the spinal or cranial epidural space. Intracranial epidural abscesses (IEA) are complications of cranial surgery or trauma; they may also complicate otorhinolaryngological infections or other neck and thoracic procedures. Spinal epidural abscess (SEA) can have an acute and chronic presentation. This simple categorization correlates with certain clinical and laboratory manifestations, bacteriological and cerebrospinal fluid (CSF) formulae, anatomic details, and pathology.

Acute SEA is usually less than 2 weeks in duration with fever and signs of systemic inflammation from a hematogenous source. This is in contrast with subtle, afebrile, and long-standing chronic SEA that has resulted from a direct extension of vertebral osteomyelitis. Both present with back and radicular pain, but leukocytosis (in serum and CSF) is more likely in the acute form and not so much in the chronic form. Acute forms are posterior to the spinal cord, but chronic forms are commonly anterior to the cord. Gross pathology is purulent and exudative in acute, but with granulation tissue in chronic.

Pearls & Oysters

Although uncommon, an epidural abscess is a potentially devastating infection, and its neurologic complications are life-changing. The positive is that prompt diagnosis and treatment can often prevent or reverse all this.

Once diagnosed with an SEA, clinicians should treat patients with the same urgency accorded to the most critical patients. Occasionally, even with recognition and intervention, the affected patient can still suffer devastating neurological complications. The feared neurological complications of the SEA could arise from either pressure causing compression of the spinal cord or septic thrombophlebitis causing ischemic necrosis. The former mechanism is probably more common, but vascular compromise is likely responsible for the sudden deterioration of otherwise stable patients.

Physicians rarely use antibiotics alone because some patients will suffer neurologic deficit progression despite antibiotics. Complications can ensue abruptly and unpredictably, without warning. The resultant paresis or paralysis may not be reversible even if surgery is performed urgently.

Bottom Line Statement

Studies related to these entities are rare since these are emergency cases that require a quick course of action. However, from the information available, early recognition and treatment are critical. This requires suspicion from all healthcare providers, especially those who encounter patients first (primary care physicians, nurse practitioners and physician assistants). All should be familiar with these entities and at least consider them in differential diagnosis; therefore, clinicians may recognize the patients quickly and be able to manage them promptly. Whenever there is doubt about the diagnosis, consult a neurosurgeon as soon as possible.

Medico-Legal Traps

Delayed Diagnosis Due to Non-Specific Symptoms

- Epidural abscesses often present with non-specific symptoms like back pain or fever, which can easily be mistaken for less serious conditions such as musculoskeletal pain or viral infections. Failing to recognize the underlying severity can lead to devastating neurological outcomes, including paralysis.

- **Thumb Rule Consideration:** Always consider an epidural abscess in patients presenting with persistent back pain, fever, or neurologic deficits, especially in those with risk factors like recent surgery, immunosuppression, or IV drug use. Immediate imaging such as MRI is critical.

Mismanagement of Initial Antimicrobial Therapy

- In some cases, antibiotics alone may not suffice, and a delay in considering surgical intervention can lead to irreversible damage. Administering inappropriate antibiotics without a proper source control plan may also increase the risk of progression to paralysis or other neurological deficits.
- **Thumb Rule Consideration:** Prompt initiation of broad-spectrum antibiotics is crucial, but always consult with a neurosurgeon early to evaluate for the need for surgical decompression, especially if neurological symptoms worsen or persist despite treatment.

Failure to Recognize Risk Factors Leading to Misdiagnosis

- High-risk patients, such as those with diabetes, recent spinal trauma, or immunocompromised conditions, are more prone to developing an epidural abscess. Overlooking these risk factors may result in delayed imaging and treatment, increasing the risk of permanent neurological injury.
- **Thumb Rule Consideration:** Maintain a high index of suspicion in high-risk patients presenting with back pain and fever, and do not delay diagnostic imaging even if initial symptoms appear mild.

Inadequate Follow-Up Post-Operative Care

- Post-surgical patients can still develop recurrent or worsening abscesses, especially if the original infection was not fully cleared. Poor follow-up or a lack of ongoing monitoring can lead to a missed recurrence, with catastrophic consequences.
- **Thumb Rule Consideration:** Ensure regular post-operative imaging and clinical evaluations in patients treated for epidural abscesses to detect potential recurrence or complications early.

Failure to Involve a Multidisciplinary Team Early

- The complex nature of epidural abscesses often requires collaboration between infectious disease specialists, neurologists, neurosurgeons, and radiologists. Delaying or failing to involve the necessary specialists can compromise the effectiveness of treatment.

- **Thumb Rule Consideration:** Early and coordinated care involving a multidisciplinary team is essential for managing epidural abscesses, particularly in high-risk cases or when neurological symptoms are present.

REFERENCES

- Chow F. Brain and Spinal Epidural Abscess. Continuum (Minneap Minn). 2018 Oct;24(5, Neuroinfectious Disease):1327-1348.

  Vakili M, Crum-Cianflone NF. Spinal Epidural Abscess: A Series of 101 Cases. Am J Med. 2017 Dec;130(12):1458-1463.

  Boody BS, Tarazona DA, Vaccaro AR. Evaluation and Management of Pyogenic and Tubercular Spine Infections. Curr Rev Musculoskelet Med. 2018 Dec;11(4):643-652.

  Babu JM, Patel SA, Palumbo MA, Daniels AH. Spinal Emergencies in Primary Care Practice. Am J Med. 2019 Mar;132(3):300-306.

  Ziu M, Dengler B, Cordell D, Bartanusz V. Diagnosis and management of primary pyogenic spinal infections in intravenous recreational drug users. Neurosurg Focus. 2014 Aug;37(2):E3.

  Reihsaus E, Waldbaur H, Seeling W. Spinal epidural abscess: a meta-analysis of 915 patients. Neurosurg Rev. 2000 Dec;23(4):175-204; discussion 205.

  Yao Y, Hong W, Chen H, Guan Q, Yu H, Chang X, Yu Y, Xu S, Fan W. Cervical spinal epidural abscess following acupuncture and wet-cupping therapy: A case report. Complement Ther Med. 2016 Feb;24:108-10.

  Eggart MD, Greene C, Fannin ES, Roberts OA. A 14-Year Review of Socioeconomics and Sociodemographics Relating to Intracerebral Abscess, Subdural Empyema, and Epidural Abscess in Southeastern Louisiana. Neurosurgery. 2016 Aug;79(2):265-9.

  Rosero EB, Joshi GP. Nationwide incidence of serious complications of epidural analgesia in the United States. Acta Anaesthesiol Scand. 2016 Jul;60(6):810-20.

  Grieve JP, Ashwood N, O'Neill KS, Moore AJ. A retrospective study of surgical and conservative treatment for spinal extradural abscess. Eur Spine J. 2000 Feb;9(1):67-71.

EXTENSOR CARPI ULNARIS TENDINITIS

The extensor carpi ulnaris muscle is one of the extensor muscles of the forearm located in the superficial layer of the posterior compartment of the forearm. It shares this compartment with the brachioradialis, the extensor carpi radialis longus, the extensor carpi radialis brevis, the extensor digitorum, and the extensor digiti minimi. All of these muscles share a common origin on the lateral epicondyle via the common extensor tendon. As all of these muscles near their distal insertion sites, they are secured by the extensor retinaculum.

Sawyer E, Tadi P. Anatomy, Shoulder and Upper Limb, Forearm Extensor Carpi Ulnaris Muscle. [Updated 2019 Mar 19]. In: StatPearls [Internet]. Treasure Island (FL): StatPearls Publishing; 2019 Jan.

Clinical Description

The extensor carpi ulnaris muscle is an elongated fusiform muscle located in the posterior compartment of the forearm and primarily functions to extend and adduct the wrist. It spans between the elbow and the base of the little finger. The extensor carpi ulnaris muscle belongs to the superficial group of extensors of the forearm along with brachioradialis, anconeus, extensor carpi radialis longus, extensor carpi radialis brevis, extensor digitorum, and extensor digiti minimi.

Its origin lies in the lateral epicondyle of the distal humerus and the posterior aspect of the ulna. It inserts onto the dorsal base of the fifth metacarpal after passing through the sixth compartment of the extensor retinaculum. It receives its innervation from the posterior interosseous nerve and gets its blood supply from the ulnar artery.

Accessory tendinous slips of the extensor carpi ulnaris are present in some individuals, potentially predisposing them to injury. It can potentially prolong the symptoms of extensor carpi ulnaris syndrome, increase the risk of tendinopathy and dislocation of the muscle, and functionally limit the wrist and fifth digit.

There are three variants of the accessory slip, types A, B, and C. Type A has been the most commonly identified and inserts into the base of the fifth metacarpal. Type B inserts onto the midshaft of the fifth metacarpal, and Type C inserts onto the fifth metacarpal head. It is an accessory digiti minimi functionally that arises from the extensor carpi ulnaris.

Pearls & Oysters

For testing the extensor carpi ulnaris muscle's function or instability, ask the patient to pronate the forearm and extend the fingers. Place your hand along the medial border of the hand to provide resistance against the movement. The extended wrist is then adducted against resistance. The muscle can be seen and felt in the proximal part of the forearm, and its tendon can be palpated proximal to the head of the ulna if the muscle is acting normally.

Bottom Line Statement

The extensor carpi ulnaris is an essential muscle in the activity of the wrist and forearm that contributes not only to the extension and adduction of the wrist but also to its medial stability. It is most commonly injured in athletes subject to forceful wrist movements. Repetitive flexion and extension of the wrist can lead to tenosynovitis due to the irritation of the tendon and the sheath that holds it in place. Overuse can also lead to tendinopathy of the muscle's tendon, in which there can be thickening and painful stiffness of the tendon with minimal structural damage. Continued excessive stress on the tendon can cause structural damage, which can lead to a partial tear.

Medico-Legal Traps

Misdiagnosis as Golfer's or Tennis Elbow

- ECU tendinitis is often misdiagnosed as medial or lateral epicondylitis due to the overlapping symptoms of forearm and wrist pain. This can lead to incorrect treatments, such as steroid injections or physical therapy targeted at the wrong location, delaying proper recovery and worsening symptoms.
- **Thumb Rule Consideration:** Always differentiate ECU tendinitis from golfer's or tennis elbow by focusing on the location of pain. For ECU tendinitis, pain is located along the ulnar side of the wrist rather than around the epicondyles. MRI or ultrasound can confirm tendon involvement.

Failure to Identify Accessory Tendinous Slips

- Accessory tendinous slips of the extensor carpi ulnaris, which are present in some patients, may predispose them to injury or prolong their symptoms. Failure to identify these anatomical variations can result in incomplete treatment or improper surgical repair if surgery is needed.
- **Thumb Rule Consideration:** Be aware of possible accessory tendon slips, and use imaging techniques such as ultrasound or MRI to evaluate tendon structure comprehensively, especially in patients with persistent

symptoms.

Underestimating the Impact of Repetitive Stress

- ECU tendinitis is common in athletes or individuals who perform repetitive wrist movements, such as tennis players or manual laborers. Failure to recognize the impact of repetitive stress or overuse can result in prolonged symptoms and potential tendon rupture if activity modifications are not implemented.
- **Thumb Rule Consideration:** Educate patients on the importance of rest, proper technique, and activity modification to reduce repetitive stress on the tendon, especially in high-risk occupations or sports.

Delayed Surgical Referral for Tendon Subluxation

- ECU tendinitis can sometimes involve tendon subluxation or dislocation, which may not be adequately treated with conservative management. Delaying a surgical referral in such cases may lead to long-term dysfunction and chronic pain.
- **Thumb Rule Consideration:** In cases of ECU subluxation, early referral to a hand surgeon is essential if conservative treatments fail to restore stability and reduce pain. Imaging with dynamic ultrasound can help confirm subluxation.

Inadequate Rehabilitation After Treatment

- Even after proper diagnosis and treatment, failing to provide adequate rehabilitation can result in recurrent injuries or incomplete recovery. In particular, neglecting wrist strengthening and flexibility exercises can predispose the tendon to further strain or injury.
- **Thumb Rule Consideration:** Ensure that patients undergo a structured rehabilitation program focusing on wrist strengthening, range of motion, and flexibility to prevent re-injury and promote complete recovery.

REFERENCES

- Campbell D, Campbell R, O'Connor P, Hawkes R. Sports-related extensor carpi ulnaris pathology: a review of functional anatomy, sports injury and management. Br J Sports Med. 2013 Nov;47(17):1105-11.
- Lung BE, Ekblad J, Bisogno M. StatPearls [Internet]. StatPearls Publishing; Treasure Island (FL): Jul 25, 2022. Anatomy, Shoulder and Upper Limb, Forearm Brachioradialis Muscle.
- Lung BE, Siwiec RM. StatPearls [Internet]. StatPearls Publishing; Treasure Island (FL): Jun 28, 2022. Anatomy, Shoulder and Upper Limb, Forearm Flexor Carpi Ulnaris Muscle.
- Glover NM, Murphy PB. StatPearls [Internet]. StatPearls Publishing; Treasure Island (FL): Aug 29, 2022. Anatomy, Shoulder and Upper Limb, Radial Nerve.
- Pınar Y, Gövsa F, Bilge O, Celik S. Accessory tendon slip arising from the extensor carpi ulnaris and its importance for wrist pain. Acta Orthop Traumatol Turc. 2012;46(2):132-5.
- Hinds RM, Gottschalk MB, Melamed E, Capo JT, Yang SS. Accessory Slip of the Extensor Carpi Ulnaris: A

Cadaveric Assessment. J Wrist Surg. 2016 Nov;5(4):273-276.]

- Nakashima T. An accessory extensor digiti minimi arising from extensor carpi ulnaris. J Anat. 1993 Feb;182 (Pt 1)(Pt 1):109-12.
- Inoue G, Tamura Y. Recurrent dislocation of the extensor carpi ulnaris tendon. Br J Sports Med. 1998 Jun;32(2):172-4.

FABELLA SYNDROME

Consistent posterolateral pain during exercise might indicate the presence of a fabella syndrome. Resecting the fabella can be indicated and is a minor surgical procedure with minimal risk. Despite good results in the literature posterolateral knee pain can persist and prevent return to a high level of sports.

Tabira Y, Saga T, Takahashi N, Watanabe K, Nakamura M, Yamaki K-I. Influence of a fabella in the gastrocnemius muscle on the common fibular nerve in Japanese subjects. Clin Anat (New York, N.Y.) 2012;26(7):893–902. doi:10.1002/ca.22153.

Clinical Description

The fabella is a sesamoid bone in the posterolateral capsule of the human knee joint. The presence of the fabella in humans varies widely and is reported in the literature to range from 20% to 87%.

The fabella is located in the posterior aspect of the knee where lines of tensile stress intersect.

It articulates with the posterior part of the articular surface of the lateral femoral condyle and is embedded in the muscular fibres of the gastrocnemius muscle.

Anteriorly the fabella is bordered by the posterior capsule of the knee joint and posteriorly it is situated at the endpoint of the oblique popliteal ligament and the lateral gastrocnemius tendon. In addition the fabellofibular ligament (or lig. of Vallois) runs to its distal insertion at the fibular head.

Recent anatomic studies suggest that the presence of a fabella is higher in the Asian population.

Functionally, the fabella is believed to have a role similar to the patella in redirecting extension forces of the knee joint from one point to another whereas the fabella redirects forces on the flexor side.

Posterolateral knee pain can be associated with the presence of a fabella and this incidence may be referred to as a fabella syndrome.

It is characterized by periodic pain in the posterolateral aspect of the knee.

Pain increases with extension of the knee causing tension by pressing the fabella onto the lateral femoral condyle. Symptoms may also be present in cases in which the fabella remains non ossified as a cartilaginous structure.

Another major symptom caused by a fabella may be palsy of the common fibular (CF) nerve. The CF nerve has been shown to be significantly reduced in diameter in relation to the fabella compared to proximally.

Ultrasound imaging may provide valuable information regarding the posterolateral structures of the knee including the presence of a fabella.

Lateral radiographs of the knee as well as MRI Imaging are able to reveal the position of a fabella in relation to the posterolateral femoral condyle.

Pearls & Oysters

The problems occurring are described to be a quartet of symptoms such as "intermittent posterolateral mechanical knee pain, pain accentuation by full knee extension, localized tenderness with compression of the fabella against its corresponding condylar surface, and immediate and persistent relief with fabellectomy".

This quartet introduced by Weiner in 1977 confirms the indication for surgery after already having performed it due to an eradication of pain following excision.

Bottom Line Statement

The incidence of the fabella syndrome appears to be higher in Asian population. Presenting complaints are commonly posterolateral knee pain and CF nerve palsy.

There are limited publications about the fabella syndrome, its function and the consequence of its presence or absence is still not clear.

According to literature posterolateral knee pain caused by the presence of a fabella can be eradicated by both non-operative and surgical excision. There however were cases in which this pain persisted postoperatively.

As postoperative success is uncertain the patient should be informed of all treatment options as well as the risks and benefits. Other causes for posterolateral knee pain need to be excluded carefully before suggesting surgery.

Medico-Legal Traps

Misdiagnosis as Other Posterolateral Knee Conditions

- Fabella syndrome may present with symptoms that overlap with common conditions like lateral meniscus injury, iliotibial band syndrome, or common fibular nerve compression. Misdiagnosis can delay proper treatment and lead to unnecessary procedures, exacerbating the patient's condition.

- **Thumb Rule Consideration:** Always rule out other causes of posterolateral knee pain using imaging techniques like lateral radiographs or MRI before concluding the diagnosis of fabella syndrome.

Failure to Recognize Fabella's Impact on the Common Fibular Nerve

- The presence of a fabella can compress the common fibular nerve, leading to nerve palsy. Failure to detect or address this nerve involvement can result in permanent nerve damage, with symptoms like foot drop or chronic weakness.
- **Thumb Rule Consideration:** Evaluate for nerve involvement in patients with posterolateral knee pain using nerve conduction studies or ultrasound, particularly if the pain is accompanied by neurological deficits.

Delayed Diagnosis Due to Non-Ossified Fabella

- In some patients, the fabella remains as a cartilaginous structure, making it less visible on standard radiographs and leading to delayed or missed diagnoses. This can result in prolonged pain and suffering for the patient.
- **Thumb Rule Consideration:** Use ultrasound or MRI imaging to detect cartilaginous fabella in patients with unresolved posterolateral knee pain, especially when radiographs are inconclusive.

Inadequate Patient Counseling Regarding Postoperative Outcomes

- While fabellectomy is commonly performed to relieve pain, some patients continue to experience pain postoperatively. Failure to properly inform patients about the uncertain prognosis of surgical intervention can lead to legal liability.
- **Thumb Rule Consideration:** Fully inform patients about the potential risks, benefits, and uncertainties of surgery, including the possibility of persistent pain, before proceeding with a fabellectomy.

Overlooking Non-Surgical Treatment Options

- Rushing into surgery without adequately exploring non-surgical options such as physical therapy, corticosteroid injections, or orthotics can be a legal pitfall. If surgery is not successful, patients may claim they were not offered less invasive treatments.
- **Thumb Rule Consideration:** Exhaust all conservative management options before suggesting surgery. Ensure that the patient understands and consents to surgical intervention only after non-operative measures have been fully explored.

REFERENCES

- Pritchett JW. The incidence of fabellae in osteoarthrosis of the knee. J Bone Jt Surg. 1984;66:1379–1380.
- Minowa T, Murakami G, Kura H, Suzuki D, Han S-H, Yamashita T. Does the fabella contribute to the reinforcement of the posterolateral corner of the knee by inducing the development of associated ligaments? J Orthop Sci Off J Japanese Orthop Assoc. 2004;9:59–65.
- Kawashima T, Takeishi H, Yoshitomi S, Ito M, Sasaki H. Anatomical study of the fabella, fabellar complex and its clinical implications. Surg Radiol Anat SRA. 2007;29:611–616. doi: 10.1007/s00276-007-0259-4.
- Müller W. Knee - Form, Funct Ligament Reconstr. New York: Springer Verlag Berlin Heidelberg; 1982. The knee - form, function and ligament reconstruction. 40, 96, 98, 192, 249, 252.
- Zeng S-X, Dong X-L, Dang R-S, Wu G-S, Wang J-F, Wang D, Huang H-L, Guo X-D. Anatomic study of fabella and its surrounding structures in a Chinese population. Surg Radiol Anat SRA. 2012;34:65–71.
- Ehara S. Potentially symptomatic fabella: MR imaging review. Jpn J Radiol. 2013;32(1):1–5. doi:10.1007/s11604-013-0253-1.
- Weiner DS, Macnab I. The "fabella syndrome": an update. J Pediatr Orthop. 1982;2:405–408. doi: 10.1097/01241398-198210000-00010.
- Zenteno Chávez B, Morales Chaparro IF, De La Torre IG. Fabella syndrome in a high performance runner. Case presentation and literature review. Acta Ortop Mex. 2010;24:264–266.
- Robertson A, Jones SCE, Paes R, Chakrabarty G. The fabella: a forgotten source of knee pain? Knee. 2004;11:243–245. doi: 10.1016/S0968-0160(03)00103-0.
- Legendre P, Fowles JV, Godin C. Chondromalacia of the fabella: a case report. Can J Surg J Can Chir. 1986;29:102–103.
- Kuur E. Painful fabella. A case report with review of the literature. Acta Orthop Scand. 1986;57:453–454. doi: 10.3109/17453678609014771.
- Benthien JP, Brunner A. A symptomatic sesamoid bone in the popliteus muscle (cyamella) Musculoskelet Surg. 2010;94:141–144. doi: 10.1007/s12306-010-0083-6.

FEMORAL NEUROPATHY

The femoral nerve is the largest nerve of the lumbar plexus. It originates from the dorsal divisions of the L2-L4 ventral rami. It has a role in motor and sensory processing in the lower limbs. It controls:

The major hip flexor muscles, as well as knee extension muscles.

Sensation over the anterior and medial thigh, as well as medial leg down to the hallux (great toe).

Refai NA, Tadi P. Anatomy, Bony Pelvis and Lower Limb, Thigh Femoral Nerve. StatPearls [Internet]. 2020 Oct 27.Available: https://www.ncbi.nlm.nih.gov/books/NBK556065/(accesseed 17.1.2022)

Clinical Description

There are various causes of femoral neuropathy, including compression by tumors or abscesses, stretch injuries to the nerve caused by extreme movements of the hip, direct trauma to the nerve during surgery or cardiac catheterization, and vascular lesions of the nerve due to diabetes.

Patients with femoral neuropathy may experience radiating pain in the anterior thigh and midcalf, as well as weakness in the quadriceps muscle, which can result in significant functional deficits. This weakness can cause the patient to be unable to fully extend the knee, leading to a risk of falls. In addition, weakness in the hip flexors can make it difficult to walk up stairs. It is important for healthcare professionals to properly diagnose and treat femoral neuropathy in order to alleviate these symptoms and improve the patient's quality of life.

Differentiating femoral neuropathy from L4 radiculopathy can be challenging based on clinical presentation alone. While there may be some subtle differences in the symptoms experienced by patients with these conditions, it can be difficult to distinguish between them without further testing. For example, L4 radiculopathy may present with sensory changes and weakness in the dorsiflexors of the foot, while femoral neuropathy may not. Additionally, intrapelvic or retroperitoneal tumors or hematomas may compress the lumbar plexus and present with similar symptoms to femoral neuropathy. It is important for healthcare professionals to consider these potential differential diagnoses and utilize additional diagnostic tools, such as imaging tests, to accurately diagnose and treat these conditions.

Pearls & Oysters

It is essential for the clinician to consider and rule out potential causes of femoral neuropathy that could be harmful to the patient, such as uncontrolled diabetes or retroperitoneal or pelvic tumors. While performing a femoral nerve block, the main side effect to be aware of is postblock ecchymosis and hematoma. There is also a risk of needle-induced trauma to the femoral nerve during the procedure. To minimize this risk, it is recommended to advance the needle slowly and then withdraw it slightly away from the nerve to avoid causing any damage. It is important for healthcare professionals to take these precautions in order to ensure the safety and well-being of their patients.

Bottom Line Statement

It is important to differentiate femoral neuropathy from lumbar plexopathy and radiculopathy of the nerve roots, as these conditions can present with similar symptoms. In some cases, lumbar radiculopathy and femoral nerve entrapment may occur together in a condition known as the "double crush syndrome," which is most commonly seen with median nerve entrapment at the wrist.

Injection of the femoral nerve can be a simple and safe technique for evaluating and treating painful conditions related to the femoral nerve. However, it is essential to perform a careful neurological examination on all patients before beginning a femoral nerve block, especially in patients with clinical symptoms of diabetes or significant femoral neuropathy. This will help to identify any preexisting neurological deficits that may be attributed to the nerve block later on. By considering these factors, healthcare professionals can ensure the best possible outcome for their patients.

Medico-Legal Traps

Misdiagnosis Between Femoral Neuropathy and L4 Radiculopathy

- Both conditions present with similar symptoms, such as anterior thigh pain and quadriceps weakness, making it difficult to distinguish between them. Misdiagnosis can delay appropriate treatment, potentially worsening the patient's condition and leading to further complications such as falls or muscle atrophy.
- **Thumb Rule Consideration:** Always use imaging and electrodiagnostic studies to differentiate between femoral neuropathy and L4 radiculopathy before confirming a diagnosis.

Failure to Identify Underlying Causes Like Tumors or Hematomas

- Femoral neuropathy can result from compressive forces such as retroperitoneal tumors, hematomas, or abscesses. Failing to identify these underlying causes can result in life-threatening delays in diagnosis and treatment.

- **Thumb Rule Consideration:** Always conduct a thorough diagnostic workup, including imaging, to exclude serious underlying conditions like tumors or vascular lesions in cases of unexplained femoral neuropathy.

Nerve Block-Related Injuries

- While performing femoral nerve blocks, inadvertent trauma to the nerve can occur, leading to worsening of the neuropathy. If the nerve is damaged during the procedure, the patient could file a claim for medical negligence.
- **Thumb Rule Consideration:** Ensure proper technique during nerve blocks by using ultrasound guidance and advancing the needle cautiously, avoiding direct needle contact with the nerve.

Failure to Recognize Double Crush Syndrome

- The coexistence of lumbar radiculopathy and femoral nerve entrapment can complicate diagnosis and treatment. Failure to recognize this can result in incomplete treatment, leaving the patient with unresolved pain and weakness.
- **Thumb Rule Consideration:** Consider the possibility of double crush syndrome in patients with concurrent radicular symptoms and femoral nerve compression, and treat both issues comprehensively.

Overlooking Diabetes as a Cause

- Diabetic patients are at an increased risk of femoral neuropathy, yet this can sometimes be overlooked if the healthcare provider focuses solely on mechanical causes. This can lead to delayed diagnosis and suboptimal management.
- **Thumb Rule Consideration:** Always assess for underlying diabetes or other systemic conditions when evaluating femoral neuropathy, especially in patients with a history of metabolic disorders.

REFERENCES

- Busis NA: Femoral and obturator neuropathies, Neurol Clin 17:633–653, 1999.
- Hsin HT, Hwang JJ: Isolated femoral nerve neuropathy after intra-aortic balloon pump treatment, J Formos Med Assoc 106:S29–S32, 2007.
- Parmer SS, Carpenter JP, Fairman RM, et al: Femoral neuropathy following retroperitoneal hemorrhage: case series and review of the literature, Ann Vasc Surg 20:536–540, 2006.
- Seijo-Martínez M, Castro del Río M, Fontoira E, Fontoira M: Acute femoral neuropathy secondary to an iliacus muscle hematoma, J Neurol Sci 209:119–122, 2003.

FIBULOCALCANEAL PAIN SYNDROME

The characteristics of the syndrome are pain at the lateral side of the ankle. "The pain is most severe when standing, walking on uneven ground or during the movements of supination and adduction of the foot'." People suffering from the sinus tarsi syndrome also have a feeling of instability (functional instability) in the hind foot.

When the syndrome is a result of an inverted ankle sprain there is a major chance the lateral collateral ligaments of the ankle are also damaged, since the ligaments in the sinus tarsi are the last ones to tear with a traumatic ankle sprain.

Taillard W, Meyer JM, Garcia J, Blanc Y. The Sinus Tarsi Syndrome. International Orthopaedics (SICOT) 1981; 5:117-130 (level: A1)

Clinical Description

Fibulocalcaneal pain syndrome is the result of injury to the fibulocalcaneal ligament, usually caused by sudden inversion of the ankle, as when stepping off a high curb.

The fibulocalcaneal ligament, which is also known as the calcaneofibular ligament, runs from the apex of the fibular malleolus downward and slightly backward to a tubercle on the lateral surface of the calcaneus, and is susceptible to strain from acute injury secondary to repetitive microtrauma to the ligament resulting from overuse or misuse, such as long-distance running on soft or uneven surfaces. Patients with fibulocalcaneal pain syndrome report pain anterior and inferior to the lateral malleolus. Inversion of the ankle joint exacerbates the pain.

Point tenderness is felt just below the lateral malleolus on physical examination. With acute trauma, ecchymosis over the ligament may be noted. Passive inversion of the ankle joint exacerbates the pain. Coexistent bursitis and arthritis of the ankle and subtalar joint may be present and confuse the clinical picture. Stress fractures of the foot also occur with increased frequency in runners, and this must be considered in all patients thought to have fibulocalcaneal pain syndrome.

Avulsion fractures of the calcaneus, the talus, the lateral malleolus, and the base of the fifth metatarsal can mimic the pain of injury to the fibulocalcaneal ligament. Bursitis, tendinitis, and gout of the midtarsal joints may coexist with ligament strain and may confuse the diagnosis. Tarsal tunnel syndrome may occur after ankle trauma and may further confuse the clinical picture.

Pearls & Oysters

Failure to identify occult fractures of the ankle and foot may result in significant morbidity. Radionucleotide bone scanning and MRI of the ankle should be performed on all patients experiencing unexplained ankle and foot pain, especially if trauma is present. The major complication of the previously mentioned injection technique is infection. This complication should be exceedingly rare if strict aseptic technique is followed. Approximately 25% of patients report a transient increase in pain after injection of the fibulocalcaneal ligament, and patients should be warned of this possibility. Injection around strained ligaments always should be done gently to avoid further damage to the already compromised ligament.

Bottom Line Statement

It is estimated that approximately 25,000 individuals in the United States sprain their ankle every day. Although viewed as benign by the lay public, ankle sprains can result in significant permanent pain and disability. The major ligaments of the ankle joint include the deltoid, anterior talofibular, calcaneofibular, and posterior talofibular ligaments, which provide most of the strength to the ankle joint. Injection of the fibulocalcaneal ligament is extremely effective in the treatment of pain secondary to fibulocalcaneal ligament strain. Coexistent arthritis, bursitis, and tendinitis also may contribute to medial ankle pain and may require additional treatment with more localized injection of a local anesthetic and depot steroid. The use of physical modalities, including local heat and gentle range-of-motion exercises, should be introduced several days after the patient undergoes the injection technique for ankle pain. Vigorous exercises should be avoided because they would exacerbate the symptoms. Simple analgesics and NSAIDs may be used concurrently with this injection technique.

Medico-Legal Traps

Misdiagnosis of Ankle Sprains as Simple Ligament Strain

- Fibulocalcaneal pain syndrome (caused by damage to the calcaneofibular ligament) is often mistaken for simple ankle sprains. This can result in patients receiving inadequate treatment and developing chronic ankle instability or long-term pain.
- **Thumb Rule Consideration:** Always rule out associated ligament tears, occult fractures, or other complex injuries with appropriate imaging like MRI or bone scans, especially in athletes or trauma cases.

Overlooking Occult Fractures

- Fractures of the calcaneus, talus, lateral malleolus, or fifth metatarsal can mimic fibulocalcaneal ligament injury. Failure to identify these fractures can lead to serious complications like malunion, chronic pain, or disability.
- **Thumb Rule Consideration:** Always consider occult fractures in patients with persistent ankle pain following inversion injuries and use radionucleotide bone scanning or MRI to confirm the diagnosis.

Failure to Recognize Coexistent Conditions

- Coexistent conditions such as bursitis, tendinitis, gout, or tarsal tunnel syndrome can complicate the clinical picture of fibulocalcaneal pain syndrome. Misdiagnosing the primary cause can lead to ineffective treatment plans.
- **Thumb Rule Consideration:** Perform a thorough differential diagnosis and consider overlapping conditions that may contribute to ankle pain and dysfunction before finalizing the treatment plan.

Improper Injection Techniques

- Injections are commonly used to treat ligament strain, but incorrect or overly aggressive injections can worsen the condition or cause infection. This could result in further legal complications if aseptic technique is not strictly followed.
- **Thumb Rule Consideration:** Use a gentle injection technique and ensure strict aseptic procedures. Inform patients of the possibility of transient pain increases post-injection.

Ignoring Post-Injection Complications and Rehabilitation

- Failure to monitor and follow up after injection therapy, including proper rehabilitation, can result in persistent pain or recurrent injuries. If patients are not adequately instructed on post-injection care and exercises, long-term recovery may be compromised.
- **Thumb Rule Consideration:** Implement and oversee a comprehensive post-injection rehabilitation plan, including gentle range-of-motion exercises and gradual reintroduction to physical activities, to minimize complications and promote recovery.

REFERENCES

- Helgeson K. Examination and Intervention for Sinus Tarsi Syndrome. North American Journal of Sports Physical Therapy 2009 February; 4(1):29-37 (level: A1)
- Rosenberg ZS, Beltran J, Bencardino JT. From the RSNA Refrecher Courses. MR Imaging of the Ankle and Foot. RadioGraphics 2000; 20:153-179 (level: A1)

- Meir Nyska, Gideon Mann, editors. The unstable ankle. Chapter 14: Sinus Tarsi Syndrome. United States: Human Kinetics Publishers, Inc. 2002. p144-120
- Akiyama K, Takakura Y, Tomita Y, Sugimoto K, Tanaka Y, Tamai S. Neurohistology of the sinus tarsi and sinus tarsi syndrome. J Orthop Sci. 1999;4(4)p:299-303.
- Roemer FW, Jomaah N, Niu J, Almusa E, Roger B, D'Hooghe P, Geertsema C, Tol JL, Khan K, Guermazi A. Ligamentous Injuries and the Risk of Associated Tissue Damage in Acute Ankle Sprains in Athletes. Am J Sports Med. 2014 Jul;42(7):1549-57.
- MyFootShop. Sinus Tarsi Syndrome. http://www.myfootshop.com/detail.asp?Condition=Sinus%20 Tarsi%20Syndrome (accessed 28/11/2010)
- American Academy of Podiatric Sports Medicine. Sinus Tarsi Syndrome. http://www.aapsm.org/sinus_tarsi_syndrome.html (accessed 27/11/2010)
- Lektrakul N, Chung CB, Lai Ym, Theodorou DJ, Yu J, Haghighi P, Trudell D,fckLRResnick D. Tarsal sinus: arthrographic, MR imaging, MR arthrographic, andfckLRpathologic findings in cadavers and retrospective study data in patients withfckLRsinus tarsi syndrome. Radiology. 2001 Jun;219(3):802-10.
- Thermann H, Zwipp H, Tscherne H. Treatment algorithm of chronic ankle andfckLRsubtalar instability. Foot Ankle Int. 1997 Mar;18(3):163-9.

FLEXOR CARPI RADIALIS TENDINITIS

The flexor carpi radialis muscle is a long, superficial muscle of the forearm that belongs to the anterior muscle group and lies in the first layer. It is a relatively thin muscle located on the anterior part of the forearm. It arises in the humerus epicondyle, close to the wrist area. It is a superficial muscle that becomes very visible as the wrist comes into flexion.

Standring S, Ellis H, Healy J, Johnson D, Williams A, Collins P, Wigley C. Gray's anatomy: the anatomical basis of clinical practice. American journal of neuroradiology. 2005 Nov;26(10):2703.

Clinical Description

The flexor carpi radialis originates from the medial epicondyle of the humerus, passes obliquely downwards to the lateral side of the forearm. The flexor carpi radialis inserts at the bases of the second and third metacarpal bones. The innervation of this muscle is provided by the Median nerve(C6-C7). The flexor carpi radialis mainly receives its blood supply (high up in the forearm) via anterior ulnar recurrent artery or posterior ulnar recurrent artery.

The main function of FCR is providing flexion of the wrist and assisting in abduction of the hand and wrist. The flexor carpi radialis (FCR) muscle has been suggested to act as a dynamic scaphoid stabilizer. Because the FCR tendon uses the scaphoid tuberosity as a pulley to reach its distal insertion onto the second metacarpal, it has been hypothesized that FCR muscle contraction generates a dorsally directed vector that resists the scaphoid from rotating into flexion.

Pearls & Oysters

Trauma to the flexor carpi radialis tendon from the injection itself is an ever-present possibility. Tendons that are highly inflamed or previously damaged are subject to rupture if they are directly injected. This complication can be greatly decreased if the clinician uses gentle technique and stops injecting immediately if significant resistance to injection is encountered. Approximately 25% of patients report a transient increase in pain after this injection technique, and patients should be warned of this possibility.

Bottom Line Statement

ECU Tendinitis is a condition common among people who play racquet sports or basketball. Baseball pitchers may suffer from this when their throwing mechanics are deficient.

Treatment for extensor carpi ulnaris tendinitis is usually simple, involving rest and treating pain. Mild cases of ECU Tendinitis can be treated with rest, splinting and non-steroidal anti-inflammatories, whereas severe instances can necessitate cortisone injection or surgery to repair the tendon and its sheath which anchors it to the ulna head and wrist (aka subsheath).

Flexor carpi radialis tendinitis is generally easily identified on clinical grounds; however, coexistent bursitis may confuse the diagnosis. Fractures of the distal radius and scaphoid and tears of the triangular fibrocartilage complex and avascular necrosis of the scaphoid also may mimic flexor carpi radialis tendinitis.

Many patients benefit from a period of rest following an injury to the extensor carpi ulnaris muscle. Your doctor may recommend a period of immobilization for 2-4 weeks following an injury. Surgical intervention may require a healing period of 6-8 weeks, followed by physical therapy. Many patients can look forward to a full recovery with full range of motion following proper medical intervention and attention to the injury.

Medico-Legal Traps

Misdiagnosis of Tendinitis as Simple Strain

- Flexor carpi radialis tendinitis is often misdiagnosed as a simple wrist strain, leading to delayed or inadequate treatment. This can result in chronic pain, decreased function, or even tendon rupture, increasing the risk of long-term disability for the patient.
- **Thumb Rule Consideration:** Always consider tendon injuries in patients presenting with wrist pain, and confirm the diagnosis with appropriate imaging techniques like ultrasound or MRI if clinical suspicion remains.

Overlooking Coexistent Pathologies

- Conditions such as fractures of the distal radius, scaphoid, triangular fibrocartilage complex tears, or avascular necrosis of the scaphoid can mimic flexor carpi radialis tendinitis. Misdiagnosing these conditions may lead to inappropriate treatment and worsen patient outcomes.
- **Thumb Rule Consideration:** Conduct a thorough differential diagnosis to rule out coexistent pathologies. Consider advanced imaging studies when clinical findings are ambiguous or not responsive to initial treatments.

Improper Injection Techniques

- Injections into or around the flexor carpi radialis tendon can result in tendon rupture if not performed correctly. Inflamed or compromised tendons are particularly vulnerable to damage during corticosteroid injections.

- **Thumb Rule Consideration:** Use a gentle injection technique, and immediately stop if significant resistance is encountered. Always inform patients of potential transient pain increases post-injection.

Failure to Address Underlying Causes of Tendinitis

- Repetitive overuse activities, poor mechanics in sports like tennis or baseball, and occupational stress are common causes of tendinitis. Failing to address these underlying issues can lead to recurrence of the condition and long-term disability.
- **Thumb Rule Consideration:** Recommend proper rehabilitation, ergonomics adjustments, and modification of activity levels to prevent recurrence. Educate the patient on proper mechanics and exercises for long-term recovery.

Delaying Surgical Intervention

- In severe or chronic cases of flexor carpi radialis tendinitis, conservative treatments may fail, and delaying surgical intervention can lead to permanent loss of function.
- **Thumb Rule Consideration:** Recognize when conservative management is no longer effective, and timely refer for surgical evaluation to prevent irreversible damage. Always discuss all treatment options with the patient, including potential risks and benefits of surgery.

REFERENCES

- Salvà-Coll G, Garcia-Elias M, Llusá-Pérez M, Rodríguez-Baeza A. The role of the flexor carpi radialis muscle in scapholunate instability. The Journal of hand surgery. 2011 Jan 1;36(1):31-6.
- Van Demark RE, Helsper E, Hayes M, Hayes M, Smith VJ. Painful Pseudotendon of the Flexor Carpi Radialis Tendon: A Literature Review and Case Report. HAND. 2017 Sep;12(5):NP78-83. Anatomy, Shoulder and Upper Limb, Forearm Radial Artery
- ACM OTA Class of 2016. MMT Flexor carpi radialis anti gravity & Flexor carpi ulnaris anti gravity. Available from: https://www.youtube.com/watch?v=iy7xdLnM_LE[last accessed 31/8/2021].
- Bishop AT, Gabel G, Carmichael SW: Flexor carpi radialis tendinitis. I. Operative anatomy, J Bone Joint Surg Am 76:1009–1014, 1994.
- Cowey AJ, Carmont MR, Tins B, Ford DJ: Flexor carpi radialis rupture reined in!, Injury Extra 38:90–93, 2007.
- Fitton JM, Shea FW, Goldie W: Lesions of flexor carpi radialis tendon and sheath causing pain at the wrist, J Bone Joint Surg Br 50:359–363, 1968.
- Gabel G, Bishop AT, Wood MB: Flexor carpi radialis tendinitis. II. Results of operative treatment, J Bone Joint Surg Am 76:1015–1018, 1994.

FOREIGN BODY SYNOVITIS

Foreign body synovitis has been neglected in the rheumatology literature. We describe 26 patients in whom arthritis, bursitis, or tenosynovitis appeared within 1 day to 7 years after an initial injury by a penetrating foreign body.

Arthritis Rheum. 1990 Dec;33(12):1753-62.

Clinical Description

Foreign body synovitis is a form of arthropathy, primarily monoarticular arthritis, resulting from an inflammatory reaction of the synovium due to a foreign object. The foreign fragments are characterized as either inorganic or organic. In this article, we will focus on foreign body synovitis from organic fragments. Typical materials that may cause organic foreign body synovitis include rose bush thorns, wood splinters, starfish, coral, sea urchin spines, and shell fragments. A common scenario is a young person who suffers a penetrating injury while working, gardening, hiking in the wilderness, or swimming. The presence of foreign objects lodged in the joint can lead to an inflammatory reaction. Foreign objects can also seed the joint with bacterial or fungal elements producing a septic arthritis. It is important to rule out septic arthritis when evaluating possible foreign body synovitis. The synovitis may be acute (hours to days after the injury), or chronic (months to years after the injury). This paper will describe the presentation, progression, diagnosis, and treatment of the two most common causes of foreign body synovitis in the Pacific Region, namely sea urchin synovitis and synovitis secondary to implantation of organic plant material.

Pearls & Oysters

A radiograph or other advanced imaging of the joint may aid in detection of a foreign body, although it is often negative and the disease process can progress even without concomitant radiographic evidence of retained foreign body. If an inflammatory process is suspected, the joint should be aspirated and sent for cell count and culture. If clinical suspicion is high enough, arthroscopic exploration and debridement should be considered. Untreated foreign body synovitis can cause serious destruction of the joint and surrounding tissue if not treated early and appropriately.

Bottom Line Statement

Foreign body synovitis secondary to implanted organic material is a common cause of monoarticular and tendon synovial tissue inflammation and should always be on the list of differential diagnoses in a patient presenting with joint swelling and erythema, even if a history of penetrating injury is not reported. If not removed and treated appropriately, acute synovitis, chronic monoarticular synovitis, chronic bursitis, chronic tenosynovitis, or a soft-tissue foreign body cyst may result.3 Common causes of foreign body synovitis in the wilderness environment include sea shell fragments, plant thorns, and sea urchin spines, with synovitis secondary to sea urchin spike implantation and implantation of organic plant material being the most commonly reported in literature.

Medico-Legal Traps

Failure to Identify Penetrating Injury

- Many cases of foreign body synovitis occur after penetrating injuries, but patients may not recall or report the injury, especially if it occurred long before symptoms arose. Missing this connection can lead to misdiagnosis as idiopathic arthritis, delaying appropriate treatment and worsening joint damage.
- **Thumb Rule Consideration:** Always ask about a history of trauma or potential exposure to foreign objects, even if the patient does not initially report it. Consider this possibility, especially in cases of unexplained monoarticular arthritis.

Overlooking Organic Foreign Bodies

- Organic materials such as thorns, wood splinters, or sea urchin spines may not show up on standard imaging. Relying solely on radiographs for diagnosis can lead to missed foreign bodies and ongoing synovitis.
- **Thumb Rule Consideration:** Use advanced imaging techniques, such as ultrasound or MRI, to assess for organic foreign bodies when clinical suspicion remains high, even if initial radiographs are negative.

Confusion with Septic Arthritis

- The inflammatory response from a foreign body can mimic septic arthritis, leading to incorrect or incomplete treatment if the possibility of a retained foreign object is not considered. Failure to rule out or treat an underlying infection can cause serious harm.
- **Thumb Rule Consideration:** Always perform joint aspiration and culture when evaluating monoarticular arthritis. Consider both septic arthritis and foreign body synovitis in the differential diagnosis, and proceed with arthroscopic exploration if infection or foreign material is suspected.

Delayed Surgical Intervention

- Prolonged synovitis from an untreated foreign body can result in permanent joint damage and functional impairment. Failure to refer for surgical debridement or exploration early can lead to unnecessary progression of the condition.
- **Thumb Rule Consideration:** If non-invasive treatments fail or if clinical suspicion for a foreign body is high, refer promptly for arthroscopy or surgical intervention to remove the foreign object and prevent further joint destruction.

Ignoring Potential Complications of Chronic Synovitis

- Chronic synovitis due to a foreign body can lead to complications such as the formation of a soft-tissue foreign body cyst or tenosynovitis. If these conditions are not recognized and treated, they can cause long-term disability.
- **Thumb Rule Consideration:** Monitor patients with chronic synovitis closely for complications, and always re-evaluate for a retained foreign body if symptoms persist despite treatment. Early intervention is critical to prevent joint and tissue damage.

REFERENCES

- Bode K S, Haggerty CJ, Krause J: Latent foreign body synovitis, J Foot Ankle Surg 46:291–296, 2007.
- Kandel L, Friedman A, Chaimski G, et al: Foreign-body synovitis mimicking sep-tic arthritis of the knee, Arthroscopy 17:993–996, 2001.
- Olenginski T P, Bush D C, Harrington T M: Plant thorn synovitis: an uncommon cause of monoarthritis, Semin Arthritis Rheum 21:40–46, 1991.
- Yewlett A, Oakley J, Makwana N, Patel H J: Retained blackthorn causing peroneal tendonitis: a case report, Foot Ankle Surg 15:205–206, 2009.
- O'Connell RL, Fageir MM, Addison A. Be aware of wood in the knee. BMJ CaseRep. 2011 Dec 13;2011.

GLOMUS TUMOR OF THE HAND

Glomus tumors were first described by Wood in 1812 as painful subcutaneous tubercles. It is an uncommon benign neoplasm involving the glomus body, an apparatus that involves in thermoregulation of cutaneous microvasculature. Glomus tumor constitutes 1%-5% of all hand tumors. It usually occurs at the subungual region and more commonly in aged women. Its classical clinical triad consists of pain, tenderness and temperature intolerance, especially cold sensitivity.

Arch Plast Surg. 2015 May; 42(3): 295–301.

Clinical Description

Glomus tumors occur relatively rarely, accounting for about 1%-5% of all hand tumors. Although they can develop in any part of the body, they commonly do so in the upper extremities-most frequently subungual areas. They are characterized by stabbing paroxysmal pain in the fingertips, tenderness, and cold intolerance.

A glomus body is an apparatus of the skin and a type of an arteriovenous anastomosis that controls the body temperature. Glomus tumors refer to hyperplasia of the glomus body. Their pathological findings were first described by Masson in 1924, being referred to as tumors that occur in the neuromyo-arterial body.

Glomus tumors are categorized into solitary and multiple types according to their clinical presentations. Solitary glomus tumors accompany pain and occur mainly in the distal extremities; multiple glomus tumors are usually painless and can develop in any part of the body. Glomus tumors require careful assessment for differential diagnosis, because they can often be misdiagnosed and followed by unsuitable treatment, due to the chronic pain in all extremities they accompany.

Pearls & Oysters

Solitary glomus tumors need to be ruled out from painful tumors, such as leiomyoma or eccrine spiradenoma. As in many cases, a diagnosis can easily be delayed for a long time while the patient suffers from severe pain because patients are easily misdiagnosed with conditions like neuropathic complaints, arthritis, or neuralgia. Therefore, they may undergo unsuitable treatment including sympathetic ganglionectomy, radicotomy, or even dismemberment. Clinicians need to be particularly careful to rule out cavernous hemangioma and blue rubber-bleb nevus syndrome from multiple glomus tumors, as they can be easily confused with one another.

Bottom Line Statement

Glomus tumors occur as some tissues of a glomus body proliferate. A glomus body is a specialized arteriovenous anastomosis responsible for thermoregulation and is located in the reticular layer of the dermis. Glomus tumors arise from deformed smooth muscle cells called glomus cells, which constitute a normal glomus body and are located in the walls of the Sucquet-Hoyer canal. These cells are present throughout the entire body. They mostly develop in the skin, but are also reported to arise in the mucous membrane or internal organs such as the stomach, lung, trachea, and bone. The most common site for glomus tumors is the hand-particularly the subungual area, the lateral aspect of the digits, and the palms.

Medico-Legal Traps

Misdiagnosis as Other Conditions

- Glomus tumors often mimic other conditions such as neuropathy, arthritis, or neuralgia. Patients may undergo inappropriate treatments like nerve blocks, sympathetic ganglionectomy, or even amputation before a proper diagnosis is made, leading to unnecessary interventions and prolonged suffering.
- **Thumb Rule Consideration:** Always consider glomus tumor in patients presenting with chronic fingertip pain, especially when cold sensitivity and localized tenderness are present. Use imaging tools like MRI to differentiate it from neuropathic or rheumatologic disorders.

Delay in Diagnosis

- Glomus tumors are often small and hidden under the nail bed or in subungual areas, making early detection difficult. Delayed diagnosis can lead to chronic pain and reduced hand function.•
- **Thumb Rule Consideration:** Suspect glomus tumor in patients with unexplained, persistent fingertip pain, particularly if accompanied by cold intolerance. Refer for appropriate diagnostic imaging, such as MRI or ultrasound, to detect small or subungual tumors.

Inadequate Surgical Management

- Incomplete surgical excision of glomus tumors can result in recurrence, leading to further surgeries and persistent symptoms. The tumors are often small and difficult to fully visualize and remove.
- **Thumb Rule Consideration:** Ensure complete excision by using

preoperative imaging to locate the tumor accurately. Employ magnification during surgery to avoid leaving residual tumor tissue, which can lead to recurrence.

Failure to Consider Differential Diagnoses

- Glomus tumors can be mistaken for other painful lesions such as leiomyomas or eccrine spiradenomas. Misidentification can result in inappropriate treatment strategies and unnecessary patient discomfort.
- **Thumb Rule Consideration:** Always include glomus tumor in the differential diagnosis of painful hand masses and rule out other similar conditions through histopathological examination if necessary.

Underestimating the Impact of Cold Intolerance

- Patients with glomus tumors frequently report cold intolerance, a symptom often overlooked in favor of addressing pain alone. Failing to recognize and manage this symptom can significantly impact the patient's quality of life post-surgery.
- **Thumb Rule Consideration:** Assess for cold intolerance during the clinical examination and inform patients that this symptom, though improved after surgery, may persist for some time.

REFERENCES

- Lee CH, Byeon JH, Rhie JW, et al. Clinical analysis of twenty cases of glomus tumor in the digits. J Korean Soc Plast Reconstr Surg. 1995;22:169–178.
- Carroll RE, Berman AT. Glomus tumors of the hand: review of the literature and report on twenty-eight cases. J Bone Joint Surg Am. 1972;54:691–703.
- Masson P. Le glomus neuro-myo-arteriel des regions tactiles et ses tumeurs. Lyon Chi. 1924;21:257–280.
- Chatterjee JS, Youssef AH, Brown RM, et al. Congenital nodular multiple glomangioma: a case report. J Clin Pathol. 2005;58:102–103.
- Vasisht B, Watson HK, Joseph E, et al. Digital glomus tumors: a 29-year experience with a lateral subperiosteal approach. Plast Reconstr Surg. 2004;114:1486–1489.
- Rohrich RJ, Hochstein LM, Millwee RH. Subungual glomus tumors: an algorithmic approach. Ann Plast Surg. 1994;33:300–304.
- Shugart RR, Soule EH, Johnson EW., Jr Glomus tumor. Surg Gynecol Obstet. 1963;117:334–340.
- Van Geertruyden J, Lorea P, Goldschmidt D, et al. Glomus tumours of the hand: a retrospective study of 51 cases. J Hand Surg Br. 1996;21:257–260.
- Rettig AC, Strickland JW. Glomus tumor of the digits. J Hand Surg Am. 1977;2:261–265.
- Beasley SW, Mel J, Chow CW, et al. Hereditary multiple glomus tumours. Arch Dis Child. 1986;61:801–802.
- Rodriguez JM, Idoate MA, Pardo-Mindan FJ. The role of mast cells in glomus tumours: report of a case of an intramuscular glomus tumour with a prominent mastocytic component. Histopathology. 2003;42:307–308.
- Hazani R, Houle JM, Kasdan ML, et al. Glomus tumors of the hand. Eplasty. 2008;8:e48.
- Takei TR, Nalebuff EA. Extradigital glomus tumour. J Hand Surg Br. 1995;20:409–412.
- Greider JL, Jr, Flatt AE. Glomus tumor associated with pacinian hyperplasia: case. J Hand Surg Am. 1982;7:113–117.

GLOMUS TUMOR OF THE SHOULDER

Glomus tumors are benign neoplasms that arise from neuromyoarterial glomus bodies, with clinical manifestations that include acute pain, cold intolerance and tenderness. Glomus tumors may occur anywhere in the skin, soft tissue or gastrointestinal tract, but are most frequently encountered in the nail bed of the hands.

White CP and Jewer DD: Atypical presentation of a glomus tumour. A case report. Can J Plast Surg. 14:237–238. 2006.

Clinical Description

Glomus tumors are neoplasms that arise from modified smooth muscle cells of the glomus body, which is a specialized form of an arteriovenous anastomosis that plays a significant role in the regulation of skin circulation. Glomus tumors were first described in 1924 by Masson, who compared the tumors with the normal glomus body and suggested that the lesion represented hyperplasia or overgrowth of this structure (3). It is now well accepted that the lesions are neoplastic.

Glomus tumors have been reported to account for 1–6% of all soft-tissue tumors and 1–5% of hand tumors. The tumors may occur during adult life at 20–40 years of age and are equally represented in males and females. In a large series by Beaton and Davis, extradigital tumors were more common in males, while subungual lesions predominantly affected females. Classic glomus tumors are typically solitary, though they may rarely occur as multiple nodules. Multiple lesions have been reported in neurofibromatosis-1. Malignant transformation is rarely reported.

Clinical manifestations include paroxysms of pain, cold sensitivity and point tenderness. In certain patients the pain is accompanied by additional signs of hyperesthesia, muscle atrophy or osteoporosis of the affected area.

Grossly, the tumor is a small purple nodule that varies between 2 and 20 mm in diameter, though tumors of >3 cm have been reported. Histologically, the tumors have variable quantities of glomus cells, blood vessels and smooth muscle cells. Accordingly, they are classified as solid glomus tumors, glomangiomas and glomangiomyomas. Solid glomus tumors are the most common subtype (73%), followed by glomangiomas (25%). Glomangiomyoma is the rarest variant with a frequency of 8% of all glomus tumors.

Pearls & Oysters

Glomus tumors are usually located in the deep dermis of the extremities and in the subungual region of the hands. Other sites are the shoulder, thigh, knee and gastrointestinal tract, including the stomach and liver.

Malignant transformation is extremely rare, but possible. Folpe et al proposed the following classification criteria for malignant glomus tumors: i) Deep location and a size of >2 cm; ii) presence of atypical mitotic figures; or iii) combination of moderate to high nuclear grade and mitotic activity (5 MFs/50 HPFs).

The typical presentation of a bluish, painful lesion in either a subungual or digital pulp location is now well recognized by clinicians. However, when the lesion is extradigital, the difficulty in forming a diagnosis often leads to delays and misdiagnosis

Bottom Line Statement

In conclusion, glomus tumors of the shoulder are not as uncommon as previously believed. On this basis, in cases of unexplained pain in this area, a glomus tumor should be considered in the differential diagnosis.

Medico-Legal Traps

Misdiagnosis Due to Uncommon Location

- Glomus tumors are most commonly associated with the hands, particularly subungual areas, leading to frequent misdiagnosis when they occur in atypical locations like the shoulder. This can result in unnecessary treatments and prolonged patient discomfort.
- **Thumb Rule Consideration:** Always consider glomus tumors in the differential diagnosis for unexplained shoulder pain, especially when classic symptoms such as cold sensitivity and tenderness are present.

Delayed Diagnosis Due to Overlooking Small Lesions

- Glomus tumors are often small, which may lead to them being overlooked during physical exams or misidentified as other soft-tissue conditions. Delayed diagnosis can result in prolonged pain and suffering for the patient.
- **Thumb Rule Consideration:** Pay close attention to persistent localized pain, especially when it worsens with cold exposure. Utilize imaging tools like MRI or ultrasound to identify small or deep-seated lesions.

Inappropriate Treatment for Unconfirmed Diagnosis

- Patients with glomus tumors of the shoulder may be subjected to unnecessary treatments such as steroid injections, physical therapy, or exploratory surgery due to an incorrect initial diagnosis, which can worsen symptoms or cause complications.
- **Thumb Rule Consideration:** Before initiating invasive treatments, ensure the diagnosis is confirmed through appropriate imaging or biopsy to avoid unnecessary procedures.

Overlooking Potential Malignant Transformation

- While rare, malignant transformation of glomus tumors is possible, and failure to recognize the potential malignancy can lead to inadequate treatment and poor outcomes.
- **Thumb Rule Consideration:** Be vigilant for signs such as rapid growth, size greater than 2 cm, or atypical features on histopathology. Refer for oncological evaluation when these signs are present.

Failure to Recognize Systemic Manifestations

- Multiple glomus tumors may be associated with conditions like neurofibromatosis, and missing this connection can lead to incomplete management of the patient's overall health.
- **Thumb Rule Consideration:** In cases of multiple glomus tumors, conduct a thorough evaluation for potential underlying syndromes such as neurofibromatosis to ensure comprehensive patient care.

REFERENCES

- White CP and Jewer DD: Atypical presentation of a glomus tumour. A case report. Can J Plast Surg. 14:237–238. 2006.PubMed/NCBI
- Takei TR and Nalebuff EA: Extradigital glomus tumour. J Hand Surg Br. 20:409–412. 1995.
- Masson P: Le glomus neuromyoartérial des régions tactiles et ses tumeurs. Lyon Chir. 21:257–280. 1924.
- Akgün RC, Güler UÖ and Onay U: A glomus tumor anterior to the patellar tendon: a case report. Acta Othop Traumatol Turc. 44:250–253. 2010.PubMed/NCBI
- Beaton LE and Davis L: Glomus tumor. Q Bull Northwest Univ Med Sch. 15:245–254. 1941.
- Moor EV, Goldberg I and Westreich M: Multiple glomus tumor: a case report and review of the literature. Ann Plast Surg. 43:436–438. 1999.
- Chiang ER and Chen TH: Multiple glomus tumors in gastrocnemius muscle: a case report. Arch Orthop Trauma Surg. 128:29–31. 2008.
- Cabral R, Santiago F and Tellechea O: Multiple glomus tumors and segmental neurofibromatosis: there are no coincidences. Dermatol Online J. 17:42011.PubMed/NCBI
- Kayal JD, Hampton RW, Sheehan DJ and Washington CV: Malignant glomus tumor: a case report and review of the literature. Dermatol Surg. 27:837–840. 2001.PubMed/NCBI
- Matsumoto K, Kakizaki H, Yagihashi N and Yagihashi S: Malignant glomus tumor in the branchial muscle of a 16-year-old girl. Pathol Int. 51:729–734. 2001.PubMed/NCBI
- Terenda T, Fujimoto J, Shirakashi Y, Kamo M and Sugiura M: Malignant glomus tumor of the palm: a case

report. J Cutan Pathol. 38:381–384. 2011.PubMed/NCBI

- Enzinger FM and Weiss SW: Perivascular tumors. Soft Tissue Tumors. 4th edition. Mosby; St Louis: pp. 985–1001. 2001
- Riddell DH and Martin RS: Glomus tumor of unusual size; case report. Ann Surg. 133:401–403. 1951.
- Rao AG, Indira D and Kamal J: Extra digital glomangioma. Indian J Dermatol. 55:397–398. 2010.
- Folpe AL, Fanburg-Smith JC, Miettinen M and Weiss SW: Atypical and malignant glomus tumors: analysis of 52 cases, with a proposal for the reclassification of glomus tumors. Am J Surg Pathol. 25:1–12. 2001.
- Abela M, Cole AS, Hill GA and Carr AJ: Glomus tumor of the scapular region. J Shoulder Elbow Surg. 9:532–533. 2000.
- Negri G, Schulte M and Mohr W: Glomus tumor with diffuse infiltration of the quadriceps muscle: a case report. Hum Pathol. 28:750–752. 1997.

GLOMUS TUMOR OF THE KNEE

Glomus tumor is a rare, benign neoplasm rising from the glomus apparatus of the skin. It occurs most frequently on fingers and toes and accounts for 1.6% of all soft tissue tumors. Clinical diagnosis may prove difficult if the tumor occurs on an extra digital location.

Rare Tumors. 2014 Oct 27; 6(4): 5588.

Clinical Description

Glomus tumor is a rare, benign neoplasm rising from the glomus apparatus in the skin. It occurs most frequently on fingers and toes and accounts for 1.6% of all soft tissue tumours. Clinical diagnosis may prove difficult if the tumor occurs on an extra digital location.

They were first clinically described by Wood in 1812, and later explained in detail by Masson; they are rare benign tumors of the Sucquet-Hoyer canals within the glomus body (a neuromyoarterial canal system that is responsible for blood flow to the skin and thermoregulation). Local hyperplasia or overgrowth of this neuroangiomatous tissue may result in tumors that produce paroxysmal pain induced either by a mechanical or thermal stimulus. These tumors occur most frequently in distal extremities, particularly in the subungual area;5 however, atypical extradigital sites, including the head and neck, lungs, mediastinum, stomach, mesentery, bowels, bone and venous system, may be observed. There are reports of multiple possible locations around the knee: subcutaneous, sub-synovial, in the patellar ligament, within the fat pad, in the popliteal area or at the fibular head. Reviews of glomus tumors in the hand have indicated a 2:1 female predominance, but extradigital glomus tumors appear to be more common in males1 These tumors are typically solitary and accompanied by the classic triad of pain, cold sensitivity and point tenderness.Symptoms are typically disproportional to the size of the tumor, and the pain mechanism still requires further elucidation. Studies suggest that the contraction of the myofilaments of the glomus cells due to cold temperatures may result in an increased intracapsular pressure that can lead to the perception of pain via transmission through unmyelinated nerve fibres. Extradigital tumours are frequently more difficult to diagnose due to the absence of classic symptoms (only 9% to 20% are initially correctly diagnosed).

Relevant differences are noted in glomus tumors in children compared with adults. In children, tumors are frequently multifocal, infiltrative, and less commonly observed in subungual locations; superficial soft tissues of the extremities are often involved. In addition, an autosomal dominant inheritance pattern may be observed, and some tumors in children may be associated with neurofibromatosis type 1. According to the World Health Organization, 3 distinctive types of glomus tumor patterns are recognized: solid type, with scarce vasculature and a minimal muscle component (the most common variant); an angiomatous type called glomangioma comprised of a prominent vascular component; and a solid type with myomatous spindle cell differentiation referred to as glomangiomyoma (with prominent vascular and smooth muscle components). Glomangiomas represent approximately 20% of all glomus tumors and 1-5% of all soft tissue tumors of the hand. Preoperative imaging studies with color Doppler ultrasonography and magnetic resonance may provide information on tumor size, shape and precise anatomic location. The differential diagnoses (both clinical and histological) may include neuromas, hemangiopericytomas, angioleiomyomas, hemangiomas and other hamartomas of the cutaneous adnexa. Immunohistochemistry can be extremely helpful, especially in tumors with an atypical histological appearance. Treatment consists of complete surgical excision.

Recurrence rates for solitary tumors range from 12% to 33%. Malignancy is extremely rare and based mainly in histologic features (atypical mitotic figures, moderate to high nuclear grade and ≥5 mitotic figures per 50 high-power field), rather than clinical findings (deep location and size >2 cm), emphasising the importance of surgical marginal resection.

Pearls & Oysters

Glomus tumors are benign lesions most commonly associated with crippling pain in the digits though they often occur in extradigital locations. In fact, over a 20 year period 61% of glomus tumors at one institution were extradigital. Patients with glomus tumors commonly suffer a delay in diagnosis irrespective of tumor location, though extradigital locations may make the diagnosis even more challenging. MRI is the imaging modality of choice though diagnosis and surgical plan can be executed with a careful history and physical alone. These tumors are relatively easy to excise given their frequent encapsulation and superficial location. Careful and complete excision can deliver permanent relief of chronic and severe pain in a simple outpatient procedure. Persistence or recurrence of symptoms could be due to inadequate resection or unrecognized synchronous satellite lesions, but a symptomatic neuroma must also be considered.

Bottom Line Statement

Patients with glomus tumors may present to a variety of health care professionals, and an accurate and prompt diagnosis is fundamental to avoid treatment delays, chronic pain syndromes or psychiatric misdiagnosis. The occurrence of glomus tumors in extradigital locations provides an even greater challenge. In the present case, the knee pain was reminiscent of many common musculoskeletal conditions, such as meniscus tears, synovitis or ligamentous strains and sprains, thereby misleading clinicians and delaying the correct diagnosis. This illustrates the importance of maintaining a high index of suspicion for the diagnosis of an extradigital glomus tumor. It also reiterates the fact that the unusual distribution of clinical signs and symptoms provides the most important clue for the precis e diagnosis.

Medico-Legal Traps

Delayed Diagnosis Due to Atypical Location

- Glomus tumors are most commonly associated with the digits, leading to delayed or missed diagnosis when they occur in less common locations such as the knee. Misdiagnosis may result in prolonged pain and inappropriate treatments.
- **Thumb Rule Consideration:** Always consider extradigital glomus tumors when a patient presents with unexplained chronic pain, especially when symptoms such as cold sensitivity or point tenderness are present.

Misinterpretation of Imaging or Failure to Use MRI

- Due to their small size and atypical location, glomus tumors in the knee may be misinterpreted or missed entirely on routine imaging like X-rays. Failing to order an MRI can lead to incorrect diagnoses such as meniscus tears or ligament injuries.
- **Thumb Rule Consideration:** Use MRI as the imaging modality of choice for suspected glomus tumors, particularly in extradigital locations where they are difficult to detect through standard imaging.

Confusion with Common Musculoskeletal Conditions

- Glomus tumors of the knee can mimic other conditions such as synovitis, meniscus tears, or ligament injuries. Clinicians may treat the patient for these more common conditions, delaying appropriate management for the actual underlying cause.
- **Thumb Rule Consideration:** Keep glomus tumors on the differential diagnosis when pain is disproportionate to clinical findings, especially

when classical symptoms like cold sensitivity are reported.

Inadequate Excision Leading to Recurrence

- Incomplete surgical excision of the glomus tumor, especially in difficult-to-reach areas like the knee, can lead to recurrence of symptoms. Failing to recognize satellite lesions may also contribute to recurrence.
- **Thumb Rule Consideration:** Ensure complete surgical excision of the tumor, including careful exploration for any satellite lesions, to prevent recurrence and persistent symptoms.

Overlooking Malignant Potential

- Although rare, malignant transformation of glomus tumors can occur, and failure to identify atypical histological features like high mitotic rates can lead to mismanagement.
- **Thumb Rule Consideration:** Perform thorough histopathological evaluation of all glomus tumors to assess for any signs of malignancy, especially when the tumor is larger than 2 cm or located in deep tissues.

REFERENCES

- Soule EH, Ghormley RK, Bulbulian AH. Primary tumors of the soft tissues of the extremities exclusive of epithelial tumors: an analysis of five hundred consecutive cases. AMA ARCH Surg 1955;70:462-74.
- Schiefer TK, Parker WL, Anakwenze OA, et al. Extradigital glomus tumors: a 20-year experience. Mayo Clin Proc 2006; 81:1337-44.
- Wood W. On painful subcutaneous tubercle. Edin Med J 1812;8:283-91.
- Masson P. Le glomos neuromyoarterial des regions tactile et les tumeurs. Lyon Chir 1924;21:257-80.
- Kale SS, Rao VK, Bentz ML. Glomus tumor of the index finger. J Craniofac Surg 2006;17:801-4.
- Tuncali D, Yilmaz AC, Terzioglu A, et al. Multiple occurrences of diferente histologic types of the glomus tumor. J Hand Surg 2004;1:161.
- Kato S, Fujii H, Yoshida A, Hinoki S. Glomus tumor beneath the plica synovialis in the knee: a case report. Knee 2007;14:164-6.
- Waseem M, Jari S, Paton RW. Glomus tumor, a rare cause of knee pain: a case report. Knee 2002;9:161-3.
- Okahashi K, Sugimoto K, Iwai M, et al. Glomus tumor of the lateral aspect of the knee joint. Arch Orthop Trauma Surg 2004;124:636-8.
- Maxwell GP, Curtis RM, Wilgis EF. Multiple digital glomus tumors. J Hand Surg (Am) 1979;4:363-7.
- Tsuneyoshi M, Enjoji M. Glomus tumor. A clinicopathologic and electron microscopicb study. Cancer 1982;50:1601-7.
- Van Geertruyden J, Lorea P, Goldschmidt D, et al. Glomus tumor of the hand: a retrospective study of 51 cases. J Hand Surg (Br) 199621:257-60.
- Weiss SW, Goldblum JR, Perivascular tumors. Enzinger and Weiss's Soft Tissue tumors. 5thMaryland Heights: Mosby; 2007. 751-756.
- Rohrich RJ, Hochstein LM, Millwee RH. Subungual glomus tumors: an algorithmic approach. Ann Plast Surg 1994;33:300-4.

GLOSSOPHARYNGEAL NEURALGIA

Glossopharyngeal neuralgia consists of recurring attacks of severe pain in the back of the throat, the area near the tonsils, the back of the tongue, part of the ear, and/or the area under the back of the jaw. The pain is due to malfunction of the 9th cranial nerve (glossopharyngeal nerve). The glossopharyngeal nerve helps move the muscles of the throat and carries information from the throat, tonsils, and tongue to the brain.

Ko MW, Prasad S. Headache, facial pain, and disorders of facial sensation. In: Liu GT, Volpe NJ, Galetta SL, eds. Liu, Volpe, and Galetta's Neuro-Ophthalmology. 3rd ed. Philadelphia, PA: Elsevier; 2019:chap 19.

Clinical Description

The cause is often unknown but sometimes is an abnormally positioned artery that puts pressure on (compresses) the glossopharyngeal nerve. People have brief attacks of excruciating pain, affecting one side of the tongue or throat and sometimes an ear. Doctors diagnose the disorder based on what the pain is like and whether a local anesthetic applied to the back of the throat eliminates the pain. Glossopharyngeal neuralgia, a rare disorder, usually begins after age 40 and occurs more often in men.

The vagus (10th cranial) nerve malfunctions at the same time because the vagus nerve and the glossopharyngeal (9th cranial) nerve exit the skull together. Thus, the problem affecting the glossopharyngeal nerve usually also affects the vagus nerve. The vagus nerve helps control the heartbeat. When the vagus nerve malfunctions, the pulse may be abnormal, and abnormal heart rhythms (arrhythmias) may occur. The glossopharyngeal nerve helps move the muscles of the throat and carries information from the throat, tonsils, and tongue to the brain. The cause is often unknown but sometimes is an abnormally positioned artery that puts pressure on (compresses) the glossopharyngeal nerve. The disorder is rare, with less than 1 case reported per year among 100,000 people in the United States. It tends to occur more often in adults over age 40, but it may be present at any age. It appears to affect men more than women.

Pearls & Oysters

Glossopharyngeal neuralgia is a rare disorder that causes severe pain in the throat, tongue, and ear. It is considered a medical emergency because the pain can be so severe that it may lead to suicide. If a dull ache remains after the intense, paroxysmal pain of glossopharyngeal neuralgia subsides, this may be indicative of persistent compression of the nerve by a structural lesion such as a brainstem tumor or schwannoma. Glossopharyngeal neuralgia is rare in people younger than 30 years old, unless it is associated with multiple sclerosis. In such cases, an MRI should be performed to identify demyelinating disease. Treatment of glossopharyngeal neuralgia may include medications to control the pain, such as anticonvulsants and tricyclic antidepressants, as well as procedures such as nerve blocks or surgery to remove the cause of the compression. It is important to seek medical attention as soon as possible if you experience symptoms of glossopharyngeal neuralgia.

Bottom Line Statement

Glossopharyngeal nerve block is a procedure that involves injecting a local anesthetic around the glossopharyngeal nerve to block pain in the throat, tongue, and ear. The major complications associated with this procedure are related to trauma to the internal jugular and carotid artery, including hematoma formation and intravascular injection of local anesthetic with subsequent toxicity. Dysphagia (difficulty swallowing) may occur if the glossopharyngeal nerve is damaged, and dysphonia (difficulty speaking) may occur if the vagus nerve is inadvertently blocked. Reflex tachycardia (rapid heartbeat) may also occur due to vagal nerve block, and weakness of the tongue and trapezius muscle may occur if the hypoglossal and spinal accessory nerves are inadvertently blocked. There is also a risk of infection, especially in immunocompromised patients with cancer. It is important to seek medical attention if you experience any complications after a glossopharyngeal nerve block.

Medico-Legal Traps

Misdiagnosis Due to Overlapping Symptoms

- Glossopharyngeal neuralgia shares symptoms with other conditions like trigeminal neuralgia or otologic disorders, leading to misdiagnosis and inappropriate treatments. This can delay effective management and exacerbate the patient's condition.
- **Thumb Rule Consideration:** Always consider glossopharyngeal neuralgia in patients presenting with severe throat, ear, or tongue pain, especially if paroxysmal in nature, and use diagnostic nerve blocks to confirm the diagnosis.

Failure to Identify Underlying Structural Lesions

- Glossopharyngeal neuralgia can result from nerve compression by tumors or vascular abnormalities. Failing to investigate the cause, especially if symptoms persist after treatment, can result in missing critical diagnoses such as brainstem tumors or schwannomas.

- **Thumb Rule Consideration:** Perform an MRI when symptoms persist or when there is a dull ache between paroxysmal pain attacks, to rule out structural lesions like tumors or vascular malformations compressing the nerve.

Ignoring Cardiovascular Implications

- Due to the proximity of the glossopharyngeal and vagus nerves, malfunction of the vagus nerve may cause serious cardiovascular complications, such as abnormal heart rhythms. Ignoring these symptoms can lead to life-threatening situations.
- **Thumb Rule Consideration:** Always monitor heart rate and rhythm in patients with glossopharyngeal neuralgia, especially during acute episodes of pain or after administering nerve blocks.

Inappropriate Use of Nerve Blocks

- While glossopharyngeal nerve blocks can relieve pain, improper technique can cause severe complications such as injury to the carotid artery or jugular vein, leading to hematomas or local anesthetic toxicity. Inadvertent blockade of adjacent nerves can cause dysphagia, dysphonia, or tongue weakness.
- **Thumb Rule Consideration:** Ensure that nerve blocks are performed with meticulous attention to anatomical landmarks, and always warn patients of potential complications such as difficulty swallowing or speaking.

Delayed Surgical Intervention

- Surgical intervention is often necessary for cases unresponsive to medical therapy. Delaying surgery when conservative treatments fail can result in prolonged suffering and risk of worsening nerve damage.
- **Thumb Rule Consideration:** Consider early referral for surgical consultation in patients with severe, refractory glossopharyngeal neuralgia, particularly if pain relief from medications is inadequate or side effects are intolerable.

REFERENCES

- Miller JP, Burchiel KJ. Microvascular decompression for trigeminal neuralgia. In: Winn HR, ed. Youmans and Winn Neurological Surgery. 7th ed. Philadelphia, PA: Elsevier; 2017:chap 174.
- Narouze S, Pope JE. Orofacial pain. In: Benzon HT, Raja SN, Liu SS, Fishman SM, Cohen SP, eds. Essentials of Pain Medicine. 4th ed. Philadelphia, PA: Elsevier; 2018:chap 23.
- Koopman JS, Dieleman JP, Huygen FJ, de Mos M, Martin CG, Sturkenboom MC: Incidence of facial pain in the general population. Pain 2009; 147: 122–127.

- Waldman SD: Glossopharyngeal nerve block. In Waldman SD, editor: Atlas of interventional pain management, ed 3, Philadelphia, 2009, Saunders, pp 93–97.

GLUTEUS MAXIMUS PAIN SYNDROME

Deep gluteal syndrome describes the presence of pain in the buttock caused from non-discogenic and extrapelvic entrapment of the sciatic nerve. Several structures can be involved in sciatic nerve entrapment within the gluteal space. A comprehensive history and physical examination can orientate the specific site where the sciatic nerve is entrapped, as well as several radiological signs that support the suspected diagnosis. Failure to identify the cause of pain in a timely manner can increase pain perception, and affect mental control, patient hope and consequently quality of life.

J Hip Preserv Surg. 2015 Jul; 2(2): 99–107.

Clinical Description

The diagnosis of deep gluteal syndrome is based upon a comprehensive history and physical examination of the hip. The lumbar spine plays an important role in hip pain. Hence, a differentiation of problems coming from the spine should be performed during the history and physical examination. Once the lumbar pathology is ruled out using specific tests and spine imaging, the physical examination should be directed toward the deep gluteal space as a cause of posterior pain.

Patients with sciatic nerve entrapment often have previous history of trauma and symptoms of sit pain, radicular pain of the lower back or hip and paresthesias of the affected leg. Patients may present with neurological symptoms of abnormal reflexes or motor weakness. Some symptoms may mimic a hamstring tear or intra-articular hip pathology such as aching, burning sensation or cramping in the buttock or posterior thigh.

The factors or positions that increase or decrease the pain can dictate the diagnostic approach. A sitting pain is usually associated with sciatic entrapment beneath the piriformis muscle. A walking pain lateral to the ischium is associated with ischiofemoral impingement, in which the lesser trochanter rubs the lateral border of the ischium.

Posterior hip pain could originate from intrapelvic problems, hence a focused urologic and gynecologic history should be addressed in order to detect any suggestive sign of intrapelvic entrapment such as cyclic variations in pain. High resolution imaging of the pelvis or abdomen assists in identifying any type of endometrioma or vascular entrapment of the sciatic nerve in the intra-abdominal region.

osterior hip pain commonly presents in a chronic fashion significantly affecting the quality of life. Therefore, a psychological evaluation before any treatment is recommended for patients complaining of chronic pain >6 months, who are using narcotics, and have a significantly impaired social function. Psychological strategies for diagnosing depression and anxiety disorders related with chronic pain have shown high specificity and reliability. These factors could affect the outcomes and the satisfaction of the patient and the surgeon.

Pearls & Oysters

Injections of trigger points in the gluteus maximus muscle can be a useful technique for managing pain, but it is important that the procedure be performed by a clinician who is well-trained in regional anatomy and experienced in interventional pain management techniques. The proximity of the sciatic nerve to the injection site means that there is a risk of damage to the nerve if the procedure is not performed correctly. Additionally, some patients may experience a transient increase in pain after the injection of trigger points. The use of long needles may also increase the risk of damage to retroperitoneal organs.

Bottom Line Statement

Gluteus maximus pain syndrome is a condition characterized by pain in the gluteus maximus muscle, which is the largest muscle in the buttocks. This diagnosis is typically made through a combination of clinical history, physical examination, radiography, and MRI. There are a number of other conditions that may cause pain similar to that seen in gluteus maximus pain syndrome, including lumbosacral radiculopathy and plexopathy, stress fractures of the pelvis and hip, muscle strain, inflammatory arthritis, and disorders of the lumbar spinal cord, roots, plexus, and nerves. Intrapelvic tumors may also present with symptoms similar to those of gluteus maximus pain syndrome.

Trigger point injections are a procedure in which a needle is used to inject a small amount of medication into specific points in the muscles known as trigger points. These injections can be an effective treatment for myofascial pain syndrome, a type of chronic pain that affects the muscles and surrounding soft tissues. To minimize the risk of complications, it is important to follow proper sterile technique and to use universal precautions to avoid infection. Common side effects of trigger point injections may include needle-induced trauma to the injection site and underlying tissues, ecchymosis (bruising), and hematoma (blood clot) formation. To reduce the risk of these complications, it is important to avoid using overly long needles and to apply pressure to the injection site immediately after the procedure. Tricyclic antidepressants, such as amitriptyline and nortriptyline, are often used to treat myofascial pain syndrome, although the precise mechanism of action is not fully understood.

Medico-Legal Traps

Misdiagnosis Due to Overlapping Conditions

- Gluteus maximus pain syndrome shares symptoms with other conditions like lumbosacral radiculopathy, pelvic fractures, or sciatica, leading to frequent misdiagnosis. Incorrect treatment based on a misdiagnosis can lead to prolonged suffering and worsening of the condition.
- **Thumb Rule Consideration:** Always differentiate between spine-related pathologies and deep gluteal syndrome using a combination of clinical history, physical exam, and imaging like MRI.

Overlooking Neurological Involvement

- Gluteus maximus pain syndrome can often involve sciatic nerve entrapment. Failure to assess for nerve involvement through proper neurological examination may result in missing cases of sciatic neuropathy, delaying critical interventions.
- **Thumb Rule Consideration:** Conduct a thorough neurological examination, including testing for abnormal reflexes and motor weakness, especially in patients presenting with radicular pain or paresthesia in the lower extremities.

Inaccurate Trigger Point Injections

- Improperly performed trigger point injections into the gluteus maximus can damage the sciatic nerve or underlying organs, leading to severe complications. Inexperienced clinicians performing the procedure may also inadvertently cause retroperitoneal damage.
- **Thumb Rule Consideration:** Ensure that trigger point injections are done by clinicians trained in regional anatomy, using the appropriate needle size, and always with attention to sciatic nerve proximity.

Failure to Rule Out Intrapelvic Causes

- Some posterior hip pain might be due to intrapelvic problems such as tumors or endometriosis. Neglecting to evaluate intrapelvic causes can delay accurate diagnosis and treatment, leading to progressive pathology.
- **Thumb Rule Consideration:** Always perform a focused urologic and gynecologic history and consider high-resolution pelvic imaging to rule out intrapelvic causes when treating chronic gluteal pain.

Ignoring Psychological Factors in Chronic Pain

- Patients with chronic gluteus maximus pain often suffer from related psychological conditions like depression or anxiety, especially if the pain has persisted for over six months. Failure to address these psychological aspects can negatively impact treatment outcomes and patient satisfaction.
- **Thumb Rule Consideration:** Incorporate psychological evaluation into the treatment plan for patients with chronic pain lasting more than six months, particularly if narcotics are involved or social function is impaired.

REFERENCES

- Robinson DR. Pyriformis syndrome in relation to sciatic pain. Am J Surg 1947; 73: 355–8.
- Filler AG, Haynes J, Jordan SE, et al. Sciatica of nondisc origin and piriformis syndrome: diagnosis by magnetic resonance neurography and interventional magnetic resonance imaging with outcome study of resulting treatment. J Neurosurg Spine 2005; 2: 99–115.
- Martin HD, Shears SA, Johnson JC, et al. The endoscopic treatment of sciatic nerve entrapment/deep gluteal syndrome. Arthroscopy 2011; 27: 172–81.
- Puranen J, Orava S. The hamstring syndrome: a new diagnosis of gluteal sciatic pain. Am J Sports Med 1988; 16: 517–21.
- Young IJ, van Riet RP, Bell SN. Surgical release for proximal hamstring syndrome. Am J Sports Med 2008; 36: 2372–8.
- Cox JM, Bakkum BW. Possible generators of retrotrochanteric gluteal and thigh pain: the gemelli-obturator internus complex. J Manipulative Physiol Ther 2005; 28: 534–8.
- Meknas K, Kartus J, Letto JI, et al. Surgical release of the internal obturator tendon for the treatment of retro-trochanteric pain syndrome: a prospective randomized study, with long-term follow-up. Knee Surg Sport Traumatol Arthrosc 2009; 17: 1249–56.
- Labropoulos N, Tassiopoulos AK, Gasparis AP, et al. Veins along the course of the sciatic nerve. J Vasc Surg 2009; 49: 690–6.

GLUTEUS MEDIUS SYNDROME

Deep gluteal syndrome describes the presence of pain in the buttock caused from non-discogenic and extrapelvic entrapment of the sciatic nerve. Several structures can be involved in sciatic nerve entrapment within the gluteal space. A comprehensive history and physical examination can orientate the specific site where the sciatic nerve is entrapped, as well as several radiological signs that support the suspected diagnosis. Failure to identify the cause of pain in a timely manner can increase pain perception, and affect mental control, patient hope and consequently quality of life.

J Hip Preserv Surg. 2015 Jul; 2(2): 99–107.

Clinical Description

Myofascial pain syndrome is a type of chronic pain that affects the muscles and surrounding soft tissues. It is characterized by the presence of trigger points, which are localized areas of tenderness within the affected muscle. The gluteus medius muscle, which is responsible for hip abduction and rotation, is prone to the development of myofascial pain syndrome. This type of pain is often the result of repetitive microtrauma from activities such as running or overuse of exercise equipment, or it may be caused by blunt trauma to the muscle. Myofascial pain syndrome is often misdiagnosed or attributed to other organ systems, leading to extensive evaluations and ineffective treatment. The pain of myofascial pain syndrome is often referred to other areas of the body, and patients with myofascial pain syndrome involving the gluteus medius may experience primary pain along the posterior iliac crest that is referred down the buttocks and into the posterior lower extremity. In addition to local and referred pain, patients with gluteus medius syndrome may also exhibit an involuntary withdrawal of the stimulated muscle, known as the jump sign, upon mechanical stimulation of the trigger point.

Myofascial pain syndrome is a chronic muscle pain disorder that is characterized by the presence of trigger points in the muscle tissue. These trigger points are identifiable by the presence of taut bands of muscle fibers when palpated and can cause pain, muscle weakness, and fatigue. While the exact cause of myofascial pain syndrome remains unknown, it is thought to be related to microtrauma or injury to the affected muscle. This microtrauma may be the result of a single injury or repetitive microtrauma, as well as chronic muscle deconditioning.

In addition to muscle trauma, there are several other factors that may increase the risk of developing myofascial pain syndrome. These include participating in unaccustomed physical activity, poor posture, previous injuries, and psychological or behavioral abnormalities such as chronic stress and depression. Poor nutritional status may also contribute to the development of myofascial pain syndrome. The gluteus medius muscle is particularly prone to stress-induced myofascial pain syndrome. Treatment options for myofascial pain syndrome may include medications, physical therapy, and trigger point injections.

Pearls & Oysters

At the present time, among 200 international cases have addressed extrapelvic deep gluteal syndrome and complications continue to be extremely low. To help avoid post-surgical stretch injury, it is recommended that intra-articular work be performed separately from extra-articular work. Due to the length of time from diagnosis to treatment and recovery, the psychological toll of the pain cycle can be frustrating. Complications have involved hematomas brought on by early post-operative use of NSAIDs with excessive post-operative activity. Concomitant pudendal nerve and sciatic nerve complaints are often resolved, however in two of those 200 cases the pudendal complaints worsened.

Bottom Line Statement

Gluteus medius syndrome is a condition that affects the gluteus medius muscle, which is a muscle in the buttocks. It is a common disorder, but it is often misdiagnosed and may coexist with other somatic (physical) and psychological disorders. Therefore, it is important to perform a thorough evaluation to identify any underlying disease processes in patients who are suspected of having gluteus medius syndrome. The treatment of gluteus medius syndrome may involve a combination of medications, physical therapy, and other modalities, depending on the specific underlying cause of the disorder.

Medico-Legal Traps

Misdiagnosis as Lumbar or Hip Pathology

- Gluteus medius syndrome is often misdiagnosed as lumbar spine disorders, hip pathology, or sciatica, leading to inappropriate treatment. The pain patterns of gluteus medius syndrome overlap with other conditions, causing clinicians to focus on more obvious sources of pain while ignoring the underlying muscle issue.
- **Thumb Rule Consideration:** Always perform a thorough musculoskeletal examination, including palpation of the gluteal muscles

and assessment for trigger points, to rule out gluteus medius syndrome before proceeding with imaging studies focused solely on the spine or hips.

Failure to Recognize Psychological Contributors

- Chronic pain from gluteus medius syndrome can lead to psychological issues such as depression and anxiety, but these are often overlooked in clinical evaluations. Ignoring the psychological impact can exacerbate the pain cycle, delay recovery, and result in poor treatment outcomes.
- **Thumb Rule Consideration:** Incorporate psychological screening for depression, stress, and anxiety in patients with chronic gluteal pain, especially those unresponsive to conventional treatment.

Overlooking the Role of Trigger Points

- Trigger points in the gluteus medius can be mistaken for nerve or joint pain, leading to inappropriate treatments like nerve blocks or unnecessary surgeries. Clinicians who are unfamiliar with myofascial pain syndromes may miss the presence of these localized areas of tenderness.
- **Thumb Rule Consideration:** Always evaluate for myofascial pain by palpating the gluteus medius muscle for trigger points and considering myofascial pain syndrome as a differential diagnosis in patients with unexplained hip and buttock pain.

Inadequate Post-Operative Care

- In cases requiring surgery, improper post-operative care, such as early return to activity or the use of NSAIDs, can result in complications like hematomas or worsening of symptoms, particularly pudendal or sciatic nerve irritation.
- **Thumb Rule Consideration:** Advise patients on appropriate rest, the cautious use of NSAIDs, and gradual return to activity after surgery to minimize complications and promote effective recovery.

Failure to Rule Out Extrapelvic Nerve Entrapments

- Entrapment of the sciatic or pudendal nerves in the deep gluteal space can co-exist with gluteus medius syndrome but may be overlooked, leading to unresolved pain even after treatment of the muscle. This can result in delayed or incomplete relief for the patient.
- **Thumb Rule Consideration:** Always consider and evaluate for extrapelvic nerve entrapment, such as sciatic or pudendal nerve involvement, when diagnosing gluteus medius syndrome, especially in patients with persistent or atypical symptoms.

REFERENCES

- McCrory P, Bell S. Nerve entrapment syndromes as a cause of pain in the hip, groin and buttock. Sports Med 1999; 27: 261–74.
- Robinson DR. Pyriformis syndrome in relation to sciatic pain. Am J Surg 1947; 73: 355–8.
- Filler AG, Haynes J, Jordan SE, et al. Sciatica of nondisc origin and piriformis syndrome: diagnosis by magnetic resonance neurography and interventional magnetic resonance imaging with outcome study of resulting treatment. J Neurosurg Spine 2005; 2: 99–115.
- Martin HD, Shears SA, Johnson JC, et al. The endoscopic treatment of sciatic nerve entrapment/deep gluteal syndrome. Arthroscopy 2011; 27: 172–81.
- Puranen J, Orava S. The hamstring syndrome: a new diagnosis of gluteal sciatic pain. Am J Sports Med 1988; 16: 517–21.
- Young IJ, van Riet RP, Bell SN. Surgical release for proximal hamstring syndrome. Am J Sports Med 2008; 36: 2372–8.
- Cox JM, Bakkum BW. Possible generators of retrotrochanteric gluteal and thigh pain: the gemelli-obturator internus complex. J Manipulative Physiol Ther 2005; 28: 534–8.
- Meknas K, Kartus J, Letto JI, et al. Surgical release of the internal obturator tendon for the treatment of retro-trochanteric pain syndrome: a prospective randomized study, with long-term follow-up. Knee Surg Sport Traumatol Arthrosc 2009; 17: 1249–56.
- Labropoulos N, Tassiopoulos AK, Gasparis AP, et al. Veins along the course of the sciatic nerve. J Vasc Surg 2009; 49: 690–6.
- Papadopoulos SM, McGillicuddy JE, Albers JW. Unusual cause of "piriformis muscle syndrome". Arch Neurol 1990; 47: 1144–6.
- Beauchesne RP, Schutzer SF. Myositis ossificans of the piriformis muscle: an unusual cause of piriformis syndrome. J Bone Joint Surg Am 1997; 79: 906–10.

HAMSTRING TENDINITIS-PROXIMAL

Hamstring tendonitis is an inflammation of the hamstring tendons. It usually results from overuse or not stretching before and after you run or play. Hamstring tendonitis is also more common among older athletes and in running and cutting sports.

Naugle KM, Fillingim RB, Riley JL 3rd. A meta-analytic review of the hypoalgesic effects of exercise. J Pain. 2012 Dec;13(12):1139-50.

Clinical Description

Proximal hamstring tendinopathy (PHT) is commonly seen in long distance runners and athletes taking part in sprinting or hurdles. It is also common among athletes taking part in sports such as football and hockey, which involves a change of direction activities. Proximal hamstring tendinopathy is also referred to as hamstring origin tendinopathy or high hamstring tendinopathy. It can also affect people who do not participate in sport.It is characterised by deep, localised pain in the region of the ischial tuberosity. Pain is usually worse during or after activities such as running, lunging, squatting and sitting. This condition can include tendon degeneration, partial tearing and peritendinous inflammatory reactions. Proximal Hamstring Tendinopathy-related Sciatic Nerve Entrapment (PHTrSNE) is a neuropathy caused by fibrosis interposed between the semimembranosus tendon and the sciatic nerve, at the level of the ischial tuberosity.

One of the most important muscle groups in running is the hamstrings muscle group. The hamstrings are active at various stages in the gait cycle, particularly in knee flexion and hip extension. The hamstrings muscles share a common origin on the lateral aspect of the ischial tuberosity. Semitendinosus and the long head of biceps femoris share a conjoined tendon originating from the lateral facet. The origin of Semimembranosus is deeper. Various locations of hamstring tendon pathology have been reported. The semimembranosus is one of the most commonly affected parts of the hamstring muscles in proximal hamstring tendinopathy. Other studies found a variety of locations such as the common hamstring tendon, biceps femoris, semimembranosus and semitendinosus.

The junction between the tendons of the hamstrings and the ischial tuberosity is the area affected by high hamstring tendinopathy. The tendon's thickness, fibrousness and poor blood supply are the causes of difficult healing. The muscles contain a higher proportion of type 2 muscle fibres than the other muscles of the lower extremity; suggesting high intrinsic force generation.

During running, the hamstrings have three main functions. First, they decelerate knee extension at the end of the forward swing phase of the gait cycle. Through an eccentric contraction, the hamstrings decelerate the forward momentum (i.e, leg swing) at approximately 30° short of full knee extension. This action helps provide dynamic stabilization to the weight bearing knee. Second, at foot strike, the hamstrings elongate to facilitate hip extension through an eccentric contraction, thus further stabilizing the leg for weight bearing. Third, the hamstrings assist the gastrocnemius in paradoxically extending the knee during the take-off phase of the running cycle.

Proximal hamstring tendinopathy is regarded as insertional tendinopathy. Compression of the tendon at its attachment during hip flexion/adduction is hypothesized to be an important etiological factor,but the evidence is limited. Other contributing factors may be the presence of a shearing force between the hamstring attachment and the ischial tuberosity and the increased displacement of the proximal hamstring tendon with an increased hip flexion angle.

Pearls & Oysters

Return to sports can be gradually introduced when the athlete is able to cope with the loading requirements of the sport with minimal symptom aggravation (i.e. VAS 0 -3 of 10 with pain settling within 24 hours on load tests). The exercise progressions form stepping stones for return to sport, but it is important to not just add these exercises to the normal training volume on resumption, as this can lead to overloading and aggravation of symptoms. Be careful with the introduction of hill training as well as speed training sessions, as these can easily exacerbate symptoms. In team sports, there may be more complex loading requirements. This needs a more detailed assessment and a graded return to sport will usually consist of gradual exposure to activity prior to return to full competition.

Bottom Line Statement

HHT is a painful condition that is often challenging to medically manage. While eccentric exercise has been thoroughly studied with other tendinopathies, the research for hamstring tendinopathy is limited. ASTYM has also been proposed as a treatment for tendinopathy and it is thought to work by stimulating the patient's body to normalize tissue structure following an increase in fibroblast recruitment and activation.

Medico-Legal Traps

Misdiagnosis as Sciatica or Lumbar Pathology

- Proximal hamstring tendinitis often presents with symptoms similar to sciatica or lower back issues, leading to misdiagnosis. Patients with PHT may be subjected to unnecessary spinal imaging and treatments like lumbar injections, without addressing the real source of pain.
- **Thumb Rule Consideration:** Always include a comprehensive musculoskeletal assessment of the hamstring and gluteal regions when evaluating patients with posterior thigh pain, especially if lumbar imaging is negative.

Failure to Recognize Tendon Degeneration

- Chronic cases of PHT can involve tendon degeneration, yet clinicians may overlook this and assume the issue is purely inflammatory. This can lead to the overuse of anti-inflammatory treatments, such as corticosteroid injections, which may worsen tendon degeneration over time.
- **Thumb Rule Consideration:** Consider imaging studies like MRI or ultrasound to assess the condition of the tendon and avoid relying solely on anti-inflammatory treatments in chronic cases.

Overaggressive Rehabilitation

- Returning athletes to sports or physical activities too quickly can exacerbate symptoms and delay recovery. This often occurs due to pressure from athletes or insufficiently individualized rehabilitation protocols.
- **Thumb Rule Consideration:** Implement a gradual return-to-sport program that is tailored to the athlete's pain tolerance and recovery progression, and monitor closely for signs of overload, particularly with exercises like sprinting or hill running.

Ignoring the Role of Hip Flexion and Compression

- Hip flexion and compression at the attachment point of the hamstring tendon are significant contributors to PHT, yet this factor may be ignored during treatment. Overemphasis on general strengthening exercises without considering specific biomechanical contributors can hinder recovery.
- **Thumb Rule Consideration:** Focus on exercises that minimize excessive hip flexion and compression, and use movement modifications to protect the tendon from further irritation during rehabilitation.

Failure to Identify Coexisting Nerve Entrapment

- PHT can coexist with sciatic nerve entrapment due to fibrosis near the ischial tuberosity. Clinicians may treat the tendinopathy while missing nerve involvement, leading to unresolved or worsening symptoms.
- **Thumb Rule Consideration:** Evaluate for signs of sciatic nerve entrapment in all cases of PHT, especially in chronic or treatment-resistant cases, and consider diagnostic nerve blocks or advanced imaging if nerve involvement is suspected.

REFERENCES

- Fredericson M, Moore W, Guillet M, Beaulieu C. High hamstring tendinopathy in runners: meeting the challenges of diagnosis, treatment, and rehabilitation. The Physician and sports medicine. 2005 Jan 1;33(5):32-43.
- Jesus JF, Bryk FF, Moreira VC, Nakaoka GB, Reis AC, Lucareli PR. Gluteus Maximus inhibition in proximal hamstring tendinopathy. MedicalExpress. 2015 Aug;2(4)..
- Lempainen L, Johansson K, Banke IJ et al. Expert opinion: diagnosis and treatment of proximal hamstring tendinopathy. Muscles Ligaments Tendons J. 2015;5: 23 - 28
- Goom TS, Malliaras P, Reiman MP, Purdam CR. Proximal Hamstring Tendinopathy: Clinical Aspects of Assessment and Management. J Orthop Sports Phys Ther. 2016 Jun;46(6):483-93
- Zissen MH, Wallace G, Stevens KJ, Fredericson M, Beaulieu CF. High hamstring tendinopathy: MRI and ultrasound imaging and therapeutic efficacy of percutaneous corticosteroid injection. American Journal of Roentgenology. 2010 Oct;195(4):993-8.
- Philippon MJ1, Ferro FP, Campbell KJ, Michalski MP, Goldsmith MT, Devitt BM, Wijdicks CA, LaPrade RF. A qualitative and quantitative analysis of the attachment sites of the proximal hamstrings. Knee Surg Sports Traumatol Arthrosc. 2015 Sep;23(9):2554-61.
- Benazzo F, Marullo M, Zanon G, Indino C,Pelillo F. Surgical management of chronic proximal hamstring tendinopathy in athletes: a 2 to 11 years of follow-up. J Orthop Traumatol. 2013 Jun; 14(2): 83–89.
- High hamstring tendinopathy injuries – Signs, symptoms and research-backed treatment solutions for a literal pain in the butt. Available from:accessed from http://runnersconnect.net/running-injury-prevention/high-hamstring-tendinopathy-injuries-a-pain-in-the-butt/ on 27/04/2019.
- Cook JL, Purdam CR. Is tendon pathology a continuum? A pathology model to explain the clinical presentation of load-induced tendinopathy. British journal of sports medicine. 2009 Jun 1;43(6):409-16.
- Hamming MG, Philippon MJ, Rasmussen MT, Ferro FP, Turnbull TL, Trindade CA, LaPrade RF, Wijdicks CA. Structural properties of the intact proximal hamstring origin and evaluation of varying avulsion repair techniques: an in vitro biomechanical analysis. The American journal of sports medicine. 2015 Mar;43(3):721-8.
- Harvey MA, Singh H, Obopilwe E, Charette R, Miller S. Proximal Hamstring Repair Strength: A Biomechanical Analysis at 3 Hip Flexion Angles. Orthop J Sports Med. 2015;3(4):2325967115576910
- Chumanov ES, Heiderscheit BC, Thelen DG. Hamstring musculotendon dynamics during stance and swing phases of high-speed running. Med Sci Sports Exerc. 2011;43(3):525-32.

HEADACHE ASSOCIATED WITH TEMPORAL ARTERITIS

Headache is the most common complaint in cranial or temporal arteritis. The major symptoms of central nervous system arteritis are multifocal neurological symptoms following stroke, in combination with headache and some degree of encephalopathy, with and without seizures. CNS-vasculitis may be part of a systemic autoimmune disease or the only manifestation of angiitis (isolated or primary angiitis of the central nervous system – PACNS).

Ad Hoc Committee on Neuropsychiatric Lupus Nomenclature. (1999). The American College of Rheumatology nomenclature and case definitions for neuropsychiatric lupus. Arthritis and Rheumatism, 42, 599–608.

Clinical Description

Temporal arteritis (TA), also called giant cell arteritis (GCA) or cranial arteritis, is a systemic inflammatory vasculitis of medium and large-sized arteries occurring most frequently in adults. TA leads to ischemic optic neuropathy with potentially irreversible vision loss on the affected side with potential contralateral involvement.•

Giant cell arteritis (GCA) is a disease of blood vessels, may occur together with polymyalgia rheumatica (pain and stiffness in the neck, shoulder, and hip). GCA occurs only in older adults, those over age of 50, and can cause swelling and thickening of the arteries located on each side of the head called the temporal artery.

If GCA affects blood flow to the eye, loss of vision can occur. Prompt detection and treatment of GCA can prevent loss of vision. As the name suggests, headache associated with temporal arteritis is located primarily in the temples, with secondary pain often located in the frontal and occipital regions. A disease of the sixth decade and beyond, temporal arteritis affects whites almost exclusively, and there is a 3:1 female gender predominance. Temporal arteritis is also known as giant cell arteritis because of the finding of giant multinucleated cells that infiltrate arteries containing elastin, including the temporal, ophthalmic, and external carotid arteries. Approximately half of patients with temporal arteritis also have polymyalgia rheumatica.

Pearls & Oysters

Failure to recognize, diagnose, and treat temporal arteritis promptly may result in the permanent loss of vision. Failure to diagnose the headache associated with temporal arteritis correctly may put the patient at risk if an intracranial pathological condition or demyelinating disease (which may mimic the clinical presentation of temporal arteritis) is overlooked. MRI of the brain is indicated in all patients thought to have headaches associated with temporal arteritis. Failure to diagnose glaucoma, which also may cause intermittent ocular pain, may result in permanent loss of sight.

Bottom Line Statement

The management of temporal arteritis is with an interprofessional team that consists of an internist, neurologist, rheumatologist, ophthalmologist, nursing staff, pharmacist, and surgeon. Education is the essential step as patients need to know the complications of this disorder and the need for close monitoring related to both the condition and its treatment. All patients should be urged to follow up with an ophthalmologist to ensure that vision loss is not occurring. Anyone with weakness, loss of vision, difficulty with gait, dysphagia, or speech problems should immediately seek medical assistance. The pharmacist should educate the patient on corticosteroid compliance and the potential side effects. Nursing will often be the patient's first point of contact for questions and can also coordinate activities and information sharing between the various disciplines involved in care. All patients should understand that they may develop problems with other blood vessels in the future despite treatment.

Medico-Legal Traps

Delayed Diagnosis Leading to Vision Loss

- One of the most severe complications of temporal arteritis (TA) is permanent vision loss due to ischemic optic neuropathy. Misdiagnosing the headache associated with TA as a common tension or migraine headache can delay the necessary corticosteroid treatment, resulting in irreversible blindness.
- **Thumb Rule Consideration:** Always consider temporal arteritis in patients over 50 presenting with new-onset headache, jaw claudication, scalp tenderness, or visual symptoms, and order prompt ESR/CRP blood tests and temporal artery biopsy.

Confusing TA with Other Intracranial Conditions

- Headaches from temporal arteritis may mimic intracranial conditions such as brain tumors or demyelinating diseases like multiple sclerosis. Overlooking TA in favor of these other diagnoses can lead to unnecessary imaging studies or treatments, while missing the crucial inflammatory cause.

- **Thumb Rule Consideration:** Include TA in differential diagnoses for elderly patients with atypical or persistent headaches and obtain MRI if other neurological symptoms or intracranial pathology are suspected, but prioritize temporal artery evaluation.

Inappropriate Use of Imaging Without Biopsy

- Relying solely on imaging such as MRI to diagnose TA can result in misdiagnosis, as imaging often cannot confirm the vasculitis present in temporal arteritis. Failing to perform a temporal artery biopsy when needed can lead to legal consequences due to improper diagnosis.
- **Thumb Rule Consideration:** Temporal artery biopsy remains the gold standard for diagnosing TA. Do not omit this essential diagnostic tool, even if imaging is inconclusive, particularly in high-risk patients.

Failure to Treat Polymyalgia Rheumatica Coexisting with TA

- Approximately 50% of patients with temporal arteritis also have polymyalgia rheumatica (PMR). Overlooking the diagnosis of PMR or inadequately treating it can prolong symptoms, lead to functional disability, and delay treatment of the systemic inflammation.
- **Thumb Rule Consideration:** Screen all patients diagnosed with TA for symptoms of PMR, including shoulder and hip stiffness, and ensure the treatment plan covers both conditions.

Inadequate Monitoring of Corticosteroid Therapy Side Effects

- Long-term corticosteroid use, which is often required for managing TA, has significant side effects like osteoporosis, diabetes, and hypertension. Failure to monitor and address these side effects can result in patient harm and potential litigation.
- **Thumb Rule Consideration:** Ensure close monitoring of corticosteroid side effects through regular blood pressure checks, bone density scans, and blood glucose assessments, and involve a multidisciplinary team to mitigate complications.

REFERENCES

- Trial of Tocilizumab in Giant-Cell Arteritis J.H. Stone, K. Tuckwell, S. Dimonaco, M. Klearman, M. Aringer, D. Blockmans, E. Brouwer, M.C. Cid, B. Dasgupta, J. Rech, C. Salvarani, G. Schett, H. Schulze-Koops, R. Spiera, S.H. Unizony, and N. Collinson. NEJM, 377: 2017: 317-328.
- Pearce JM. Sir Jonathan Hutchinson (1828-1913) and an early description of temporal arteritis. J Neurol Neurosurg Psychiatry. 1994 Feb;57(2):216.
- HORTON BT. Temporal arteritis; report of 39 cases. Proc Annu Meet Cent Soc Clin Res U S. 1946 Nov 1-2;19:78.
- Nordborg E. Epidemiology of biopsy-positive giant cell arteritis: an overview. Clin Exp Rheumatol. 2000 Jul-Aug;18(4 Suppl 20):S15-7.

- Alberts M. Temporal arteritis: improving patient evaluation with a new protocol. Perm J. 2013 Winter;17(1):56-62.
- Koster MJ, Matteson EL, Warrington KJ. Large-vessel giant cell arteritis: diagnosis, monitoring and management. Rheumatology (Oxford). 2018 Feb 01;57(suppl_2):ii32-ii42.
- Waldman SD: Connective tissue diseases. In Waldman SD, editor: Pain review, Philadelphia, 2009, Saunders, pp 431–448.

HYOID SYNDROME

A condition characterized by both dental and non-dental referral sites, this degenerative injury of the middle pharyngeal constrictor muscle is confirmed by photomicroscopic evidence of insertion tendinosis. The hyoid bone has been identified with a specific, although not well recognized, pain syndrome for over 40 years. The painful symptoms are generally caused by trauma at the greater cornu of the hyoid bone with the pain radiating to other sites.

Brown LA. Hyoid bone syndrome. South Med J. 1954. 47:1088-91.

Clinical Description

The hyoid bone (hyoid) is a small U-shaped (horseshoe-shaped) solitary bone, situated in the midline of the neck anteriorly at the base of the mandible and posteriorly at the fourth cervical vertebra. Its anatomical position is just superior to the thyroid cartilage. It is closely linked with an extended tendon-muscular complex but not specifically interconnected to any adjacent bones and hence is considered by many anatomists and anthropologists to be an unconventional bone. It is anchored in the anterior triangle of the neck by muscles from the larynx, pharynx, tongue, and the floor of the mouth. The name hyoid derives from the Greek word "hyodeides," which means "shaped like the letter Upsilon." Although dubbed as an unconventional bone, the hyoid being a part of the hyoid-larynx complex is indeed a bone of clinical and forensic significance.

The condition is not well known in medicine and dentistry for at least two reasons:

(1) the diffuse and seemingly unrelated radiation of symptoms and

(2) the apparent absence of histopathologic evidence of injury.

Hyoid bone syndrome was first described by Brown in 1954, and later by Steinmann, Kopstein, Lim, and Ernest. The syndrome represents a group of confounding head and neck symptoms that may suggest carotodynia to the unsuspecting clinician. The primary site of pain is associated with the region of the greater cornu tip of the hyoid bone. Steinmann,[5] Kopstein, Lim, and Ernest have reported surgical removal of the greater cornu with remarkable resolution of pain for the affected patient. However, some clinicians deny the existence or the validity of hyoid bone syndrome because reports offer no objective evidence other than the signs, symptoms, and results of surgery.

Pearls & Oysters

Hyoid bone insertion tendinitis is also known as hyoid bone syndrome. Patients describe it as neck pain that increases with swallowing and movement of the neck. The pain is characteristically either dull or sharp, radiating to the

temporal area, posterior pharyngeal wall, sternocleidomastoid muscle, ear, and supraclavicular region. On examination, tenderness over the greater horn of the hyoid is noted upon palpation. The condition is diagnosed mainly by history and physical examination. Imaging may be used to exclude the other differential diagnoses. Medical therapy is the initial treatment of choice. It includes topical and systemic non-steroidal anti-inflammatory medications, local anaesthetics and steroid injections. If medical therapy fails, then surgery is the next consideration.

Bottom Line Statement

Trauma to the hyoid and laryngeal cartilages (thyroid cartilage and cricoid cartilage), is one of the significant signs of manual strangulation or throttling discovered during a forensic autopsy. Fractures of the hyoid-laryngeal complex are present in cases of death due to a constricting force around the neck. Forensic pathologists have intensively studied traumatic lesions of the hyoid-laryngeal complex in strangulation, including manual strangulation and ligature strangulation, and hanging. Other forms of blunt force impact to the neck can also cause fracture of the hyoid.

The damage commonly affects the greater horns or the region between the body of the hyoid and the horns. Injuries are mainly in the form of vertical or oblique fractures. Displacements of the fracture segments are also observed. Bilateral fractures of the hyoid and double fractures of one of the greater horns are not uncommon. The frequency of a fractured hyoid is more in cases of strangulation in comparison to cases of hanging. However, a hyoid fracture is present in only about a third of all homicides from strangulation. Therefore, it merits noting that an intact hyoid does not always rule out strangulation as the underlying cause of death. The hyoid is fractured more commonly in the older victims of strangulation and is less likely to occur in younger victims of strangulation in the age group 20 to 40. The differences in the age-related frequency of hyoid fracture are dependent on the degree of ankylosis of the hyoid that progresses with age. The mobility in the region of the junction between the greater horns and the body of the hyoid should not be mistaken for a fracture.

Medico-Legal Traps

Misdiagnosis Due to Diffuse Pain Radiation

- Hyoid syndrome presents with diffuse pain radiating to multiple unrelated areas such as the temporomandibular joint, ear, and neck. This can lead to misdiagnosis, often mistaken for conditions like carotodynia or temporomandibular disorders, delaying appropriate treatment.
- **Thumb Rule Consideration:** Always consider hyoid syndrome in patients presenting with neck pain that radiates to multiple areas and

worsens with swallowing, even in the absence of definitive histopathologic findings.

Overlooking Hyoid Bone Injury

- Clinicians unfamiliar with hyoid syndrome may overlook the possibility of hyoid bone or greater cornu injury in patients with neck trauma or pain. This can result in inadequate or ineffective treatment and prolonged symptoms.
- **Thumb Rule Consideration:** Palpate the greater cornu of the hyoid bone in patients with neck pain and tenderness to ensure early diagnosis and rule out conditions mimicking hyoid syndrome.

Inadequate Use of Imaging

- Imaging for hyoid syndrome is often underused, leading to missed diagnoses or over-reliance on clinical symptoms alone. This may result in untreated or improperly managed cases.
- **Thumb Rule Consideration:** Use imaging, such as CT scans or MRIs, to rule out other conditions like fractures or tumors, while understanding that hyoid syndrome is mainly diagnosed through clinical history and physical examination.

Failure to Recognize Surgical Indications

- Non-surgical treatments like NSAIDs or steroid injections often fail to relieve hyoid syndrome symptoms. Failure to recognize when surgery, such as the removal of the greater cornu, is needed can prolong patient suffering.
- **Thumb Rule Consideration:** Consider surgical intervention early if conservative treatments do not resolve symptoms within a reasonable timeframe.

Forensic Misinterpretation in Trauma Cases

- In forensic settings, failure to recognize fractures of the hyoid-laryngeal complex, especially in cases of strangulation, can lead to incorrect conclusions regarding the cause of death. Misidentifying trauma to the hyoid as natural degeneration, particularly in older individuals, is a significant legal risk.
- **Thumb Rule Consideration:** Always consider the possibility of hyoid fractures in autopsy cases involving strangulation, especially in older victims, as ankylosis of the hyoid increases with age.

REFERENCES

- Lim RY. The hyoid bone syndrome. Otolaryngol Head Neck Surg. 1982. 90:198-200.
- Ernest EA. Temporomandibular joint and craniofacial pain-an orthopedic and neurological approach to diagnosis and management. 3rd ed. Montgomery, Ala: Ernest Publications. 1986. 132.
- Steinmann EP. Styloid syndrome in absence of an elongated process. Acts. Otolaryngol. 1968. 66:347-56.
- Kopstein E. Hyoid syndrome. Arch Otolaryngol. 1975. 101:484-5.
- Lim RY. Carotodynia exposed: hyoid bone syndrome. South Med J. 1987. 80:444-6.
- Aydil, Utku; Ekinci, Özgür; Köybaşioğlu, Ahmet; Kizil, Yusuf (2007-01-04). "Hyoid bone insertion tendinitis: clinicopathologic correlation". European Archives of Oto-Rhino-Laryngology. 264 (5): 557–560.
- Khokhlov, Vladislav D. (2015-01). "Trauma to the hyoid bone and laryngeal cartilages in hanging: Review of forensic research series since 1856". Legal Medicine. 17 (1): 17–23.

HYPNIC HEADACHE

Hypnic headaches are a primary headache disorder that presents in the elderly population and usually wakes people up from sleep. It is not very common, but because it could be misdiagnosed with giant cell arteritis, small and medium intracranial vasculitis, and other conditions, it is a critical disorder to be comfortable with its presentation. To avoid the misdiagnosis of hypnic headache, it must be promptly diagnosed and treated.

Olesen J. From ICHD-3 beta to ICHD-3. Cephalalgia. 2016 Apr;36(5):401-2.

Clinical Description

Headaches and chronic pain are amongst the leading cause of morbidity and years lived with disability in the world. Headaches have been classified into various categories based on the International Classification of Headache Disorders criteria. One such headache disorder is a hypnic headache.

Hypnic headache (HH) is a rare headache syndrome that occurs exclusively during sleep, usually at the same time at night. It also has been named before the clockwise headache or alarm clock headache. It is considered a primary headache, according to the international classification of headache disorders.

HH is characterized by attacks of dull headaches that occur after the age of 50 years, at least 15 times per month, and come only during sleep with no associated autonomic symptoms. The attacks wake the patient during sleep and usually last more than 15 minutes after waking. Hypnic headache is a chronic disorder that can last for years, with no remission of headache.

Patients with migraines and hypertension are more likely to develop HH compared to others. Nearly all patients with HH had some type of motor activity, such as getting out of bed and eating, drinking, showering, or reading when awakened by the headache attack. Still, they did not typically have the restlessness that is seen with cluster headache and trigeminal autonomic cephalalgias.

Pearls & Oysters

The diagnosis of hypnic headache is essential as many differential diagnoses are very similar. History taking is the most critical step in the evaluation of these patients and also proper work up to rule out all secondary causes of such headaches like cerebral tumors, etc. All members of the healthcare team should be familiar with this condition as it is not very common, but it does occur in the real world and must be well managed.

Failure to diagnose hypnic headache correctly may put the patient at risk if an intracranial pathological condition or demyelinating disease (which may rarely mimic the clinical presentation of hypnic headache) is overlooked. MRI and MRA are indicated in all patients thought to have hypnic headache. Failure to diagnose glaucoma, which also may cause intermittent ocular pain, may result in permanent loss of sight.

Bottom Line Statement

HH is a benign, recurrent headache disorder that occurs exclusively during slumber, awakening the patient. It occurs primarily in persons older than age 50 years, although rarely younger patients are affected. The pathology, diagnostic criteria, and management of HH continue to evolve with available evidence from case reports and case series. An extensive workup for patients with a suspected diagnosis is important to rule out secondary causes or other headache disorders. Limited evidence supports the use of caffeine, lithium, indomethacin, melatonin, amitriptyline, and some anticonvulsants in the treatment of HH, although efficacy reported for each of these agents is variable, and tolerability may be a problem with some agents. Future research in the areas of neurophysiology and treatment options for HH are necessary in order to better understand, and improve outcomes for, this rare headache disorder.

Medico-Legal Traps

Misdiagnosis as a Secondary Headache

- Hypnic headache (HH) is often misdiagnosed as secondary headaches caused by conditions like giant cell arteritis, intracranial vasculitis, or brain tumors. This can lead to inappropriate treatments, unnecessary testing, and delayed intervention for the actual condition.•
- **Thumb Rule Consideration:** Always consider hypnic headache in patients over 50 presenting with nocturnal headaches that wake them from sleep and rule out secondary causes through imaging and clinical evaluation.

Failure to Differentiate from Cluster Headaches

- Hypnic headache shares some characteristics with cluster headaches, such as waking the patient from sleep, but the two differ significantly in terms of autonomic symptoms and response to treatment. Misdiagnosing HH as a cluster headache can lead to ineffective treatment strategies.
- **Thumb Rule Consideration:** Pay attention to the absence of autonomic symptoms (e.g., tearing or nasal congestion) in HH, which distinguishes it

from cluster headaches, and utilize this information for accurate diagnosis.

Overlooking Underlying Neurological Disorders

- Due to the unusual nature of hypnic headaches, healthcare professionals may overlook potential underlying neurological or vascular conditions, such as small and medium intracranial vasculitis, or even early signs of neurodegenerative disorders.
- **Thumb Rule Consideration:** Conduct thorough neurological exams and use MRI or MRA to exclude other potential causes in patients with new-onset nocturnal headaches, especially those with neurological deficits.

Delayed Recognition Due to Benign Presentation

- Hypnic headache is often benign and self-limiting, but its presentation may lead to dismissal of the symptoms as trivial, especially in elderly patients. This can result in prolonged suffering without proper management.
- **Thumb Rule Consideration:** Treat hypnic headaches seriously in patients over 50 and consider early intervention with agents like caffeine, lithium, or indomethacin to prevent chronicity and improve quality of life.

Inadequate Treatment Leading to Poor Symptom Control

- Given the rarity of hypnic headache, some healthcare providers may not be aware of the appropriate therapeutic options, leading to inadequate treatment and continued suffering.
- **Thumb Rule Consideration:** Ensure that patients with hypnic headache receive well-documented treatments, such as caffeine or low-dose lithium, to manage symptoms effectively, and monitor for side effects in elderly patients who may be sensitive to these medications.

REFERENCES

- Jain S, Malinowski M, Chopra P, Varshney V, Deer TR. Intrathecal drug delivery for pain management: recent advances and future developments. Expert Opin Drug Deliv. 2019 Aug;16(8):815-822.
- Lanteri-Minet M, Donnet A. Hypnic headache. Curr Pain Headache Rep. 2010 Aug;14(4):309-15.
- Headache Classification Subcommittee of the International Headache Society. The International Classification of Headache Disorders: 2nd edition. Cephalalgia. 2004;24 Suppl 1:9-160.
- Liang JF, Wang SJ. Hypnic headache: a review of clinical features, therapeutic options and outcomes. Cephalalgia. 2014 Sep;34(10):795-805.
- Holle D, Naegel S, Obermann M. Hypnic headache. Cephalalgia. 2013 Dec;33(16):1349-57.
- Pascual J, González-Mandly A, Martín R, Oterino A: Headaches precipitated by cough, prolonged exercise or sexual activity: a prospective etiological and clinical study, J Headache Pain 9:259–266, 2008.
- Waldman SD: Arnold Chiari malformation type I. In Waldman SD, Campbell RS, editors: Imaging of pain, Philadelphia, 2011, Saunders, pp 27–28.
- Waldman SD: Arnold Chiari malformation type II. In Waldman SD, Campbell RS, editors: Imaging of pain, Philadelphia, 2011, Saunders, pp 29–30..

ICE PICK HEADACHE

Ice pick headache, also called idiopathic or primary stabbing headache, is a unique headache type associated with ultra-brief stabs of pain, most commonly in the frontal or temporal area. It occurs predominantly in women and is estimated to affect 2-35% of the population.

Curr Pain Headache Rep. 2016 May;20(5):30.

Clinical Description

Ice pick headache is a constellation of symptoms consisting of paroxysms of tabbing jabs and jolts that occur primarily in the first division of the trigeminal nerve. It occurs predominantly in women and is estimated to affect 2-35% of the population. Unlike other headache types of short duration, such as short-lasting unilateral neuralgiform headache with conjunctival injection and tearing (SUNCT), ice pick headache is not associated with any cranial autonomic symptoms but has been known to occur with nausea, vomiting, photophobia, and dizziness. It exists in two forms: primary and secondary, with examples of secondary causes being herpes zoster meningoencephalitis, meningiomas, stroke, and multiple sclerosis.

The pain of ice pick headache occurs in irregular intervals of hours to days. Similar to cluster headache, ice pick headache is an episodic disorder that is characterized by "clusters" of painful attacks followed by pain-free periods. Episodes of ice pick headache usually occur on the same side, but in rare patients, the pain may move to the same anatomical region on the contralateral side. It occurs predominantly in women and is estimated to affect 2-35% of the population and is generally not seen before the fourth decade of life, but rare reports of children suffering from ice pick headache sporadically appear in the literature. It exists in two forms: primary and secondary, with examples of secondary causes being herpes zoster meningoencephalitis, meningiomas, stroke, and multiple sclerosis. Synonyms for ice pick headache include jabs and jolts headache and idiopathic stabbing headache.

Pearls & Oysters

Failure to correctly diagnose ice pick headache may put the patient at risk if intracranial pathological conditions or demyelinating disease, which may mimic the clinical presentation of chronic paroxysmal hemicrania, is overlooked. MRI is indicated in all patients thought to be suffering from ice pick headache. Failure to diagnose glaucoma, which also may cause intermittent ocular pain, may result in permanent loss of sight.

Bottom Line Statement

The diagnosis of ice pick headache is made by obtaining a thorough, targeted headache history. Patients suffering from ice pick headache should have a normal neurological examination. If the results of the neurological examination are abnormal, the diagnosis of ice pick headache should be discarded and a careful search for the cause of the neurological findings should be undertaken. Ice pick headaches are not something to worry about. Ice pick headaches usually do not require medical treatment and are not generally a sign of a severe underlying condition.

Medico-Legal Traps

Misdiagnosis as a Secondary Headache

- Ice pick headache (IPH) shares similar symptoms with more severe conditions like stroke, multiple sclerosis, and herpes zoster meningoencephalitis. Failing to distinguish between primary and secondary headaches can result in missed or delayed diagnoses, potentially leading to serious outcomes.
- **Thumb Rule Consideration:** Always perform a thorough neurological assessment and consider advanced imaging (e.g., MRI) to exclude secondary causes before confirming the diagnosis of primary ice pick headache.

Failure to Exclude Life-Threatening Conditions

- Given that ice pick headaches can mimic the presentation of conditions like meningioma, stroke, or demyelinating diseases, clinicians risk missing critical diagnoses by attributing the symptoms solely to idiopathic headache.
- **Thumb Rule Consideration:** If the patient has any abnormal neurological signs or persistent symptoms, investigate further for intracranial pathologies to rule out serious conditions such as tumors or vascular abnormalities.

Inadequate Documentation of Symptom Progression

- Without proper documentation of the episodic nature and detailed characteristics of the headache (e.g., pain frequency, location, and triggers), a misdiagnosis can occur, complicating future treatment or referrals.
- **Thumb Rule Consideration:** Maintain detailed records of headache episodes, including duration, frequency, location, and any associated symptoms to aid in distinguishing IPH from other headache disorders and ensure proper follow-up care.

Overlooking Secondary Causes in Younger Patients

- While ice pick headaches predominantly affect middle-aged women, rare cases in children or young adults can be related to secondary causes. Misinterpreting the headache as primary in these cases may delay appropriate interventions.
- **Thumb Rule Consideration:** In younger patients or those with atypical presentations, always evaluate for secondary causes, such as infections, structural lesions, or systemic illnesses that could manifest as ice pick headache.

Failure to Recognize Associated Ocular Symptoms

- Occasionally, ice pick headaches can be mistaken for ocular conditions, such as glaucoma, which shares intermittent pain as a symptom. Misdiagnosing or neglecting the ocular evaluation may lead to irreversible vision loss.
- **Thumb Rule Consideration:** In patients with recurring unilateral or ocular pain, include a thorough ophthalmologic assessment and ensure that glaucoma or other eye conditions are ruled out before diagnosing IPH.

REFERENCES

- Curr Pain Headache Rep. 2016 May;20(5):30.
- Cutrer FM, Boes CJ: Cough, exertional, and sex headaches, Neurol Clin 22:133–149, 2004.
- Dafer RM: Neurostimulation in headache disorders, Neurol Clin 28:835–841,2010.
- Mathew NT: Indomethacin responsive headache syndromes: headache, J Head Face Pain 21:147–150, 1981.
- Current Pain and Headache Reports volume 20, Article number: 30 (2016).

ILIOPECTINATE BURSITIS

Iliopsoas bursitis is characterized by distension of the iliopsoas muscle bursa due to synovial fluid and/or hypertrophic synovium. Hip disease is usually associated with it, however, isolated bursitis is also present. Clinically Diagnosing iliopsoas bursitis can be difficult, and imaging is usually required to differentiate iliopsoas bursitis from other inguinal masses such as lymphadenopathy, hernias, and tumors.

Radiol Case Rep. 2020 Nov; 15(11): 2149–2152.

Clinical Description

The iliopsoas (or iliopectineal) bursa is the largest synovial bursa in the body, and is present and bilateral in 98% of adults. It is located between the iliopsoas muscle and the anterior capsule of the hip, this structure is collapsed. The bursa is placed in front of the hip joint, it is adjacent to the thinnest and most vulnerable portion of the anterior capsule and reduces tendon friction over the hip joint during muscle activation and joint movement. Iliopsoas bursitis is characterized by distension of the iliopsoas muscle bursa due to synovial fluid and / or hypertrophic synovium. Hip disease is usually associated with it, however isolated bursitis is also present. In some cases iliopsoas bursitis looks like a mass in the groin or inguinal region. Diagnosing iliopsoas bursitis clinically can be difficult, and imaging is usually required to differentiate iliopsoas bursitis from other inguinal masses such as lymphadenopathy, hernias and tumors.

Pearls & Oysters

In outpatient clinics, the cases can go unnoticed by a less aware orthopedist, general surgeon, vascular surgeon, gynecologist and general practitioner. Thus, the differential diagnosis includes inflammatory and neoplastic adenopathies, neuromyofascial syndrome, iliopsoas tendinitis, lumbosacral injuries, osteitis pubis, vascular lesions such as aneurysm, pseudoaneurysm of the femoral artery, arteriovenous femoral fistula, hematoma, varicose femoral veins, psoas muscle abscess, neoplasias, femoral or inguinal hernia, cryptorchidism, anterior coxofemoral luxation, appendicitis, etc.

Bottom Line Statement

The iliopsoas bursa is normally a potential space. Communication between the iliopsoas bursa and the hip joint is present in 15% of individuals and can be congenital or acquired. Gatc and Green described the connection acquired between bursa and the joint capsule and the presence of hip pathology. One or more pathological mechanisms could contribute to this communication, including increased intra-articular pressure, friction from the overlying iliopsoas tendon, a capsule weakened by inflammation, arthritic degeneration, or osteonecrosis of the hip. Very often it can be associated with snap hip syndrome. It is a sign characterized by a snap sensation during movement and not always associated with pain. In the absence of hip diseases, inflammation and distension of the iliopsoas bursa can be caused by rheumatological diseases, gout, infection, trauma, or overuse injuries. Sometimes both described pathological conditions can be concurrent. Iliopsoas bursitis can be asymptomatic or cause various symptoms related to compression of adjacent vascular and nerve structures: lower limb edema, paresthesias, and thrombosis. Iliopsoas bursitis is an infrequent cause of hip pain. It's important note that often, iliopsoas bursitis and tendinitis are related as the inflammation of one will inevitably lead to inflammation of the other because of their proximity. This condition it is often referred to as iliopsoas syndrome. Although iliopsoas bursitis is a deep anatomical structure, it can sometimes cause swelling of the hip joint and must be placed in differential diagnosis with intraperitoneal hernias content, tumors, aneurysms of the iliac or common femoral vessels, and lymphadenopathy. In both situations, the position of the deep bursa to the iliopsoas muscle often delays the diagnosis. Differential clinical diagnosis is difficult and imaging is indispensable.

Medico-Legal Traps

Misdiagnosis of Groin or Inguinal Mass

- Iliopectinate bursitis can present as a groin mass, leading to confusion with conditions such as hernias, lymphadenopathy, or tumors. Failure to correctly diagnose iliopsoas bursitis and misinterpreting it as a more common inguinal mass can delay proper treatment.
- **Thumb Rule Consideration:** Always consider iliopsoas bursitis in the differential diagnosis of unexplained groin or inguinal masses, and utilize imaging like ultrasound or MRI for accurate differentiation.

Overlooking Hip Pathology in Bursitis Diagnosis

- Iliopectinate bursitis is often associated with underlying hip pathology, such as osteoarthritis or femoral head degeneration. Neglecting to assess the hip joint comprehensively can result in incomplete treatment of the underlying cause of the bursitis.
- **Thumb Rule Consideration:** Evaluate for concurrent hip joint disease when diagnosing iliopsoas bursitis, and investigate with appropriate

imaging to rule out hip degeneration or intra-articular pathology.

Failure to Differentiate from Vascular Lesions

- Because iliopsoas bursitis can mimic vascular conditions like aneurysms or pseudoaneurysms, incorrect diagnosis might lead to unnecessary vascular interventions or mismanagement of a non-vascular cause of pain.
- **Thumb Rule Consideration:** Include vascular imaging techniques, such as Doppler ultrasound, in the workup of suspected iliopsoas bursitis to rule out vascular complications before initiating treatment.

Neglecting Rheumatologic or Infectious Causes

- Isolated iliopsoas bursitis can occur in the absence of hip disease and may be related to systemic conditions like gout, rheumatologic disorders, or infection. Missing these contributing factors can delay targeted treatment and worsen patient outcomes.
- **Thumb Rule Consideration:** Always consider systemic causes like rheumatologic diseases, gout, or infections in cases of iliopsoas bursitis, especially when there is no clear mechanical cause or history of overuse.

Delayed Diagnosis Due to Deep Location of Bursa

- The deep anatomical position of the iliopsoas bursa often leads to a delay in diagnosis, especially when clinical symptoms are non-specific or mimic other conditions like tendinitis or neuromuscular syndromes.
- **Thumb Rule Consideration:** In cases of chronic, unexplained hip or groin pain, where no superficial cause is identified, always consider deep structures like the iliopsoas bursa, and prioritize imaging early in the diagnostic process to avoid delays.

REFERENCES

- Johnston 1 C.A., Wiley J.P., Lindsay D.M., Wiseman D.A. Iliopsoas bursitis and tendinitis. Sports Med. 1998;25(4):271–283.
- O'Connor Early recognition of iliopectineal bursitis. Surg Gynecol Obstet. 1933;57:674–684.
- Bianchi Stefano, Martinoli Carlo, Keller Alain, Bianchi-Zamorani Maria Pia. Giant iliopsoas bursitis: Sonographic findings with magnetic resonance correlations. J Clin Ultrasound. 2002;30(7):437–441.
- Ginesty E., Dromer C., Galy-Fourcade D. Iliopsoas bursopathies. A review of twelve cases. Revue du Rhumatisme English Edition. 1998;65:181.
- Pellman E., Kumari S., Greenwald R. Rheumatoid iliopsoas bursitis presenting as unilateral leg edema. J Rheumatol. 1986;13:197.
- Janus C., Hermann G. Enlargement of the iliopsoas bursa: unusual cause of cystic mass on pelvic sonogram. J Clin Ultrasound. 1982;10:133.
- Pec'ina M.M., Bojanic' I. CRC Press; Boca Raton: 1982. Overuse injuries of the musculoskeletal system; pp. 143–147.
- Salmeron I., Cardenas J.L., Ramirez-Escobas M.A. Idiopathic iliopsoas bursitis. Eur Radiol. 1999;9:175.

- Finder J.G. lliopectineal bursitis. Arch Surg. 1938;36:519–530.
- Corvino Antonio, Setola Sergio Venanzio, Sandomenico Fabio, Corvino Fabio, Catalano Orlando. Synchronous tumours detected during cancer patient staging: prevalence and patterns of occurrence in multidetector computed tomography. Pol J Radiol. 2020;85:e261–e270.
- Catelli Antonio, Pane Francesco, Liccardo Alessandro, Tafuri Domenico. Giant right-side inguinal hernia: anatomo-clinical and diagnostic considerations of a case. Acta Medica Mediterranea. 2020;36:439.
- Corvino Antonio, Caruso Martina, Varelli Carlo, Gennaro Francesca Di, Pignata Saverio, Corvino Fabio. Diagnostic imaging of parotid gland oncocytoma: a pictorial review with emphasis on ultrasound assessment. J Ultrasound. 2020;36:439.

ILIOTIBIAL BAND BURSITIS

Iliotibial band (friction) syndrome is a common cause of lateral knee pain related to intense physical activity resulting in chronic inflammation of the fat adjacent to the iliotibial band (ITB). Alternatively, the same pathology can occur over the greater trochanter and is considered the same diagnosis.

Haims A, Medvecky M, Pavlovich R, Katz L. MR Imaging of the Anatomy of and Injuries to the Lateral and Posterolateral Aspects of the Knee. AJR Am J Roentgenol. 2003;180(3):647-53.

Clinical Description

Iliotibial band syndrome (ITBS) is a common knee injury that usually presents with pain and/or tenderness on palpation of the lateral aspect of the knee, superior to the joint line and inferior to the lateral femoral epicondyle. It is considered a non-traumatic overuse injury, often seen in runners, and is often concomitant with underlying weakness of hip abductor muscles. The current theory is that this condition is likely to be caused by compression of the innervated local adipose tissue. Studies have described an 'impingement zone' occurring at, or slightly below, 30° of knee flexion during foot strike and the early stance phase of running. During this impingement period in the running cycle, eccentric contraction of the tensor fascia latae muscle and of the gluteus maximus causes the leg to decelerate, generating tension (compression) in the iliotibial band.

The iliotibial tract is a thick band of fascia that runs on the lateral side of the thigh from the iliac crest and inserts at the knee. It is composed of dense fibrous connective tissue that appears from the m. tensor fasciae latae and m. gluteus maximus. It descends along the lateral aspect of the thigh, between the layers of the superficial fascia, and inserts onto the lateral tibial plateau at a projection known as Gerdy's tubercle. In its distal portion the iliotibial tract covers the lateral femoral epicondyle and gives an expansion to the lateral border of the patella. While the iliotibial band does not have any boney attachments as it courses between the Gerdy tubercle and the lateral femoral epicondyle, this absence of attachment allows it to move anteriorly and posteriorly with knee flexion and extension.

In many instances the subjective assessment will already provide an excellent basis for suspicion of this syndrome. Activities that require repetitive activities involving knee flexion-extension are usually reported, as well as a burning pain at the level of (or just underneath) the lateral femoral epicondyle. The diagnosis in patients with this syndrome is based on different symptoms.

The main symptom of ITBS is a sharp pain on the outer aspect of the knee, particularly when the heel strikes the floor, that can radiate into the outer thigh or calf. The pain tends to be worse when running or coming down stairs. There may be an audible snapping sensation the knee bends due to the band flicks over the bony tubercle. There may also be some swelling on the outer side of the knee.

Among the characteristics, we find an exercise-related tenderness over the lateral femoral epicondyle. The patient may experience, on a regular basis, an acute, burning pain when pressure is applied on the lateral femoral epycondyle with the knee in flexion and in extension. Signs of inflammation may also be found. There is pain on the lateral aspect of the knee during running, increasing in intensity while running down hill or descending stairs and pain is typically exacerbated when running longer distances.

The first well documented cases of ITBS were performed by Lieutenant Commander James Renne, a medical corps officer who documented on 16 ITBS cases out of 1000 military recruits. The onset occurred most frequently at the lateral knee after 2 miles of running, or hiking over 10 miles. Walking with the knee extended relieved the symptoms. All of the patients had focal tenderness over the lateral femoral epicondyle at 30 of flexion, and 5 patients had an unusual palpation described as "rubbing of a finger over a wet balloon."

The prevalence of ITBS in women is estimated to be between 16% and 50% and for men between 50% and 81%.

Pearls & Oysters

Iliotibial band syndrome causes pain on the outside of the knee.

It often happens in athletes, especially distance runners. But anyone can get it.

Using incorrect sporting equipment and having a poor running stance may increase the chance of having this condition.

Most people respond to treatment such as pain medicines, ice, stretching, and strengthening exercises, and limiting the activity for a while.

Some people may need surgery to treat the condition.

Bottom Line Statement

Classically, iliotibial band syndrome is diagnosed by history and physical examination. Pain over the greater trochanter or at the lateral knee joint is the presenting symptom with point tenderness 1-2 cm above the lateral joint line. Pain is usually worse with downhill running and increases throughout an episode of activity.

MRI is reserved for when the diagnosis is unclear and to exclude other etiologies of lateral knee pain such as a meniscal tear or lateral collateral ligament injury.

Initial treatment of iliotibial band syndrome is conservative, consisting of physical therapy, anti-inflammatory medication, and steroid injections.

Surgical treatment is reserved only for those who fail conservative treatment and includes resection of the posterior aspect of the iliotibial band.

Medico-Legal Traps

Misdiagnosis with Other Knee Pathologies

- Iliotibial band bursitis can be mistaken for meniscal tears, lateral collateral ligament injuries, or other knee pathologies due to overlapping symptoms of lateral knee pain. This can lead to incorrect treatment approaches.
- **Thumb Rule Consideration:** Always perform a thorough clinical history and physical examination to differentiate between iliotibial band bursitis and other lateral knee conditions. Use imaging like MRI only when the diagnosis is unclear or to rule out other pathologies.

Failure to Address Underlying Hip Abductor Weakness

- Iliotibial band bursitis is often associated with hip abductor weakness. Focusing treatment solely on the knee without addressing the hip muscles may result in incomplete recovery or recurrence of the condition.
- **Thumb Rule Consideration:** Always assess and include strengthening exercises for the hip abductors as part of the treatment plan to prevent recurrence and ensure a holistic approach to the injury.

Overlooking the Role of Biomechanical Factors

- Poor running mechanics, incorrect footwear, or inappropriate sporting equipment are common contributing factors to iliotibial band bursitis. Failing to address these biomechanical issues may lead to chronic pain and ineffective treatment.
- **Thumb Rule Consideration:** Evaluate the patient's biomechanics, including running stance and equipment, and recommend corrective measures, such as gait retraining or proper footwear, to reduce the risk of recurrence.

Inappropriate Use of Imaging

- While MRI is useful in ruling out other knee pathologies, unnecessary imaging can delay treatment and lead to increased healthcare costs. Relying too heavily on imaging without clinical correlation may result in misdiagnosis.
- **Thumb Rule Consideration:** Reserve MRI and other advanced imaging modalities for cases where the diagnosis is unclear or to exclude other causes of lateral knee pain, such as meniscal injuries.

Failure to Educate Patients on Activity Modification

- Inadequate patient education on modifying activity levels, especially running distances or downhill running, can prolong recovery and worsen the condition. Patients may continue to engage in activities that aggravate their symptoms.
- **Thumb Rule Consideration:** Provide clear instructions on activity modification, including reducing running distances or avoiding downhill running, until symptoms improve. Tailor rehabilitation exercises to gradually reintroduce activity without exacerbating the condition.

REFERENCES

- Lavine R. Iliotibial band friction syndrome. Current Reviews in Musculoskeletal Medicine, 2010; 3(1-4) :18–22
- Fairclough J, Hayashi K, Toumi H, Lyons K, Bydder G, Phillips N, Best TM, Benjamin M. The functional anatomy of the iliotibial band during flexion and extension of the knee: implications for understanding iliotibial band syndrome. Journal of Anatomy, 2006; 208(3): 309-316
- Michael D. Clinical Testing for Extra-Articular Lateral Knee Pain: A Modification and Combination of Traditional Tests. North American Journal of Sports Physical Therapy, 2008; 3: 107–109.
- Lazenby, T & Geisler, P (2017). Iliotibial Band Impingement Syndrome: An Updated Evidence-Informed Clinical Paradigm. Published 2017/03/06 DOI: 10.13140/RG.2.2.22882.53448
- van der Worp MP, van der Horst N, de Wijer A, Backx FJ, Nijhuis-van der Sanden MW. Iliotibial Band Syndrome in Runners. Sport Medicine, 2012; 42(11):969-92
- Iliotibial tract (highlighted in green) - posterior view image - © Kenhub https://www.kenhub.com/en/library/anatomy/iliotibial-band
- Baker RL, Fredericson M. Iliotibial Band Syndrome in Runners : Biomechanical Implications and Exercise Interventions. Physical médicine and réhabilitation clinics of North America, 2016; 27(1):53-77
- van der Worp MP, van der Horst N, de Wijer A, Backx FJ, Nijhuis-van der Sanden MW. Iliotibial Band Syndrome in Runners. Sport Medicine, 2012;42(11):969-92.
- Mucha MD, Caldwell W, Schlueter EL, Walters C, Hassen A, Hip abductor strength and lower extremity running related injury in distance runners: A systematic review., Journal of Science Medicine in Sports, 2017;20(4):349-355 .
- Strauss EJ, Kim S, Calcei JG, Park D. Iliotibial band syndrome: evaluation and management. Journal of the American Academy of Orthopedic Conditions. 2011;19(12):728-36.
- Fairclough J, Hayashi K, Toumi H, Lyons K, Bydder G, Phillips N, Best TM, Benjamin M. Is iliotibial band syndrome really a friction syndrome? Journal of Science and Medicine in Sport, 2007; 10:74-76
- Physical Medicine and Rehabilitation for Iliotibial Band Syndrome Differential Diagnoses. 2016.https://emedicine.medscape.com/article/307850 (accessed on 26th of Jul 2018)

- Wong M. Pocket Orthopaedics, Evidence-Based survival guide. Jones and Bartlett Publishers, 2009 .
- Seijas R, Sallent R, Galán M, Alvarez-Diaz P, Ares O, Cugat R. Iliotibial Band Syndrome Following Hip Arthroscopy: An unreported complication, Indian Journal of Orthopaedics, 2016; 50(5): 486–491. doi: 10.4103/0019-5413.18959.
- Khaund R, Flynn SH. Iliotibial band syndrome: a common source of knee pain. American Family Physician. 2005;71(8):1545-1550.
- Bischoff C, Prusaczyk WK, Sopchick TL, Pratt NC, Goforth HW. Comparison of phonophoresis and knee immobilization in treating iliotibial band syndrome, Journal of Sports Medicine, Training and Rehabilitation, 1995, 6(1):1-6.https://doi.org/10.1080/15438629509512030
- Weckström K, Söderström J. Radial extracorporeal shockwave therapy compared with manual therapy in runners with iliotibial band syndrome, Journal of Back and Musculoskeletal Rehabilitation, 2016; 29(1):161-70. doi: 10.3233/BMR-150612.

INFRASPINATUS TENDINITIS

A thick, triangular muscle; one of the 4 muscles which comprise the Rotator Cuff of the shoulder. The infraspinatus fossa of scapula, with some fibres arising from the infraspinatous fascia which covers the muscle and separates it from Teres Major and Teres Minor. The posterior aspect of greater tuberosity of humerus, and the capsule of shoulder joint.

Gray H. Anatomy of the Human Body. Philadelphia: Lea & Febiger, 1918. Available from https://www.bartleby.com/107/123.html (accessed on 29/2/2016)

Clinical Description

Atrophy in the supraspinatus and infrapinatus muscles, usually indicates compression on the suprascapular never near the scapular notch, such compression can be seen in overhead athletes and SLAP lesions. While isolated weakness or atrophy in the infrapinatus muscle can be seen in suprascapular nerve compression in the spinoglenoid notch, compression of the nerve in the spinpglenoid notch is usually due to a ganglion cyst.

A study by Simons et al, described that infraspinatus muscle trigger points are associated with referred pain to the middle and anterior deltoid regions. Myofascial release techniques at the infraspinatus muscle may help shoulder pain.

It provides the primary muscle force for external rotation of the shoulder. Along with the rest of the Rotator Cuff muscles it provides stability to the shoulder complex.

Pearls & Oysters

The most important positive test for this injury is pain felt on resisted lateral rotation. If the tendon is injured at the deep distal end of the tendon, then there will also be pain during another test: passive elevation of the arm. This test compresses the deep fibers of the tendon between the head of the humerus and the acromion. If the tendon is injured at the superficial distal end, then there is a so-called painful arc. This test compresses superficial fibers of the tendon between the head of the humerus and the acromion when the arm is approximately 70 degrees to 110 degrees from the body. If both of these auxiliary tests cause pain, then both the deep and superficial parts of the tendon are injured. If resisted lateral rotation is the only test that causes pain, then infraspinatus tendinitis is present in the body of the tendon. The latter is fairly uncommon.

Bottom Line Statement

The most common injuries to the infraspinatus muscle are tendinitis (or tendinopathy) and a tear of the tendon. Tendinitis is an inflammation of the tendon which usually is a result of repetitive overhead reaching, pushing, or lifting with outstretched arms. Athletes who perform overhead activities such as swimming, tennis, throwing, golf, weightlifting, volleyball, and gymnastics, are also at risk. Tears in the tendon can be partial or full, and may be the result of either an acute injury or degeneration (breakdown) of the muscle over a period of time. An acute injury to the muscle can be caused by a fall, direct blow, or a rapid use of force (like pulling on a starter cable for a lawn mower). Also, it is not uncommon for an untreated tendinopathy to, overtime, result in a degenerative tear. Degenerative tears are more likely to occur when the muscle is unused and/or maintained in a stretched position over a period of time (for example, sitting with rounded shoulders). Because the muscle also acts to stabilize and compress the humeral head in the glenoid fossa, weakness may also lead to secondary issues including shoulder impingement.

Medico-Legal Traps

Misdiagnosis of Shoulder Pain Causes

- Infraspinatus tendinitis may be misdiagnosed as general shoulder pain or other rotator cuff injuries, leading to ineffective treatments like steroid injections or surgeries that target the wrong condition.
- **Thumb Rule Consideration:** Always perform specific physical tests like resisted lateral rotation and passive elevation to differentiate infraspinatus tendinitis from other rotator cuff injuries. Use imaging when necessary to confirm diagnosis.

Failure to Identify Suprascapular Nerve Compression

- Atrophy or weakness in the infraspinatus muscle could indicate suprascapular nerve compression, particularly near the spinoglenoid notch. Failure to consider nerve compression could result in delayed treatment and persistent symptoms.
- **Thumb Rule Consideration:** Evaluate for nerve compression in patients with infraspinatus weakness, especially in athletes. Early use of MRI or EMG can help identify nerve entrapment.

Overlooking Overhead Sports Activities

- Athletes, particularly those engaged in overhead sports like swimming or tennis, are at a higher risk for infraspinatus tendinitis due to repetitive stress. Ignoring their specific training patterns can result in a recurrence of the condition.

- **Thumb Rule Consideration:** Obtain a detailed history of sports activities or repetitive arm movements in patients. Incorporate sport-specific rehabilitation exercises to address biomechanical factors contributing to injury.

Neglecting Trigger Point Pain Referral

- Trigger points in the infraspinatus muscle can refer pain to other areas, such as the deltoid, leading to confusion and potential misdiagnosis as shoulder joint or deltoid pathology.
- **Thumb Rule Consideration:** Check for trigger points in the infraspinatus muscle when patients report referred shoulder or deltoid pain. Consider myofascial release techniques as part of the treatment.

Inadequate Postural Assessment and Rehabilitation

- Poor posture, especially rounded shoulders, can predispose patients to chronic infraspinatus tendinopathy, leading to muscle degeneration or tearing. Failing to correct postural issues during treatment can lead to incomplete recovery or re-injury.
- **Thumb Rule Consideration:** Always evaluate shoulder posture and provide postural correction exercises, especially in patients with chronic tendinopathy.

REFERENCES

- Williams JM, Sinkler MA, Obremskey W. Anatomy, shoulder and upper limb, infraspinatus muscle. StatPearls [Internet]. 2020 May 24.
- Moccia D, Nackashi AA, Schilling R, Ward PJ. Fascial bundles of the infraspinatus fascia: anatomy, function, and clinical considerations. Journal of anatomy. 2016 Jan;228(1):176-83.
- Wheeles CR. Infraspinatus. Available from: http://www.wheelessonline.com/ortho/infraspinatus (last accessed 29/2/2016)
- AnatomyExpert. 3D Infraspinatus- infraspinatus. Available from: http://www.anatomyexpert.com/app/structure/5510/554/ (last accessed on 29/2/2016)
- https://www.uptodate.com/contents/rotator-cuff-tendinitis-and-tear-beyond-the-basics

ISCHIAL GLUTEAL BURSITIS

Ischial bursitis (ischio-gluteal bursitis) is a condition of inflammation of the bursa, which lies between the ischial tuberosity and the gluteus maximus muscle. It presents with gluteal pain or posterior upper thigh pain following exercise or sitting for a long time.

Kubota K, Yamashita H, Mimori A. Clinical Value of FDG-PET/CT for the Evaluation of Rheumatic Diseases: Rheumatoid Arthritis, Polymyalgia Rheumatica, and Relapsing Polychondritis. Semin Nucl Med. 2017 Jul;47(4):408-424.

Clinical Description

Ischial bursitis, also known as ischio-gluteal bursitis or "weaver's bottom," is a condition where the bursa that lies between the ischial tuberosity and the gluteus maximus muscle becomes inflamed. This bursa is present physiologically to reduce the amount of frictional force generated between the gluteal muscle and the ischial tuberosity that otherwise might become damaged or irritated by this contact. This inflammation of the bursa most commonly results from prolonged pressure on the ischium, as occurs in sitting for extended periods or from the repeated movement of the gluteus maximus muscle in such activities as bicycling. These activities cause an inflammatory reaction that results in swelling and tenderness over the lower buttock and upper posterior thigh. Many other differential diagnoses have common presentations, such as sciatica and tendonitis of hamstring muscles.

Ischial bursitis is a relatively uncommon clinical condition. Although the diagnosis is often unrecognized, it may present in patients of all ages. Bursitis as whole accounts for less than one percent of total primary care visits. This condition is most common in persons with sedentary careers with constant irritation of the ischial bursa due to prolonged periods sitting on hard surfaces, which gives this condition its colloquial name, "weaver's bottom." Weaving as a profession has been around since approximately 6000 BCE, and people have been suffering from this condition for as many years.

Pearls & Oysters

Patients with ischial bursitis should not continue with activities that aggravate their pain or exacerbate it. These activities cause increased friction on the bursa, resulting in further irritation and inflammation, and potentially delaying recovery.

Bottom Line Statement

Ischial bursitis is a rare disorder that is encountered by the primary care provider, nurse practitioner, internist, or the sports physician. The diagnosis is clinical but may require exhaustive workup to rule out other disorders. The treatment is usually conservative with rest, pain relief, and physical therapy.

Cold compresses may help in the short term to minimize pain from swelling. If the pain is unbearable or unrelenting, an intrabursal corticosteroid injection with lidocaine may provide relief. The lidocaine will help by providing immediate relief from the pain by blocking the sodium channels in the surrounding tissue, inhibiting the transmission of the pain signal.

It is essential to educate the patient on lifestyle changes, including weight loss and regular exercise. Occupational and/or physical therapy may be of value in this regard. Recurrences are common in patients who lead a sedentary lifestyle.

Medico-Legal Traps

Misdiagnosis as Sciatica or Hamstring Tendonitis

- Ischial gluteal bursitis presents with symptoms similar to sciatica or hamstring tendonitis, such as posterior thigh pain, leading to potential misdiagnosis. This can result in delayed or inappropriate treatment.
- **Thumb Rule Consideration:** Always conduct a thorough physical examination, and consider imaging such as MRI or ultrasound to differentiate between ischial bursitis, sciatica, and tendonitis.

Inappropriate Treatment Following Misdiagnosis

- Incorrect diagnosis of ischial gluteal bursitis as sciatica often leads to unnecessary or ineffective treatments like nerve blocks or surgery, which do not address the underlying inflammation.
- **Thumb Rule Consideration:** Before opting for invasive interventions, ensure the correct diagnosis through clinical tests and imaging. Initial conservative treatments should focus on reducing inflammation in the bursa.

Failure to Advise Proper Rest and Activity Modification

- Patients may continue activities that worsen bursitis, such as prolonged sitting or cycling, which exacerbates inflammation and delays recovery. Failure to provide clear instructions on activity modification can result in chronic pain.
- **Thumb Rule Consideration:** Advise patients to avoid aggravating

activities, such as sitting for long periods or participating in strenuous physical exercise, until inflammation subsides.

Overlooking Underlying Risk Factors like Sedentary Lifestyle

- Sedentary individuals are at higher risk for ischial bursitis due to prolonged pressure on the bursa. Failure to address lifestyle factors can lead to recurrent episodes and chronic pain.
- **Thumb Rule Consideration:** Educate patients on lifestyle modifications, including regular exercise, posture correction, and weight management, to prevent recurrence and improve long-term outcomes.

Neglecting to Rule Out Other Pathologies with Similar Presentations

- In patients with persistent or unexplained buttock pain, ischial bursitis may be mistaken for more serious conditions, such as tumors, hernias, or vascular issues. This oversight can lead to legal consequences if more severe diagnoses are missed.
- **Thumb Rule Consideration:** Perform comprehensive imaging and diagnostic workups, including ruling out conditions like hernias, tumors, or vascular abnormalities, especially in atypical presentations.

REFERENCES

- Chen B, Rispoli L, Stitik T, Leong M. Successful Treatment of Gluteal Pain from Obturator Internus Tendinitis and Bursitis with Ultrasound-Guided Injection. Am J Phys Med Rehabil. 2017 Oct;96(10):e181-e184.
- Ekiz T, Biçici V, Hatioglu C, Yalçın S, Cingöz K. Ischial Pain and Sitting Disability Due to Ischiogluteal Bursitis: Visual Vignette. Pain Physician. 2015 Jul-Aug;18(4):E657-8.
- Navarro-Zarza JE, Villaseñor-Ovies P, Vargas A, Canoso JJ, Chiapas-Gasca K, Hernández-Díaz C, Saavedra MÁ, Kalish RA. Clinical anatomy of the pelvis and hip. Reumatol Clin. 2012 Dec-2013 Jan;8 Suppl 2:33-8.
- Guanche CA. Hamstring injuries. J Hip Preserv Surg. 2015 Jul;2(2):116-22.
- Paluska SA. An overview of hip injuries in running. Sports Med. 2005;35(11):991-1014.
- Bard H. [Periarticular pathology of the hip]. Rev Prat. 2002 Mar 15;52(6):627-31.

JUMPER'S KNEE

"Jumper's knee," also called patellar tendinopathy, is a painful condition of the knee caused by small tears in the patellar tendon that mainly occurs in sports requiring strenuous jumping. The tears are typically caused by accumulated stress on the patellar or quadriceps tendon.

Lian OB, Engebretsen L, Bahr R. Prevalence of jumper's knee among elite athletes from different sports: a cross-sectional study. Am J Sports Med. 2005 Apr;33(4):561-7.

Clinical Description

"Jumper's knee," also called patellar tendinopathy, is a painful condition of the knee, mainly activity-related, caused by small tears in the patellar tendon that mainly occurs in sports requiring strenuous jumping and results in localized patellar tendon tenderness. The tears are typically caused by accumulated stress on the patellar or quadriceps tendon. As the name implies, the condition is common in athletes from jumping sports where there is a high demand for the speed and power of leg extensors. These sports often lead to high eccentric quadriceps loadings such as volleyball, track (long and high jump), basketball, long-distance running, and skiing. The condition has a male predominance, with a more common occurrence in adolescents and young adults. Contrary to traditional belief, a jumper's knee does not involve inflammation of the knee extensor tendons. Studies dating back 40 years describe jumper's knee as a degenerative condition. Jumper's knee is a clinical diagnosis made through detailed history taking and a physical exam. Ultrasound can facilitate the diagnosis, as this imaging study is readily available and affordable. Treatment mainly revolves around conservative measures such as reducing activities that place a loading impact on the knee. Once the pain subsides, restoration of function is achieved through physical and exercise therapy. Surgery usually remains the last resort for chronic refractory cases.

Pearls & Oysters

Athletes, clinicians, coaches, and athletic trainers need to understand that the treatment for patellar tendinopathy can be a slow and sometimes frustrating process. There are multiple pitfalls to be aware of, including the failure to control pain. The athlete's beliefs about pain and pathology may influence the development and management of unresponsive tendinopathies. Because some athletes may have been told that they have weakened tendons due to tears and degeneration, and hence an increased risk of rupture, they may develop fear-avoidance behavior, which can be associated with poorer functional outcomes in individuals suffering from lower-limb tendinopathy. Over-reliance on non-invasive therapies like shockwave therapy and injections instead of including rehabilitation exercises as part of the treatment plan can also lead to complications. Failure to address the athletes' landing kinematics can also bring difficulties. Athletes should have their jump-landing mechanics retrained after adequate rehabilitation.

Bottom Line Statement

Managing patellar tendinopathy is a job for physicians trained in the care of musculoskeletal conditions along with other members of the interprofessional healthcare team. Sports medicine physicians, physiatrists, and rheumatologists provide the first line of care. Orthopedic surgeons are consulted for refractory cases or when the knee extensor tendons are partially or completely torn. A team of professionals from multiple disciplines including athletic trainers, physical therapists, sports biomechanists, and sports psychologists is needed since the condition commonly affects athletes. The orthopedic specialty nurse is often responsible for the coordination of care and follow-up and reporting concerns to the clinician.

Initially, the physical therapist must work at hand with physicians to implement a nonoperative regimen consisting of therapy with isometric or eccentric exercises as the mainstay treatment. In a level 2 study, at 12 weeks, patients undergoing an eccentric exercise program showed significant improvement compared with those undergoing a concentric exercise program. As the treatment progresses, plyometrics and sport-specific training is required to return the athlete to sport at the highest level

Alternative medical treatments have been studied at different levels of evidence, demonstrating mixed and inconclusive results. Acceptable outcomes have been obtained from surgical interventions in refractory cases.

An interprofessional team approach involving clinicians, specialists, orthopedic nursing, and therapists will yield the best results.

Medico-Legal Traps

Misdiagnosis of Patellar Tendinopathy as Patellar Tendonitis

- One common legal pitfall is diagnosing jumper's knee as an inflammatory condition (patellar tendonitis) when it is a degenerative tendinopathy. This mistake can lead to inappropriate treatments like NSAIDs or corticosteroids, which may not address the degenerative nature of the condition.

- **Thumb Rule Consideration:** Differentiate between tendonitis and tendinopathy through clinical examination and imaging (ultrasound, MRI) to ensure the correct treatment approach.

Failure to Consider Load Management in Treatment Plans

- Jumpers knee results from repetitive strain, and treatment often fails when load management strategies are neglected. Patients may return to sports too quickly or continue aggravating activities, worsening the condition and increasing the risk of a complete tendon rupture.
- **Thumb Rule Consideration:** Enforce a structured, gradual return to activity and load management plan, avoiding premature return to sports that could exacerbate the condition.

Inadequate Rehabilitation and Failure to Address Biomechanics

- Simply resting the knee without addressing underlying biomechanical issues such as improper landing techniques or muscle imbalances is a common medico-legal trap. This can result in chronic pain and recurrent injury.
- **Thumb Rule Consideration:** Ensure rehabilitation includes retraining of landing mechanics and eccentric strengthening exercises to restore proper function and prevent recurrence.

Over-reliance on Passive Treatments Without Functional Rehabilitation

- Treatments like shockwave therapy or corticosteroid injections without concurrent functional rehabilitation can fail to resolve the underlying mechanical and structural issues, prolonging the recovery process.
- **Thumb Rule Consideration:** Always integrate active rehabilitation exercises (e.g., isometric and eccentric exercises) alongside passive therapies to improve tendon health and functionality.

Failure to Inform Patients of Slow Recovery and Risks of Surgery

- Another common trap is not informing patients about the slow recovery process and potential risks of surgical intervention for jumper's knee, leading to unrealistic expectations and potential legal claims if the outcomes are not satisfactory.
- **Thumb Rule Consideration:** Educate patients about the nature of the condition, the expected recovery timeline, and the potential complications of surgical options, reserving surgery for refractory cases.

REFERENCES

- Fredberg U, Bolvig L. Jumper's knee. Review of the literature. Scand J Med Sci Sports. 1999 Apr;9(2):66-73.
- Ferretti A. Epidemiology of jumper's knee. Sports Med. 1986 Jul-Aug;3(4):289-95.
- Khan KM, Cook JL, Kannus P, Maffulli N, Bonar SF. Time to abandon the "tendinitis" myth. BMJ. 2002 Mar 16;324(7338):626-7.
- Tibesku CO, Pässler HH. [Jumper's knee--a review]. Sportverletz Sportschaden. 2005 Jun;19(2):63-71.
- van der Worp H, van Ark M, Roerink S, Pepping GJ, van den Akker-Scheek I, Zwerver J. Risk factors for patellar tendinopathy: a systematic review of the literature. Br J Sports Med. 2011 Apr;45(5):446-52.
- Rudavsky A, Cook J. Physiotherapy management of patellar tendinopathy (jumper's knee). J Physiother. 2014 Sep;60(3):122-9.
- Lian O, Engebretsen L, Ovrebø RV, Bahr R. Characteristics of the leg extensors in male volleyball players with jumper's knee. Am J Sports Med. 1996 May-Jun;24(3):380-5.
- Durcan L, Coole A, McCarthy E, Johnston C, Webb MJ, O'Shea FD, Gissane C, Wilson F. The prevalence of patellar tendinopathy in elite academy rugby: a clinical and imaging study. J Sci Med Sport. 2014 Mar;17(2):173-6.
- Schwartz A, Watson JN, Hutchinson MR. Patellar Tendinopathy. Sports Health. 2015 Sep-Oct;7(5):415-20.

KIENBÖCK'S DISEASE

Kienböck's disease is a condition where the blood supply to one of the small bones in the wrist, the lunate, is interrupted. The lunate is a carpal bone. Bone is living tissue that requires a regular supply of blood for nourishment. If the blood supply to a bone stops, the bone or parts of the bone can die. This is called osteonecrosis. A loss of blood supply to the lunate causes the bone to lose its structural support, and it will collapse, causing a painful, stiff wrist. Over time, these changes can lead to arthritis of the surrounding bones in the wrist.

Beredjiklian PK: Kienböck's disease, J Hand Surg Am 34:167–175, 2009.

Clinical Description

Kienbock's disease, or osteonecrosis of the lunate, can lead to chronic, debilitating wrist pain. Etiologic factors include vascular and skeletal variations combined with trauma or repetitive loading. In stage I Kienbock's disease, plain radiographs appear normal, and bone scintigraphy or magnetic resonance imaging is required for diagnosis. Initial treatment is nonoperative. In stage II, sclerosis of the lunate, compression fracture, and/or early collapse of the radial border of the lunate may appear. In stage IIIA, there is more severe lunate collapse. Because the remainder of the carpus is still uninvolved, treatment in stages II and IIIA involves attempts at revascularization of the lunate-either directly (with vascularized bone grafting) or indirectly (by unloading the lunate). Radial shortening in wrists with negative ulnar variance and capitate shortening or radial-wedge osteotomy in wrists with neutral or positive ulnar variance can be performed alone or with vascularized bone grafting. In stage IIIB, palmar rotation of the scaphoid and proximal migration of the capitate occur, and treatment addresses the carpal collapse. Surgical options include scaphotrapeziotrapezoid or scaphocapitate arthrodesis to correct scaphoid hyperflexion. In stage IV, degenerative changes are present at the midcarpal joint, the radiocarpal joint, or both. Treatment options include proximal-row carpectomy and wrist arthrodesis.

Pearls & Oysters

Kienböck's disease varies considerably in its severity, as well as in its rate of progression. Each patient's response to treatment depends on the degree of damage to the lunate and surrounding wrist bones. Some patients may require more than one procedure over time if the disease continues to progress.

Bottom Line Statement

Symptoms of the following disorders can be similar to those of Kienböck Disease. Comparisons may be useful for a differential diagnosis:

Carpal Tunnel Syndrome is a condition caused by compression of peripheral nerves in the wrist, affecting one or both hands. It is characterized by a sensation of numbness, tingling, burning and/or pain in the hand and wrist. Persons affected by this disorder may be awakened at night with the feeling that the hand has "gone to sleep". Various other diseases may occur in conjunction with this condition. With timely treatment, the prognosis in most cases is favorable. (For more information on this disorder, please choose "Carpal Tunnel" as your search term online.)

Sudeck's Atrophy, also known as post-traumatic osteoporosis, is marked by an acute atrophy of the bones. The wrist and ankle bones are most commonly affected, following a slight injury such as a sprain.

Juvenile Osteoporosis is marked by a porous condition or atrophy of bone tissue beginning before puberty. The exact cause has not been identified. This condition can lead to pain or fractures in many bones of the body including the wrist. Spontaneous remission may occur within several years.

Medico-Legal Traps

Misdiagnosis Due to Overlapping Symptoms with Other Conditions

- Kienböck's disease shares symptoms such as wrist pain and stiffness with other conditions like carpal tunnel syndrome or tendonitis. Misdiagnosis may delay appropriate treatment and lead to disease progression, resulting in more invasive interventions later.
- **Thumb Rule Consideration:** Always consider Kienböck's disease in cases of unexplained chronic wrist pain and stiffness. Use advanced imaging like MRI to confirm diagnosis in early stages when X-rays may appear normal.

Failure to Diagnose Early Stages (Stage I)

- Early Kienböck's disease (Stage I) may not show up on plain radiographs, leading to a missed or delayed diagnosis. This is especially problematic as early intervention could prevent progression to advanced stages where bone collapse occurs.
- **Thumb Rule Consideration:** In cases of persistent wrist pain with negative X-rays, perform MRI or bone scintigraphy to rule out early Kienböck's disease and avoid underdiagnosis.

Inadequate Consideration of Non-Operative Treatments

- Initial treatment of Kienböck's disease often involves non-operative measures like immobilization, but clinicians may rush into surgical options without exploring conservative management, particularly in early stages.•
- **Thumb Rule Consideration:** In Stage I and II, prioritize non-operative treatments such as splinting or immobilization and avoid premature surgical intervention unless disease progression is evident.

Overlooked Ulnar Variance and Its Role in Surgical Planning

- Ignoring the anatomical variation of ulnar variance (the length difference between the ulna and radius) can result in suboptimal surgical outcomes, as this factor affects both the etiology and management of the disease.
- **Thumb Rule Consideration:** Assess ulnar variance meticulously before surgical planning. Procedures such as radial shortening or osteotomy should be tailored according to the patient's ulnar variance to optimize outcomes.

Inadequate Patient Education on Disease Progression and Recurrence

- Patients may not be fully informed about the potential for recurrence or progression even after initial successful treatment. This can result in medico-legal issues if disease progression or multiple procedures are required later.
- **Thumb Rule Consideration:** Provide thorough patient education about the progressive nature of Kienböck's disease and the potential for multiple interventions over time, ensuring informed consent for both conservative and surgical treatments.

REFERENCES

- Excision of the Lunate in Kienböck's Disease. Results After Long-Term Followup. H. Kawai et al.; J Bone Joint Surg [Br] (Mar 1988; 70(2)). Pp. 287-92.
- Ulna-Minus Variance and Kienböck's Disease. P. A. Nathan et al.; J Hand Surg (Sept 1987; 12(5 pt 1)). Pp. 777-78.
- Wrist Denervation Procedures in the Treatment of Kienböck's Disease. D. Buck-Gramcko; Hand Clin (Aug 1993; 9(3)). Pp. 517-20.
- Review of Treatment Results in Kienböck's Disease. S. H. Kuschner et al.; Orthop Rev (Jun 1992; 21(6)). Pp. 717-28.
- Osteomalacia of the Lunate Bone-Indications for and Limitations of Radial Shortening and Ulnar Lengthening. M. Fishcer et al.; Orthopade (Feb 1993; 22(1)). Pp. 52-56.
- Long-Term Results of 9 Cases of Elongation of the Ulna in Treatment of Kienböck's Disease. P. Ducarmois et al.; Ann Chir Main Memb Supter (1997; 16(1)). Pp. 16-24.
- Kienböck's Disease: Treatment by Implantation of Vascular Pedicle and Bone Grafting. M. S. Moneim et al.;

Iowa Orthop J (1998; 18). Pp. 67-73.

- Kienböck Disease and Negative Ulnar Variance. M. Bonzar et al.; J Bone Joint Surg Am (Aug 1998; 80(8)). Pp. 1154-57.
- Arthroscopic Evaluation of Radial Osteotomy for Kienböck's Disease. K. Watanabe et al.; J Hand Surg (Sept 1998; 23(5)). Pp. 899-903.

LEVATOR ANI PAIN SYNDROME

Levator ani syndrome is a condition characterized by burning pain or tenesmus of the rectal or perineal area, caused by spasm of the levator ani muscle.The genesis of the syndrome is unknown; however, inflammation of the arcus tendon is a possible cause of levator ani syndrome.

Recenti Prog Med. 2011 May;102(5):196-201. doi: 10.1701/659.7668.

Clinical Description

The levator ani muscle plays a vital role in supporting the pelvic region, elevating the pelvic floor and compressing the urethra and vagina. It also helps maintain the anorectal angle by pulling the anorectal junction forward. This muscle originates at the posterior surface of the pubic bone, the obturator internus fascia, and the ischial spine, and inserts on the anococcygeal raphe and coccyx. It is innervated by the branches of the ventral primary rami of spinal nerves S3-4. However, the levator ani muscle can be prone to trauma and wear and tear from overuse or misuse, potentially leading to myofascial pain syndrome. This chronic pain condition is characterized by the presence of trigger points on physical examination, which may be referred to other areas of the body and often misdiagnosed or attributed to other organ systems. Myofascial pain syndrome in the levator ani muscle may manifest with a trigger point along the rectum or perineum and may be the result of microtrauma or chronic deconditioning of the agonist and antagonist muscle unit. The exact pathophysiology of myofascial trigger points is not fully understood, but various theories suggest that they may be the result of microtrauma to the affected muscle.

There are a range of factors that may contribute to the development of myofascial pain syndrome, including muscle trauma, unaccustomed physical activity, poor posture, previous injuries, poor nutrition, and psychological or behavioral abnormalities such as chronic stress and depression. The levator ani muscle may be particularly susceptible to stress-induced myofascial pain syndrome. This condition often causes stiffness and fatigue, leading to functional disability and complicating its treatment. It may occur as a standalone condition or in conjunction with other painful conditions, including radiculopathy and chronic regional pain syndromes. Effective treatment of myofascial pain syndrome must take into account any coexisting psychological or behavioral abnormalities, such as depression.

Pearls & Oysters

Digital massage, sitz baths, muscle relaxants, electrogalvanic stimulation and biofeedback have all been reported to be effective in treating LAS and cause no harm. However, none of these treatment modalities have been evaluated further with controlled trials. Surgical division of puborectalis muscle should be avoided due to side effects.

Bottom Line Statement

Chronic proctalgia is defined by chronic or recurrent episodes of rectal pain or aching lasting at least 20 minutes in the absence of structural or systemic disease explanation for the pain syndrome. Digital rectal examination distinguishes between levator ani syndrome where the patient reports tenderness on palpation of the pubo-rectalis muscle and unspecified functional anorectal pain where no pain can be elicited. There is no consensus on its etiology, but chronic tension of the pelvic floor muscles is the most common view. Diagnosis is focused on excluding organic diseases potentially responsible for the pain. A number of small sized, non-controlled trials have evaluated different treatments for chronic proctalgia with frustrating results for both patients and physicians. A recent well designed, prospective, randomized, controlled trial has evaluated the three most commonly prescribed treatments to relax pelvic floor muscles in chronic proctalgia: biofeedback, electrogalvanic stimulations and digital massage of the levator ani. The study has provided unequivocal evidence that biofeedback is effective treatment for chronic proctalgia, but its efficacy is limited to levator ani syndrome. In these patients a paradoxical contraction of the pelvic floor muscles on attempted defecation has been documented in most cases and its therapeutic reversal do correlate with clinical benefit. Similar data have been also reported in constipation secondary to obstructed defecation. Electrogalvanic stimulation is somewhat effective and may be considered where high biofeedback expertise is not available. No treatment has been proven effective in unspecified functional anorectal pain where analgesic and antidepressant drugs retain a role in the absence of randomized, controlled trials.

Medico-Legal Traps

Failure to Differentiate from Other Pelvic Conditions

- Levator ani syndrome (LAS) shares symptoms with other pelvic floor disorders, such as chronic prostatitis, interstitial cystitis, or even gastrointestinal issues. Misdiagnosis can lead to inappropriate treatments, causing prolonged patient suffering and unnecessary interventions.
- **Thumb Rule Consideration:** Always consider LAS in patients with chronic pelvic pain. Rule out other pelvic and anorectal disorders through comprehensive history, clinical examination, and appropriate imaging studies to avoid misdiagnosis.

Neglecting Psychological Factors

- Chronic pain syndromes like LAS often have a psychological component, including stress, anxiety, and depression, which, if unaddressed, can result in treatment failure or delayed recovery. Ignoring these factors may expose clinicians to medico-legal liability if patients experience prolonged pain.
- **Thumb Rule Consideration:** Incorporate psychological evaluation in the management of LAS. Educate patients about the influence of stress and mental health on chronic pain, and offer behavioral or psychological therapies when necessary.

Invasive Treatments Without Conservative Measures

- Some clinicians may opt for aggressive treatments, such as surgical interventions, without first exhausting non-invasive approaches like digital massage, biofeedback, or electrogalvanic stimulation. This can lead to complications and expose clinicians to legal challenges if non-invasive options were not adequately trialed first.
- **Thumb Rule Consideration:** Always begin with conservative treatments like biofeedback, pelvic floor relaxation, and sitz baths before considering invasive surgical options. Surgery should be reserved only for refractory cases with informed patient consent.

Failure to Diagnose Trigger Points or Myofascial Pain

- Many cases of LAS involve myofascial trigger points, but failure to recognize and treat these trigger points can lead to mismanagement. A superficial examination might overlook this, causing unnecessary delays in effective treatment.
- **Thumb Rule Consideration:** Conduct a thorough physical exam, including palpation of the pelvic floor muscles for trigger points. Employ myofascial release techniques, and consider trigger point injections if conservative therapies fail.

Inadequate Documentation of Treatment Efforts

- Poor documentation of diagnostic processes, treatment plans, and patient communications can lead to legal challenges if the patient's condition deteriorates. This is especially important in chronic pain syndromes, where multiple treatment options may need to be trialed.
- **Thumb Rule Consideration:** Ensure detailed documentation of all diagnostic steps, treatment trials, patient education, and follow-up. Clearly note patient responses to each therapy, particularly in cases of treatment failure or adverse outcomes.

REFERENCES

- Arnold LM: The pathophysiology, diagnosis and treatment of fibromyalgia, Psychiatr Clin North Am 33:375–408, 2010.
- Bradley LA: Pathophysiology of fibromyalgia, Am J Med 122(Suppl 1):S22–S30, 2009.
- Imamura M, Cassius DA, Fregni F: Fibromyalgia: from treatment to rehabilitation, Eur J Pain Suppl 3:117–122, 2009.
- Shobeiri SA, Chesson RR, Gasser RF: The internal innervation and morphology of the human female levator ani muscle, Am J Obstet Gynecol 199:686.e1–686.e6, 2008.
- Singh K, Reid WMN, Berger LA: Magnetic resonance imaging of normal levator ani anatomy and function, Obstet Gynecol 99:433–438, 2002.

LIVER PAIN

The clinical presentation of liver pain is directly related to whether the pain is mediated via the sympathetic or somatic nervous system or both. In patients with sympathetically mediated pain, the abdominal examination may reveal hepatomegaly with tenderness to palpation of the liver. Primary tumor or metastatic disease also may be identified. The remainder of the abdominal examination is nondescript. Auscultation over the liver fails to reveal a friction rub in most cases. As mentioned, the patient may report ill-defined pain in the supraclavicular region.

Waldman SW, Feldstein GS, Donohoe CD, Waldman KA: The relief of body wall pain secondary to malignant hepatic metastases by intercostal nerve block with bupivacaine and methylprednisolone, J Pain Symptom Manage 3:39–43, 1988.

Clinical Description

Liver pain is a common clinical occurrence, but it is often poorly diagnosed and treated. The liver can serve as a source of pain in and of itself through the sympathetic nervous system and via referred pain secondary to peritoneal irritation through the intercostal and subcostal nerves. Pain that emanates from the liver itself tends to be ill defined and may be referred primarily to the epigastrium. It is dull and aching and is mild to moderate in severity. The pain can be related to swelling of the liver and concomitant stretching of the liver capsule or distention of the veins, as is seen with portal obstruction. This pain is carried via sympathetic fibers from the celiac ganglion that enter the liver along with the hepatic artery and vein. This type of liver pain responds poorly to adjuvant analgesics. Occasionally, hepatic enlargement causes diaphragmatic irritation, which produces pain that is referred to the ipsilateral supraclavicular and shoulder region. This referred pain is known as Kehr's sign and is transmitted via the phrenic nerve and is often misdiagnosed.Referred liver pain is caused by mechanical irritation and inflammation of the inferior pleura and peritoneum. This pain is somatic and carried primarily by the lower intercostal and subcostal nerves. This somatic pain is sharp and pleuritic and is moderate to severe in intensity. It responds more favorably to nonsteroidal antiinflammatory drugs (NSAIDs) and opioid analgesics in contrast to sympathetically mediated liver pain.

Pain of hepatic origin must be taken seriously. It is often the result of an underlying serious disease, such as biliary malignancy, portal hypertension, or hepatic metastatic disease. Pain emanating from the liver is often mistaken for pain of cardiac or gallbladder origin and can lead to visits to the emergency department and unnecessary cardiac and gastrointestinal workups. If trauma has occurred, liver pain may coexist with rib fractures or fractures of the sternum itself that can be missed on plain radiographs and may require radionucleotide bone scanning for proper identification.

Neuropathic pain involving the chest wall may be confused or coexist with liver pain. Examples of neuropathic pain include diabetic polyneuropathies and acute herpes zoster involving the lower thoracic and upper lumbar nerves. The possibility of diseases of the structures of the inferior mediastinum and retroperitoneum is ever present, and these diseases sometimes can be difficult to diagnose. Pathological processes that inflame the pleura, such as pulmonary embolus, infection, and Bornholm's disease, may mimic or coexist with pain of hepatic origin.

Pearls & Oysters

The major problem in the care of patients thought to have liver pain is the failure to identify potentially serious pathological processes of the thorax or upper abdomen. Given the proximity of the pleural space, pneumothorax after intercostal nerve block is a possibility. The incidence of the complication is less than 1%, but it occurs with greater frequency in patients with chronic obstructive pulmonary disease. Although uncommon, infection, including liver abscess, remains an ever-present possibility, especially in an immunocompromised patient with cancer. Early detection of infection is crucial to avoid potentially life-threatening sequelae.

Bottom Line Statement

Liver pain is often poorly diagnosed and treated. Correct diagnosis of the cause of liver pain and the nerves subserving the pain is necessary to treat this painful condition properly and to avoid overlooking serious intrathoracic or intraabdominal pathological processes. Intercostal nerve block is a simple technique that can produce dramatic relief for patients with liver pain thought to be somatically mediated. Celiac plexus block is technically more demanding and should be performed only by clinicians well versed in the technique and potential complications.

Medico-Legal Traps

Misdiagnosis of Referred Pain

- Liver pain can often be mistaken for cardiac, gastrointestinal, or musculoskeletal pain, leading to unnecessary and invasive workups such as cardiac catheterization or gastrointestinal endoscopies. This misdiagnosis can delay appropriate treatment and cause harm to the patient.

- **Thumb Rule Consideration:** Always consider liver pain as a differential diagnosis in cases of right upper quadrant or shoulder pain, especially when there is no clear cardiac or gastrointestinal cause.

Failure to Recognize Underlying Serious Pathologies

- Liver pain may be a symptom of serious conditions like hepatic malignancies, metastases, or portal hypertension. If these are not correctly identified, patients may suffer from delayed or inadequate treatment. Missing a diagnosis of liver metastases, for example, could have dire consequences for cancer progression.
- **Thumb Rule Consideration:** When liver pain is reported, conduct thorough imaging (ultrasound, CT, or MRI) and clinical evaluations to rule out malignancies, metastases, or other life-threatening conditions.

Incorrect Nerve Block Application

- Intercostal nerve blocks, commonly used to treat liver pain, come with risks like pneumothorax, especially in patients with chronic lung conditions. Improper technique or lack of knowledge about complications can lead to further patient harm.
- **Thumb Rule Consideration:** Ensure nerve blocks, particularly intercostal or celiac plexus blocks, are performed by experienced clinicians, with thorough knowledge of potential complications like pneumothorax or infection.

Overlooking Neuropathic and Thoracic Conditions

- Neuropathic conditions like herpes zoster or polyneuropathy can present with pain similar to liver pain. Failure to differentiate between neuropathic pain and liver pain can lead to mismanagement, such as prescribing inappropriate medications or therapies.
- **Thumb Rule Consideration:** Consider neuropathic conditions and thoracic pathologies in cases where liver pain does not respond to standard treatment. Perform appropriate diagnostic tests like nerve conduction studies or thoracic imaging when necessary.

Inadequate Assessment of Infectious Processes

- Liver abscesses or other infections in immunocompromised patients can present with liver pain. Failure to detect and treat these infections early can result in severe complications, including sepsis or liver failure.

- **Thumb Rule Consideration:** In patients presenting with liver pain and risk factors such as immunosuppression or recent travel, always consider infections, and conduct appropriate lab tests and imaging to rule out liver abscess or related infectious processes.

REFERENCES

- Goodman CC: Screening for medical problems in patients with upper extremity signs and symptoms, J Hand Ther 23:105–126, 2010.
- Hansen L, Sasaki A, Zucker B: End-stage liver disease: challenges and practice implications, Nurs Clin North Am 45:411–426, 2010.
- Khoury GF, Stein C, Ramming KP: Neck and shoulder pain associated with hepatic arterial chemotherapy using an implantable infusion pump, Pain 32:275–277, 1988.
- Tsunekawa K, Matsuda R, Ohgushi N, Ogasawara A: Ohnishi: Basic problems of the pain from the gallbladder and liver, Pain 30(Suppl 1):S24, 1987.
- Waldman SW, Feldstein GS, Donohoe CD, Waldman KA: The relief of body wall pain secondary to malignant hepatic metastases by intercostal nerve block with bupivacaine and methylprednisolone, J Pain Symptom Manage 3:39–43, 1988.

LUMBAR MYOFASCIAL PAIN SYNDROME

Myofascial pain syndrome (MPS) is common among patients with musculoskeletal pain problems. MPS is a pain condition originating from muscle and surrounding fascia. Patients usually present with localized pain in a restricted area or referred pain of various patterns. Moreover, the physical examinations may reveal trigger points (TrPs) on the involved muscles. MPS can be divided into the acute and chronic forms. Acute MPS frequently resolves spontaneously or after simple treatments. However, chronic MPS are usually worse in prognosis, and the symptoms can last for 6 months or longer. This referred pain often is misdiagnosed or attributed to other organ systems, leading to extensive evaluations and ineffective treatment. Patients with myofascial pain syndrome involving the muscles of the low back often have referred pain into the hips, sacroiliac joint, and buttocks.

Saxena A, Chansoria M, Tomar G, Kumar A. Myofascial pain syndrome: an overview. J Pain Palliat Care Pharmacother. 2015 Mar;29(1):16-21.

Clinical Description

Lumbar myofascial pain syndrome is a diagnosis made based on the presence of certain symptoms and a combination of clinical history, physical examination, radiography, and MRI. It is a diagnosis of exclusion, which means that other conditions that may cause similar symptoms, such as lumbar strain, inflammatory arthritis, and disorders of the lumbar spinal cord, roots, plexus, and nerves, must be ruled out before a diagnosis of lumbar myofascial pain syndrome can be made. Congenital abnormalities such as arteriovenous malformations and trefoil spinal canal, as well as spondylolisthesis, may also present with symptoms similar to lumbar myofascial pain syndrome and should be considered in the differential diagnosis.

Lumbar myofascial pain syndrome, which is a type of chronic muscle pain affecting the lower back, is often treated with a combination of different approaches. Physical therapy can help to correct functional abnormalities such as poor posture, and the use of heat modalities and deep tissue massage can be helpful in relieving symptoms. Nonsteroidal anti-inflammatory drugs (NSAIDs) and skeletal muscle relaxants may also be used to reduce pain and muscle spasm. If these treatments are not effective, trigger point injections of anesthetic and steroid into the affected muscle tissue may be considered. In cases where there is underlying diffuse muscle pain, sleep disturbance, and depression, tricyclic antidepressants such as nortriptyline may be prescribed, starting with a single bedtime dose of 25 mg.

Pearls & Oysters

Trigger point injections for lumbar myofascial pain syndrome involve injecting a local anesthetic and steroid into the affected muscle tissue. This procedure should only be performed by healthcare providers who are well-trained in the regional anatomy and experienced in performing interventional pain management techniques. There is a risk of transient increased pain after the injection, as well as the potential for more serious complications such as pneumothorax (collapsed lung) or damage to the retroperitoneal organs if long needles are used.

Bottom Line Statement

Lumbar myofascial pain syndrome is best managed by an interprofessional team that includes the pharmacist. There is no one treatment that works in everyone and not everyone has the same response. A pain specialist should be involved early in the care. Because many of these patients have a range of mental health disorders, a mental health consult should be obtained.

Unfortunately, the prognosis for most patients is guarded because of recurrence of pain. Many patients regularly turn to alternative health care because of the failure of conventional medicine to help them with pain relief.

Medico-Legal Traps

Misdiagnosis and Failure to Exclude Other Causes

- Lumbar myofascial pain syndrome is a diagnosis of exclusion, meaning that other conditions like lumbar strain, radiculopathy, or spinal abnormalities must first be ruled out. Misdiagnosis can lead to delayed or inappropriate treatment, worsening the patient's condition or subjecting them to unnecessary interventions.
- **Thumb Rule Consideration:** Always conduct thorough diagnostic evaluations, including imaging and neurological assessments, to rule out structural causes before diagnosing lumbar myofascial pain syndrome.

Inadequate Training in Trigger Point Injections

- Trigger point injections, commonly used for this condition, carry risks such as pneumothorax or damage to retroperitoneal organs if performed incorrectly. Improper technique or use of excessively long needles can lead to serious complications.
- **Thumb Rule Consideration:** Only trained and experienced healthcare providers should administer trigger point injections, ensuring proper

anatomical knowledge and technique to avoid complications.

Overlooking Coexisting Psychological Conditions

- Many patients with chronic lumbar myofascial pain syndrome suffer from associated mental health disorders such as depression or anxiety, which may contribute to their pain experience. Failure to address these psychological aspects may result in ineffective treatment and persistent pain.
- **Thumb Rule Consideration:** Incorporate mental health assessments and consider involving psychologists or psychiatrists as part of an interprofessional treatment plan for patients with chronic pain syndromes.

Inadequate Pain Management

- Pain management in lumbar myofascial pain syndrome can be challenging, and failure to implement a multimodal approach can result in suboptimal outcomes. Over-reliance on NSAIDs or muscle relaxants without considering physical therapy or alternative therapies can delay recovery.
- **Thumb Rule Consideration:** Use a multidisciplinary approach involving medications, physical therapy, and other modalities like massage, heat, and behavioral therapy to optimize patient outcomes.

Failure to Communicate Risks of Treatment

- Patients receiving trigger point injections or other interventional procedures must be adequately informed about the risks, including temporary pain exacerbation or potential complications. Failure to obtain informed consent or thoroughly explain these risks can lead to legal repercussions.
- **Thumb Rule Consideration:** Always provide clear communication regarding potential risks and benefits of interventions, ensuring informed consent is obtained before proceeding with treatments like trigger point injections.

REFERENCES

- Skootsky SA, Jaeger B, Oye RK. Prevalence of myofascial pain in general internal medicine practice. West J Med. 1989 Aug;151(2):157-60.
- Vázquez-Delgado E, Cascos-Romero J, Gay-Escoda C. Myofascial pain syndrome associated with trigger points: a literature review. (I): Epidemiology, clinical treatment and etiopathogeny. Med Oral Patol Oral Cir Bucal. 2009 Oct 01;14(10):e494-8.
- Shah JP, Thaker N, Heimur J, Aredo JV, Sikdar S, Gerber L. Myofascial Trigger Points Then and Now: A Historical and Scientific Perspective. PM R. 2015 Jul;7(7):746-761.
- Simons DG, Stolov WC. Microscopic features and transient contraction of palpable bands in canine muscle. Am J Phys Med. 1976 Apr;55(2):65-88.
- Hsieh YL, Yang SA, Yang CC, Chou LW. Dry needling at myofascial trigger spots of rabbit skeletal muscles modulates the biochemicals associated with pain, inflammation, and hypoxia. Evid Based Complement

Alternat Med. 2012;2012:342165.

- Zhang H, Lü JJ, Huang QM, Liu L, Liu QG, Eric OA. Histopathological nature of myofascial trigger points at different stages of recovery from injury in a rat model. Acupunct Med. 2017 Dec;35(6):445-451.
- Liu L, Huang QM, Liu QG, Ye G, Bo CZ, Chen MJ, Li P. Effectiveness of dry needling for myofascial trigger points associated with neck and shoulder pain: a systematic review and meta-analysis. Arch Phys Med Rehabil. 2015 May;96(5):944-55.
- Furlan AD, van Tulder MW, Cherkin DC, Tsukayama H, Lao L, Koes BW, Berman BM. Acupuncture and dry-needling for low back pain. Cochrane Database Syst Rev. 2005 Jan 25;(1):CD001351.
- Gerwin RD. Classification, epidemiology, and natural history of myofascial pain syndrome. Curr Pain Headache Rep. 2001 Oct;5(5):412-20.

LUNOTRIQUETRAL INSTABILITY PAIN SYNDROME

Lunotriquetral joint instability is often misdiagnosed and if left untreated can result in lunotriquetral dissociation. Although patients may lack symptoms in low grade lunotriquetral injury, when symptomatic there is a typical pattern of pain and simple tests can be performed and obtained to more specifically identify injury.

Ritt MJ, Bishop AT, Berger RA, Linscheid RL, Berglund LJ, An KN. Lunotriquetral ligament properties: a comparison of three anatomic subregions. J Hand Surg Am. 1998 May;23(3):425-31.

Clinical Description

Lunotriquetral (LT) joint instability is an often missed diagnosis and can result in LT dissociation. The reasons for undiagnosed LT joint instability are in part due to multiple confounding injuries (usually associated with high energy/ impact sports) and isolated injury to the LT ligament results in relatively normal-appearing radiographs. LT ligamentous injury is less common than other proximal, carpal row, ligamentous injury and thus, more poorly understood and diagnosed.

The earliest reported LT injury was in 1903, which was then followed by a description of carpal dissociation of the lunate and triquetrum without significant change in position in 1913. Later in the 1900s, volar intercalated segmental instability (VISI) began to be defined. In the mid to late 1900s, it was found that a cause of VISI was LT ligament dissociation.

The wrist is comprised of numerous extrinsic and intrinsic ligaments that work together to provide stability. The complex, harmonious relationship between these ligaments indicates that compromise in the integrity of one of these parts will affect the overall position and strength of the wrist. The extrinsic ligaments that are most often involved in LT instability include the dorsal radiocarpal (providing dorsal support) and the radiolunate ligament (providing volar support). The interosseous LT ligament is the main intrinsic ligamentous supporter of the LT joint. It is described as "C" shaped and is divided into 3 parts. The volar portion is the strongest and thickest portion and provides the most stability and mainly prevents volar translation. The dorsal portion limits rotational movement, and the combination of all parts of the LT intrinsic ligament prevent dorsal translation. Both of these attach to bone, while the third, weaker portion, or membranous portion, connects to the articular cartilage. The dorsal radiocarpal ligament is an extrinsic ligament that when injured will cause further instability of the LT joint by allowing the lunate to flex more easily. The radiolunate ligament is extrinsic and can be involved in advanced cases of injury.

The lunate and triquetrum have been shown to have the same movements in flexion/extension motion as well as radial/ulnar deviation. This is likely why the lunotriquetral coalition is usually an asymptomatic variant.

Pearls & Oysters

Some osseous-related pain that can mimic LT instability includes fractures of the ulnar styloid, pisiform or hamate. Injury to the triangular fibrocartilage complex, extensor carpi ulnaris, and flexor carpi ulnaris are soft tissue injuries that can also mimic LT instability. Some vascular diseases that can mimic LT instability include Kienbock syndrome or hypothenar hammer syndrome. Neurological diseases that should be considered include ulnar nerve entrapment and ulnar dorsal sensory branch neuritis.

Bottom Line Statement

Lunotriquetral instability frequently poses a diagnostic dilemma as many injuries could be a mimic of this pathology. Patients will present with general wrist pain to an urgent care facility or emergency department. There is usually no apparent deformity, and the pain is generalized over the ulnar region of the wrist. With non-specific signs such as these, an accurate and precise physical exam is vital in correctly identifying the abnormality. Often this will require a team of specialists which include an emergency physician, orthopedic surgeon, and radiologist for accurate diagnosis.

Imaging of the wrist will almost always be involved with generalized ulnar-sided wrist pain. A well-trained x-ray technician will aid by obtaining quality imaging for more accurate diagnoses by the radiologist. If no findings on the initial radiographs are present, MR imaging of the wrist can be obtained, and a well trained MRI technician is also utilized for a radiologist to make a diagnosis of LT ligamentous injury.

If intervention is indicated once the diagnosis of LT instability is made, an orthopedic surgeon and their staff including nurses, surgery technicians, and accompanying anesthesiologists will be involved for proper surgical fixation.

Almost always, even if surgery is not indicated, physical therapists will help with recovery of mobility, functioning and with pain relief. Physical therapists can also guide orthopedic surgeons in determining improvement or lack thereof for decisions on intervention with more invasive stabilization procedures.

Medico-Legal Traps

Failure to Recognize or Diagnose Early

- Lunotriquetral (LT) instability is often misdiagnosed or missed due to its subtle presentation and the fact that initial radiographs may appear normal. This delay can result in the progression of the condition to LT dissociation or VISI (volar intercalated segment instability), leading to more complex treatment needs and possible permanent dysfunction.
- **Thumb Rule Consideration:** Always perform detailed physical exams and consider advanced imaging, such as MRI, if initial radiographs fail to show definitive signs, especially in patients with ulnar-sided wrist pain.

Confounding Diagnoses and Overlooking Mimicking Conditions

- Many conditions mimic LT instability, such as fractures of the ulnar styloid, pisiform, or hamate, as well as injuries to the triangular fibrocartilage complex (TFCC) and extensor carpi ulnaris. Misdiagnosis or failure to consider these differential diagnoses can lead to inappropriate treatment and prolonged pain for the patient.
- **Thumb Rule Consideration:** Maintain a broad differential diagnosis, including soft tissue, neurological, and vascular conditions. Utilize comprehensive clinical exams and imaging to rule out mimics.

Inadequate Physical Examination and History-Taking

- Given the subtle presentation, LT instability can be missed if a thorough physical examination is not performed. Standardized wrist examination protocols are often not fully employed, leading to missed signs of instability, such as a positive LT ballotment test or pain with wrist extension.
- **Thumb Rule Consideration:** Ensure that specific tests like the LT ballotment test, Watson test, and assessment for localized ulnar wrist pain are performed to aid in diagnosis.

Failure to Collaborate with Specialists

- LT instability often requires a multidisciplinary approach for accurate diagnosis and management. A failure to collaborate with radiologists, orthopedic surgeons, and physical therapists may result in delayed or improper treatment.
- **Thumb Rule Consideration:** Always refer patients with persistent wrist pain or instability signs to a specialist team, including radiologists for advanced imaging and orthopedic surgeons for possible surgical intervention.

Inadequate Post-Diagnosis Care and Follow-up

- Once diagnosed, improper or insufficient rehabilitation and failure to follow up can result in chronic pain or decreased wrist function. Physical therapy is critical in regaining mobility and function, but lack of adherence to prescribed therapy or monitoring can lead to long-term disability.
- **Thumb Rule Consideration:** Ensure comprehensive rehabilitation planning, including regular follow-ups with physical therapists, to monitor recovery progress and adjust treatment as needed to prevent chronic dysfunction.

REFERENCES

- Shin AY, Battaglia MJ, Bishop AT. Lunotriquetral instability: diagnosis and treatment. J Am Acad Orthop Surg. 2000 May-Jun;8(3):170-9.
- Ritt MJ, Bishop AT, Berger RA, Linscheid RL, Berglund LJ, An KN. Lunotriquetral ligament properties: a comparison of three anatomic subregions. J Hand Surg Am. 1998 May;23(3):425-31.
- Weiss LE, Taras JS, Sweet S, Osterman AL. Lunotriquetral injuries in the athlete. Hand Clin. 2000 Aug;16(3):433-8.
- Geissler WB, Burkett JL. Ligamentous sports injuries of the hand and wrist. Sports Med Arthrosc Rev. 2014 Mar;22(1):39-44.
- Mayfield JK, Johnson RP, Kilcoyne RK. Carpal dislocations: pathomechanics and progressive perilunar instability. J Hand Surg Am. 1980 May;5(3):226-41.
- Geissler WB, Freeland AE, Savoie FH, McIntyre LW, Whipple TL. Intracarpal soft-tissue lesions associated with an intra-articular fracture of the distal end of the radius. J Bone Joint Surg Am. 1996 Mar;78(3):357-65.

MANUBRIOSTERNAL JOINT PAIN

Osteoarthritis of the manubriosternal joint is a rare cause of chest pain. The diagnosis is difficult, and other serious causes of chest pain have to be ruled out first.

Cureus. 2015 Nov; 7(11): e370.

Clinical Description

Osteoarthritis of MSJ is an uncommon cause of chest pain, and hence, awareness and high index of awareness about this rare condition is crucial in reaching a diagnosis. However, other major underlying medical conditions must be ruled out before making the diagnosis and planning the operative treatment for OA of the MSJ.

An early onset of OA of the MSJ can be attributed to repetitive stress on this joint. In this patient, the repetitive stress was caused due to the lifting of heavy weights due to his profession (manual labourer) and may be the cause of the localized osteoarthritis of the MSJ. Localized symptoms and physical signs, in addition to imaging findings, often give clues to its diagnosis. Radiographic findings are often difficult to interpret, especially in early stages, and higher imaging modalities, such as CT or MRI scan, may be able to help in early diagnosis of OA of the MSJ.

The manubriosternal joint is a cartilaginous joint (symphysis) where only a thin layer of hyaline cartilage covers the articular surfaces with an intervening fibrocartilage disc. Cavitation in the disc is a common phenomenon (30%); therefore, although this joint may degenerate like a synovial joint, this joint remains a symphysis. It is more commonly involved in inflammatory arthritides, including rheumatoid arthritis (RA) and gouty, psoriatic arthritis among others. The symphysis at the MSJ limits anteroposterior displacement and allows only a small range of angulatory movement between longitudinal axes of the body of the sternum and manubrium. Hence, arthrits of the MSJ rarely gives rise to symptoms.

Arthrodesis of a joint is a known treatment option for advanced OA by various different techniques. Litchman, et al. had performed an arthrodesis in a case of post-traumatic OA of the MSJ, where they did a resection of the joint and performed a reverse sliding bone graft to fix the joint across and claimed to achieve a 'satisfactory outcome'. However, their patient could not return to heavy manual work postoperatively. Shewring and Carvell performed an arthrodesis of MSJ for a patient with gouty arthritis, using cancellous bone grafts only (without joint fixation). Al-Dahiri and Pallister were the first to publish a case report of an arthrodesis of the MSJ for OA using double locking compression plates with good results. The potential complications in the use of implants for arthrodesis of this joint include implant prominence due to the subcutaneous nature of the joint. Also, the MSJ is in close proximity to vital structures in the mediastinum and, hence, care needs to be taken to avoid injury to these structures and also ensure no possibility of implant migration.

A locking plate provides good stability to the construct as the screws lock in the plate. Since, the MSJ cannot be immobilized firmly by a cast or a brace, the plate fixation, therefore, seems to be an excellent option of fixing the MSJ. The locking plates offer specialized advantages over normal compression plates as they have minimal chances of implant migration. Also, since the screws are locked on the plate and need not have purchase at the far cortex, smaller screws can be used for fixation. This helps in decreasing the possibility of damage to important neurovascular structures behind the far cortex, especially in places like the MSJ. These plates offer further advantages such as the very little likelihood of loosening and migration of the metal work. We preferred to use a cervical locking plate because of its thin profile to avoid hardware prominence over the sternum. Bone grafting further enhances the chance of fusion in such cases and, hence, is a preferred choice along with locking plate. Preoperative planning using the CT scan images to measure screw length and drill stop depth in order to provide safety to the underlying vital structure in this surgery was crucial..

Pearls & Oysters

Preoperative images of the CT scan helped us to measure the thickness of the bone and the screw length. OA of the MSJ can be treated successfully by arthrodesis when the conservative treatment fails. A cervical locking plate may be a satisfactory and safe technique for fusion, but requires good preoperative planning. The cervical locking plate provides durable pain relief and bony fusion of the MSJ.

Bottom Line Statement

The manubriosternal joint should be considered as a differential for anterior chest pain in young males when all other differential diagnoses are ruled out. It more often affects young individuals involved in heavy manual labour. Initial management includes the use of NSAIDs and local steroid injection. In the presence of severe osteoarthritis and failed conservative means, arthrodesis should be considered. Arthrodesis using the locking plate and screws entails careful preoperative planning due to the proximity of vital structures. If well planned, the surgery can have satisfactory long-term results for this unusual diagnoses.

Medico-Legal Traps

Failure to Recognize Rare Causes of Chest Pain

- Due to the rarity of osteoarthritis (OA) of the manubriosternal joint, physicians may overlook this diagnosis when evaluating anterior chest pain, leading to unnecessary cardiac or gastrointestinal investigations and delayed treatment.•
- **Thumb Rule Consideration:** Always consider MSJ osteoarthritis in patients with localized anterior chest pain, especially young males or individuals engaged in heavy manual labor, after ruling out serious cardiopulmonary conditions.

Misdiagnosis of Non-Cardiac Chest Pain

- MSJ pain can be misdiagnosed as other conditions like costochondritis, pectoral muscle strain, or even gastrointestinal issues, due to its presentation near the sternum. This leads to ineffective treatment, prolonged pain, and patient dissatisfaction.
- **Thumb Rule Consideration:** Conduct a thorough clinical examination, including palpation of the MSJ and obtaining advanced imaging (CT or MRI), to rule out more common conditions and confirm the diagnosis.

Inappropriate Surgical Intervention

- Arthrodesis for MSJ osteoarthritis is a technically demanding procedure with risks, especially in the subcutaneous area near vital mediastinal structures. Inadequate preoperative planning or improper hardware choice could lead to implant migration, neurovascular injury, or unsatisfactory fusion.
- **Thumb Rule Consideration:** Preoperative imaging, including CT scans, should guide screw length and implant choice. Select locking plates to minimize migration risk and avoid damage to critical structures.

Overlooking Conservative Treatments

- Immediate surgical intervention without attempting conservative measures such as NSAIDs, physical therapy, or local steroid injections can lead to legal implications, especially if conservative approaches could have relieved symptoms.
- **Thumb Rule Consideration:** Always initiate conservative treatment options first, including NSAIDs and steroid injections, before considering surgical arthrodesis for advanced osteoarthritis.

Complications from Postoperative Care

- Improper postoperative management, such as inadequate immobilization or failure to monitor for implant migration, could result in poor outcomes or additional surgeries. Postoperative complications are common if not monitored carefully.
- **Thumb Rule Consideration:** Post-surgery, provide clear rehabilitation protocols, regular imaging follow-ups, and patient education on activity limitations to ensure proper recovery and avoid recurrence or complications.

REFERENCES

- Di Cesare PE, Haudenschild DR, Samuels J, Abramson SB. Kelley's Textbook of Rheumatology, 9th edition. 2, Part 15. Philadelphia: Elsevier Saunders; 2013. Pathogenesis of osteoarthritis; pp. 1617–1635.
- Symptomatic manubriosternal joint involvement in rheumatoid arthritis. Doube A, Clarke AK. Ann Rheum Dis. 1989;48:516.
- Post-traumatic degenerative arthrosis in the manubriosternal joint. Litchman HM, Silver CM, Simon SD, Tamura H. Clin Orthop Relat Res. 1969;67:111–115.
- Arthrodesis for recurrent manubriosternal gout. Shewring DJ, Carvell JE. J Bone Joint Surg Br. 1991;73:341.
- Arthrodesis for osteoarthritis of the manubriosternal joint. Al-Dahiri A, Pallister I. Eur J Cardiothorac Surg. 2006;29:119–121.
- Al-Dahiri A, Pallister I: Arthrodesis for osteoarthritis of the manubriosternal joint, Eur J Cardiothorac Surg 29:119–121, 2006.
- Ellis H: The superior mediastinum, Anaesth Intens Care Med 10:360–361, 2009.
- Lyons I, Saha S, Arulampalam T: Manubriosternal joint dislocation: an unusual risk of trampolining, J Emerg Med 39:596–598, 2010.
- Stochkendahl MJ, Christensen HW: Chest pain in focal musculoskeletal disorders, Med Clin North Am 94:259–273, 2010.
- Waldman SD: Manubriosternal joint syndrome. In Waldman SD, editor: Pain review, Philadelphia, 2009, Saunders, pp 247–248.

METATARSALGIA

Metatarsalgia is a general term for pain in the area of the metatarsophalangeal joints. This is often seen in clinical practice, the deformity and pain can deteriorate gait function and decrease quality of life.

Park CH, Chang MC. Forefoot disorders and conservative treatment. Yeungnam University Journal of Medicine. 2019 May;36(2):92.

Clinical Description

The most important and relevant anatomy is the forefoot and the metatarsal. The metatarsus of the foot consists of five long bones, which are called the metatarsals.

Metatarsals:

Comprised of: proximal base; shaft; distal head.

Proximally connected to the tarsal bones and distally to the phalanges.

Named I to V medially to laterally, from the dorsal surface of the foot.

Convex on their dorsal surfaces but concave on their plantar surfaces

Along with the tarsals, help form the arches of the foot, which are essential in both weight-bearing and walking.

The joints between the head of the metatarsals and the respective proximal phalanx are called the metatarsophalangeal joint (MTP).

These joints form the ball of the foot, and the ability to move in these joints is very important for normal walking.

In addition, the bases of the metatarsals articulate with each other to form intermetatarsal joints.

Pearls & Oysters

Metatarsalgia is a condition in which the ball the foot becomes painful and inflamed.

Causes include - activities that involve running and jumping, foot deformities and shoes that are too tight or too loose.

Generally not serious.

Conservative measures such as ice and rest, often relieve symptoms. Wearing

proper footwear with shock-absorbing insoles or orthoses may prevent or minimize future problems with metatarsalgia.

Bottom Line Statement

Metatarsal pain occurs under the ball of the foot, just in front of the toes. It can result from structural features a person is born with, an injury, excessive pressure due to high-impact sports, a medical condition, and many other factors.

Home remedies include:

resting the foot

applying ice

performing exercises to stretch the muscles and relax the feet

doing low-impact exercise

taking over-the-counter drugs to manage pain and inflammation

In some cases, a doctor may recommend stronger pain relief, immobilization of the bones, or surgery.

The outlook will depend on the cause. Often, home remedies and rest are enough to relieve pain, but pain that results from arthritis or another medical condition may need ongoing care.

Medico-Legal Traps

Failure to Identify Underlying Structural Issues

- Metatarsalgia can be caused by structural abnormalities such as high arches, flat feet, or deformities like hammertoes. If these are not identified and treated, the pain may persist or worsen, potentially leading to claims of mismanagement.
- **Thumb Rule Consideration:** Always perform a thorough clinical and radiological examination to assess any underlying structural abnormalities, and consider orthotics early in the treatment plan to address the biomechanical cause.

Overlooking Footwear as a Primary Cause

- Improper footwear is one of the most common causes of metatarsalgia. Failure to counsel patients on footwear choices can delay recovery or cause recurrence, resulting in patient dissatisfaction and potential legal issues.

- **Thumb Rule Consideration:** Educate patients on the importance of proper, well-fitted footwear with adequate cushioning and shock absorption, and recommend custom orthoses if necessary.

Delaying Referral to Specialists

- If conservative treatments fail, delayed referral to specialists (orthopedists or podiatrists) for further evaluation and intervention can lead to prolonged pain and disability for the patient. This delay can be construed as negligence in care.
- **Thumb Rule Consideration:** If symptoms do not improve after 6-8 weeks of conservative management, consider early referral to a specialist for further diagnostic workup and possible surgical intervention.

Inadequate Documentation of Conservative Management

- In cases where surgery becomes necessary, inadequate documentation of failed conservative treatments (rest, ice, NSAIDs, and physical therapy) can lead to medico-legal challenges, as patients may claim they were pushed too early into surgery.
- **Thumb Rule Consideration:** Keep detailed records of all conservative measures attempted, including patient compliance and response to treatments, to ensure a clear progression of care if surgery is needed.

Failure to Rule Out Systemic Causes

- Metatarsalgia can sometimes be caused by systemic conditions like arthritis, gout, or diabetes. Overlooking these conditions can lead to improper treatment and further complications, which could result in liability claims.
- **Thumb Rule Consideration:** Always evaluate for systemic causes of foot pain through a detailed medical history, lab tests (for gout, diabetes), and imaging when appropriate, to avoid missing an underlying systemic condition.

REFERENCES

- Mercks manual. MTP joint pain Available from:https://www.merckmanuals.com/professional/musculoskeletal-and-connective-tissue-disorders/foot-and-ankle-disorders/metatarsophalangeal-joint-pain (last accessed 25.6.2020)
- Doty, Jesse F., and Michael J. Coughlin. "Metatarsophalangeal joint instability of the lesser toes." The Journal of Foot and Ankle Surgery 53.4 (2014): 440-445.
- Espinosa, Norman, Ernesto Maceira, and Mark S. Myerson. "Current concept review: metatarsalgia." Foot & ankle international 29.8 (2008)
- https://www.kenhub.com/en/library/anatomy/metatarsal-bones
- Radiopedia Metatarsalgia Available from:https://radiopaedia.org/articles/metatarsalgia (last accessed 25.6.2020)
- Brukner P. Brukner & Khan's clinical sports medicine. North Ryde: McGraw-Hill; 2012.

- G. McPoil Thomas and Schuit Dale. "Management of metatarsalgia secondary to biomechanical disorders". Physical Therapy 66(6): 970-2; July 1986.
- Sobel Ellen, D.P.M., Ph. D., C.PED. and Levitz Steven, D.P.M.; "Metatarsalgia : Diagnosis and Manangement, Etiologies and Differential diagnoses". Podiatry Management.
- Espinosa, Norman, Ernesto Maceira, and Mark S. Myerson. "Current concept review: metatarsalgia." Foot & ankle international 29.8 (2008).

MIDTARSAL JOINT PAIN

Midtarsal Joint Sprains are usually the result of the stress of jumping and landing causing pain and swelling. Midtarsal Joint Sprains are a graded condition ranging from mild to severe. There is little written about this subject in literature and is often not well known by orthopaedic surgeons in general.

J Clin Orthop Trauma. 2020 May-Jun; 11(3): 399–405.

Clinical Description

A joint sprain refers to damage or tearing to the connective ligament tissue that stretches over a joint. Ligaments help hold joints together and keep their movements restricted within a desired range. This provides essential stability when joints are placed under the pressures of muscle action and external ground resistance forces.

A joint sprain can cause instability within the joint that may lead to greater damage if left untreated. Our experienced physiotherapists at Physio.co.uk can assess the sprain and address your specific issues with targeted treatments.

Mid-tarsal joint sprains usually result from the pressures of jumping and landing, consequently they are most commonly seen amongst people playing sports. The ligaments affected are responsible for stabilising the joints in the foot between the Talus, Calcaneus, Navicular and Cuboid bones. Specifically they are called the Calcaneocuboid ligament and the Calcaneonavicular ligament. Part of these ligaments join in a 'Y' shape across the joint which is referred to as the bifurcate ligament. Damage to any of the ligament tissues will produce very similar symptoms and require the same treatment approach.

Injuries to the transverse tarsal joint (Chopart joint) occur when the foot and ankle is flexed, twisted (inverted/everted) and loaded at the same time. Therefore athletes, such as football players and gymnasts, are at risk of a Chopart's joint sprain. Patients will present with immediate pain and swelling on the top (dorsal) and outside (lateral) of the foot. The Chopart's joint plays a significant role in balance and stability of the foot. Patients will usually not be able to weight-bear after a major transverse tarsal joint injury. Patients may also have bruising over the Chopart's joint and this bruising can extend to the sole of the foot within a few days of the injury.

Pearls & Oysters

Midfoot arthritis can be debilitating, and a successful union is linked to a satisfactory outcome which most authors report to be on the range of 90%.

The hardware appropriate for each case should be carefully chosen but the surgeon should not deviate from the key principles of careful patient selection, pre-operative planning, adequate joint preparation and a stable fixation.

Bottom Line Statement

The transverse tarsal joint, also called the midtarsal or Chopart's joint, is made up of the joints between the calcaneus and cuboid, and the talus and navicular. It is the joint that connects the hindfoot to the midfoot. A sprain is the most common injury to the transverse tarsal joint and occurs when some or all of the ligaments holding the joint together are torn. The most common mechanism of this injury is an inward twisting and loading of the foot -somewhat similar to the mechanism that causes an ankle sprain. Patients will have significant pain and will often be unable to weight-bear. Diagnosing a transverse tarsal joint injury is made through a combination of patient history, physical examination, and x-ray imaging. Treatment involves rest, anti-inflammatory medications (if tolerated), and immobilization in a cast or walker boot. After the pain and swelling has settled (often a number of weeks) formal physical therapy can be started. Transverse joint sprains typically do not require surgery, although some injuries to Chopart's joint have associated fractures or dislocation and may require surgery. Although a transverse tarsal joint injury/sprain and an ankle sprain occur via a somewhat similar mechanism with a roughly similar area of injury the length of recovery is usually much longer in patients who have suffered a transverse tarsal joint injury.

Medico-Legal Traps

Failure to Recognize the Severity of the Sprain

- Midtarsal joint injuries can be graded from mild to severe. A failure to recognize severe sprains or associated fractures early on can lead to delayed treatment, chronic instability, and long-term disability, resulting in potential claims of negligence.
- **Thumb Rule Consideration:** Always evaluate midtarsal injuries with a thorough clinical examination and imaging (X-ray, MRI) to differentiate between sprains, fractures, or ligamentous tears, ensuring appropriate treatment is provided from the start.

Misdiagnosis as Ankle Sprain

- Midtarsal joint sprains can be mistaken for ankle sprains due to similar mechanisms of injury and overlapping symptoms. This misdiagnosis may lead to inadequate treatment, potentially resulting in prolonged recovery or complications.

- **Thumb Rule Consideration:** Always consider the possibility of a midtarsal injury in patients with foot and ankle pain, especially if there is difficulty in weight-bearing or swelling over the dorsal midfoot. Order appropriate imaging and perform a detailed examination of the midfoot.

Delayed Surgical Intervention in Severe Cases

- In cases where fractures or dislocations are associated with midtarsal sprains, delayed surgical intervention can worsen the prognosis and lead to permanent disability, opening the door to medico-legal claims.
- **Thumb Rule Consideration:** If imaging reveals fractures, dislocations, or severe ligamentous damage, consult an orthopedic surgeon early. Timely surgical intervention is crucial to prevent long-term complications such as midfoot arthritis.

Inadequate Post-Injury Rehabilitation

- Failure to provide a structured rehabilitation plan can result in chronic instability, pain, or stiffness, potentially leading to claims of improper management or negligence in aftercare.
- **Thumb Rule Consideration:** Ensure patients receive a tailored rehabilitation plan post-immobilization, including physical therapy to restore strength, flexibility, and stability, particularly after a transverse tarsal joint injury.

Neglecting to Inform Patients of Prolonged Recovery Time

- Midtarsal joint injuries often have a longer recovery period than ankle sprains. Failing to properly inform patients of this can lead to dissatisfaction and potential legal claims for unrealistic expectations.
- **Thumb Rule Consideration:** Clearly communicate the expected duration of recovery and rehabilitation, emphasizing that transverse tarsal injuries often require more extended recovery periods, and ensure proper follow-up appointments for monitoring progress.

REFERENCES

- Jaffe W.L., Gannon P.J., Laitman J.T. Paleontology, embryology, and anatomy of the foot. In: Jahss M.H., editor. Disorders of the Foot and Ankle: Medical and Surgical Management. Saunders; Philadelphia, PA: 1991. pp. 3–34.
- Jahss M.H. Disorders of the anterior tarsus, midtarsus, and Lisfranc's joint: the anterior tarsus, midtarsus, and Lisfranc's joint. In: Jahss M.H., editor. Disorders of the Foot and Ankle: Medical and Surgical Management. Saunders; Philadelphia, PA: 1991. pp. 1284–1332.
- Sayeed S.A., Khan F.A., Turner N.S., 3rd, Kitaoka H.B. Midfoot arthritis. Am J Orthop (Belle Mead NJ) 2008 May;37(5):251–256.
- Cavanagh P.R., Rodgers M.M., Iiboshi A. Pressure distribution under symptom-free feet during barefoot

standing. Foot Ankle. 1987;7(3):262–276.

- Patel Amar, Rao Smita PT., Nawoczenski Deborah PT., Flemister Adolf S., DiGiovanni Benedict, Baumhauer Judith F. Midfoot Arthritis. J. Am. Acad. Orthop. Surg. 2010;18(7):417–425. July.
- Ouzounian T.J., Shereff M.J. In vitro determination of midfoot motion. Foot Ankle. 1989;10(3):140–146.
- Lakin R.C., DeGnore L.T., Pienkowski D. Contact mechanics of normal tarsometatarsal joints. J Bone Joint Surg Am. 2001;83(4):520–528.
- Komenda G.A., Myerson M.S., Biddinger K.R. Results of arthrodesis of the tarsometatarsal joints after traumatic injury. J Bone Joint Surg. 1996;78-A:1665–1676.

MULTIPLE MYELOMA

Multiple myeloma (MM) is a plasma cell malignancy in which monoclonal plasma cells proliferate in bone marrow, resulting in an overabundance of monoclonal paraprotein (M protein), destruction of bone, and displacement of other hematopoietic cell lines. First described in 1848, MM is part of a spectrum of diseases ranging from monoclonal gammopathy of unknown significance (MGUS) to plasma cell leukemia.

Dimopoulos M, Kyle R, Fermand JP, Rajkumar SV, San Miguel J, et al. Consensus recommendations for standard investigative workup: report of the International Myeloma Workshop Consensus Panel 3. Blood. 2011 May 5. 117 (18):4701-5.

Clinical Description

Presenting signs and symptoms of multiple myeloma (MM) include bone pain, pathologic fractures, weakness, anemia, infection (often pneumococcal), hypercalcemia, spinal cord compression, and renal failure. In approximately 30% of cases, MM is discovered through routine blood screening when patients are being evaluated for unrelated problems. Typically, a large gap between the total protein and the albumin levels observed on an automated chemistry panel suggests a problem (ie, protein minus albumin equals globulin).

In one third of patients, MM is diagnosed after a pathologic fracture occurs; such fractures commonly involve the axial skeleton. Two thirds of patients complain of bone pain, commonly with lower back pain. This bone pain is frequently located in the back, long bones, skull, and/or pelvis.

Patients may also complain of nonspecific constitutional symptoms related to hyperviscosity and hypercalcemia.

Bone pain is the most common presenting symptom in MM. Most case series report that 70% of patients have bone pain at presentation. The lumbar spine is one of the most common sites of pain.

Pathologic fractures are very common in MM; 93% of patients have more than one site of bony involvement. A severe bony event is a common presenting issue.

The symptoms that should alert physicians to consider spinal cord compression are back pain, weakness, numbness, or dysesthesias in the extremities. Because spinal cord compressions in MM occur at multiple levels, comprehensive evaluation of the spine is warranted. Patients who are ambulatory at the start of therapy have the best likelihood of preserving function and avoiding paralysis.

Confusion, somnolence, bone pain, constipation, nausea, and thirst are the presenting symptoms of hypercalcemia. This complication may be present in as many as 30% of patients with MM at presentation. In most solid malignancies, hypercalcemia carries an ominous prognosis, but in MM, its occurrence does not adversely affect survival.

Pearls & Oysters

Renal failure and insufficiency are seen in 25% of patients with MM, and may reflect any of the following:

Myeloma kidney syndrome with multiple etiologies

Amyloidosis with light chains

Nephrocalcinosis due to hypercalcemia

Anemia, neutropenia, or thrombocytopenia is due to bone marrow infiltration of plasma cells. Thrombosis and Raynaud phenomenon due to cryoglobulinemia may be present.

Radiculopathy and/or cord compression may occur because of skeletal destruction and nerve compression.

Bacterial infection may develop; it is the leading cause of death in patients with myeloma. The highest risk is in the first 2-3 months of chemotherapy.

Purpura, retinal hemorrhage, papilledema, coronary ischemia, seizures, and confusion may occur as a result of hyperviscosity syndrome.

Hypercalcemia may cause polyuria and polydipsia, muscle cramps, constipation, and a change in the patient's mental status.

Bottom Line Statement

Guidelines on the management of multiple myeloma complications by the European Myeloma Network include the following recommendations :

Whole body low-dose computed tomography is more sensitive than conventional radiography in depicting osteolytic disease and thus is recommended as the novel standard for the detection of lytic lesions in myeloma.

Myeloma patients with adequate renal function and bone disease at diagnosis should be treated with zoledronic acid or pamidronate.

Symptomatic patients without lytic lesions on conventional radiography can be treated with zoledronic acid, but its advantage is not clear for patien ts with no bone involvement on computed tomography or magnetic resonance imaging.

In asymptomatic myeloma, bisphosphonates are not recommended.

Zoledronic acid should be given continuously, but it is not clear if patients who achieve at least a very good partial response benefit from its continuous use.

Treatment with ESAs may be initiated in patients with persistent symptomatic anemia (hemoglobin < 10g/dL) in whom other causes of anemia have been excluded.

Erythropoietic agents should be stopped after 6-8 wk if no adequate hemoglobin response is achieved.

For renal impairment, bortezomib-based regimens are the current standard of care.

For the management of treatment-induced peripheral neuropathy, drug modification is needed.

Vaccination against influenza is recommended; vaccination against• Streptococcus pneumoniae and• Haemophilus influenzae is appropriate, but efficacy is not guaranteed due to suboptimal immune response.

Prophylactic acyclovir (or valacyclovir) is recommended for patients receiving proteasome inhibitors, or autologous or allogeneic transplantation.

Medico-Legal Traps in Managing Multiple Myeloma

Delayed Diagnosis of Spinal Cord Compression

- Multiple myeloma (MM) patients commonly present with bone pain, particularly in the spine, which can lead to spinal cord compression if not promptly identified. Missing early signs like back pain or weakness may result in irreversible paralysis, leading to allegations of negligence.

- **Thumb Rule Consideration:** Always evaluate spinal symptoms such as back pain, weakness, or numbness thoroughly in MM patients and consider urgent imaging for timely diagnosis of potential spinal cord compression.

Failure to Recognize Hypercalcemia

- Hypercalcemia is present in about 30% of MM cases and can cause confusion, somnolence, and constipation. Failing to recognize and treat hypercalcemia can result in life-threatening complications such as renal failure or coma, potentially leading to malpractice claims.
- **Thumb Rule Consideration:** Be vigilant for symptoms of hypercalcemia (confusion, bone pain, polyuria), check serum calcium levels, and initiate prompt treatment to prevent serious complications.

Inadequate Monitoring of Renal Function

- Renal failure affects 25% of MM patients and can result from various causes including myeloma kidney, hypercalcemia, and amyloidosis. Failing to monitor renal function appropriately can lead to worsening renal impairment and medico-legal issues.
- **Thumb Rule Consideration:** Regularly monitor kidney function in MM patients, especially those with risk factors like hypercalcemia, and manage renal impairment with appropriate interventions such as hydration and bortezomib-based therapy.

Missed or Inadequate Management of Infections

- Infection is the leading cause of death in MM patients, especially during the first few months of chemotherapy. Neglecting preventive measures like vaccination or failing to address early signs of infection may result in serious patient harm and potential legal action.
- **Thumb Rule Consideration:** Ensure that MM patients receive prophylactic antibiotics, vaccinations (influenza, pneumococcal), and close monitoring for signs of infection, particularly during chemotherapy.

Improper Use of Bisphosphonates

- Zoledronic acid and other bisphosphonates are recommended for patients with bone involvement in MM. However, prolonged or inappropriate use can lead to complications like osteonecrosis of the jaw. Mismanagement of bisphosphonate therapy can result in legal claims for causing avoidable harm.
- **Thumb Rule Consideration:** Use bisphosphonates judiciously, based

on imaging-confirmed bone involvement, and follow up closely to monitor for adverse effects like osteonecrosis, adjusting treatment as necessary.

REFERENCES

- [Guideline] National Comprehensive Cancer Network. NCCN Clinical Practice Guidelines in Oncology, Multiple Myeloma. Available at http://www.nccn.org/professionals/physician_gls/pdf/myeloma.pdf. Version 4.2022 — December 14, 2021; Accessed: March 3, 2022.
- Rajkumar SV. Myeloma today: Disease definitions and treatment advances. Am J Hematol. 2016 Jan. 91 (1):90-100.
- Palumbo A, Rajkumar SV. Treatment of newly diagnosed myeloma. Leukemia. 2009 Mar. 23(3):449-56.
- Bensinger WI. Role of autologous and allogeneic stem cell transplantation in myeloma. Leukemia. 2009 Mar. 23(3):442-8. [Full Text].
- van Nieuwenhuijzen N, Spaan I, Raymakers R, Peperzak V. From MGUS to Multiple Myeloma, a Paradigm for Clonal Evolution of Premalignant Cells. Cancer Res. 2018 May 15. 78 (10):2449-2456. [Full Text].
- Kuehl WM, Bergsagel PL. Molecular pathogenesis of multiple myeloma and its premalignant precursor. J Clin Invest. 2012 Oct. 122 (10):3456-63. [Full Text].
- Raab MS, Podar K, Breitkreutz I, Richardson PG, Anderson KC. Multiple myeloma. Lancet. 2009 Jul 25. 374(9686):324-39.
- Ludwig H, Drach J, Graf H, Lang A, Meran JG. Reversal of acute renal failure by bortezomib-based chemotherapy in patients with multiple myeloma. Haematologica. 2007 Oct. 92(10):1411-4.
- Zucchelli P, Pasquali S, Cagnoli L, Ferrari G. Controlled plasma exchange trial in acute renal failure due to multiple myeloma. Kidney Int. 1988 Jun. 33(6):1175-80.
- Key Statistics About Multiple Myeloma. American Cancer Society. Available at http://www.cancer.org/cancer/multiplemyeloma/detailedguide/multiple-myeloma-key-statistics. January 12, 2021; Accessed: February 3, 2021.
- Koutros S, Baris D, Bell E, Zheng T, Zhang Y, Holford TR, et al. Use of hair colouring products and risk of multiple myeloma among US women. Occup Environ Med. 2009 Jan. 66 (1):68-70. [Full Text].
- Wadhera RK, Kyle RA, Larson DR, et al. Incidence, clinical course, and prognosis of secondary monoclonal gammopathy of undetermined significance in patients with multiple myeloma. Blood. 2011 Sep 15. 118(11):2985-7.

NECK-TONGUE SYNDROME

Neck-tongue syndrome (NTS) is a headache disorder often initiated by rapid axial rotation of the neck resulting in unilateral neck and/or occipital pain and transient ipsilateral tongue sensory disturbance.

Curr Pain Headache Rep. 2016 Apr;20(4):27.

Clinical Description

Neck–tongue syndrome (NTS) is a rarely reported disorder. Plausible speculations on its pathophysiology have recently been described in case reviews. It is characterised by brief attacks of occipital pain and ipsilateral hemiglossal dysaesthesia elicited by abrupt neck rotation. Although NTS can occur without obvious abnormalities, associated pathological changes include degenerative spondylosis, ankylosing spondylitis, psoriatic arthritis and loose ligaments of joint capsules.

According to the ICHD-3 (International Classification of Headache Disorders, third edition) criteria, to be diagnosed as having NTS, a person must display: **(A)** at least two episodes fulfilling criteria B–D; **(B)** sharp or stabbing unilateral pain in the upper neck and/or occipital region with concurrent abnormal sensation and/or posture of the ipsilateral tongue (may or may not be simultaneous dysaesthesia); **(C)** episodes triggered by sudden neck turning; **(D)** symptoms lasting from seconds to several minutes; **(E)** clinical features not better accounted for by another ICHD-3 diagnosis. Imaging is primarily used to search for secondary causes amenable to more aggressive medical treatment or surgical intervention.

Pearls & Oysters

Because of the rarity of neck-tongue syndrome, it is often misdiagnosed. Further complicating the confusion many of the pathological processes that mimic neck-tongue syndrome are also difficult to diagnose, especially diseases of the hypopharynx. Neck-Tongue syndrome typically has pediatric or adolescent onset, suggesting that ligamentous laxity during growth and development may facilitate transient subluxation of the lateral atlantoaxial joint with sudden head turning. Familial cases suggest a genetic predisposition in some individuals. Neck-Tongue syndrome should be re-instated in the International Classification of Headache Disorders.

Bottom Line Statement

Neck-tongue syndrome (NTS) is characterised by unilateral headache triggered by head turning and accompanied by dysaesthesia of the ipsilateral hemitongue.

The pain of NTS is in the distribution of the C2 nerve root. NTS is rarely reported but may be more frequent than hitherto surmised. Conservative management, including physiotherapy and minor cervical adjustment, may be the preferred initial treatment.

Medico-Legal Traps

Misdiagnosis and Delay in Diagnosis

- Neck-Tongue Syndrome (NTS) is rare and often misdiagnosed due to its unusual presentation and lack of familiarity among clinicians. This can lead to inappropriate treatments or prolonged suffering. Patients could claim negligence if diagnostic delays result in exacerbation of symptoms or unnecessary investigations.
- **Thumb Rule Consideration:** Maintain a high index of suspicion for NTS in patients with sharp neck pain and transient tongue dysaesthesia following neck rotation. Use clinical history and ICHD-3 diagnostic criteria to confirm the condition and avoid unnecessary delays.

Failure to Rule Out Serious Underlying Conditions

- Given that NTS can be associated with other conditions such as degenerative spondylosis, ankylosing spondylitis, or ligamentous laxity, failure to investigate potential secondary causes can expose clinicians to legal risks. If these conditions are missed, it could lead to significant complications such as spinal cord involvement or chronic pain.
- **Thumb Rule Consideration:** Always conduct imaging studies (e.g., MRI or CT) to exclude secondary causes, particularly in patients with other risk factors like systemic inflammatory conditions or cervical spine instability.

Inappropriate or Invasive Treatment

- Without clear diagnostic confirmation, initiating aggressive treatments like surgery or inappropriate medications can result in complications. This may lead to legal claims for unnecessary procedures or adverse outcomes, especially if conservative management could have sufficed.
- **Thumb Rule Consideration:** Prioritize conservative treatments such as physiotherapy and cervical adjustments for NTS. Invasive procedures should be reserved only for cases where secondary causes (e.g., structural abnormalities) are confirmed and conservative measures fail.

Neglecting Pediatric or Genetic Considerations

- NTS often presents in pediatric or adolescent patients, with familial cases suggesting a genetic predisposition. Failure to recognize the genetic or developmental aspects could result in inadequate care or complications from inappropriate interventions, particularly in younger patients.
- **Thumb Rule Consideration:** In pediatric cases, consider ligamentous laxity and potential familial predisposition when evaluating NTS. Avoid overly aggressive treatments in younger patients without thorough investigation of genetic or structural causes.

Failure to Provide Adequate Patient Education

- Due to the chronic and recurrent nature of NTS, not educating the patient about preventive strategies (e.g., avoiding sudden neck movements) and long-term management may result in ongoing discomfort or injury. This could lead to claims of inadequate care or negligence.
- **Thumb Rule Consideration:** Provide comprehensive education on the nature of NTS, its triggers, and the importance of posture and gradual neck movements to reduce symptom recurrence. Encourage regular follow-ups to monitor progress and adjust treatment as needed.

REFERENCES

- Orrell RW , Marsden CD . The neck-tongue syndrome. J Neurol Neurosurg Psychiatry 1994;57:348–52.
- Hu N , Dougherty C . Neck-Tongue Syndrome. Curr Pain Headache Rep 2016;20:27 https://doi.org/.
- Cephalalgia. 2018 Feb;38(2):374-382.
- Gelfand AA , Johnson H , Lenaerts ME , et al . Neck-Tongue syndrome: A systematic review. Cephalalgia 2018;38:374–82.
- Cassidy JD , Diakow PRP , De Korompay VL , et al . Treatment of neck-tongue syndrome by spinal manipulation: a report of three cases. Pain Clin 1986;1:41–6.
- Maheshwari PK , Pandey A . Unusual headaches. Ann Neurosci 2012;19:172–6.
- Headache Classification Committee of the International Headache Society (IHS). The International Classification of Headache Disorders: 3rd edition. Cephalalgia 2018;38:1–211.

NERVUS INTERMEDIUS NEURALGIA

Nervus intermedius neuralgia, or geniculate neuralgia, corresponds to a clinical manifestation of sudden paroxysms of excruciating otalgia which usually lasts a few seconds to a few minutes, involving the nervus intermedius (intermediate nerve of Wrisberg).

Smith JH, Robertson CE, Garza I, Cutrer FM. Triggerless neuralgic otalgia: a case series and systematic literature review. Cephalalgia : an international journal of headache. 33 (11): 914-23.

Clinical Description

Nervus intermedius neuralgia is an extremely uncommon pain syndrome in which the pain is very similar to that of trigeminal neuralgia but in the distribution of n. intermedius. Generally it is presumed that its etiology is the cross compression of the nerve at its central-peripheral myelin junction. Few cases have been reported since the original report by Clark and Taylor in 1909. This letter describes this very uncommon pain syndrome which began as a Ramsey–Hunt Syndrome and progressed as n. intermedius neuralgia.

Nervus intermedius neuralgia typically occurs in middle-aged women. Although the exact incidence is unknown, it is considered far less common than trigeminal neuralgia.

The clinical diagnostic criteria for nervus intermedius neuralgia are defined by the International Classification of Headache Disorders 3rd edition (ICHD-3) as:

- at least three attacks of unilateral pain
- the pain is located in the auditory canal, sometimes radiating to the parieto-occipital region
- the pain has at least three of the following four characteristics
- recurring in paroxysmal attacks lasting from a few seconds to minutes
- severe intensity
- shooting, stabbing or sharp in quality
- precipitated by stimulation of a trigger in the posterior wall of the auditory canal and/or periauricular region
- no clinically evident neurological deficit
- not better accounted for by another ICHD-3 diagnosis

The ICHD-3 further comments that disorders of lacrimation, salivation and/or taste sometimes accompany the pain of nervus intermedius neuralgia, and that the pain may result in secondary psychological effects and impairment to quality of life.

Pearls & Oysters

While the most common cause of cranial neuralgia is trigeminal neuralgia, limited data are available on the incidence of NIN. However, NIN is very rare; the number of cases found between 1932 and 2012 was less than 150. Other neurological and otolaryngological etiologies should be excluded in patients with NIN, which is mostly seen in middle-aged women. Therefore, it is essential to thoroughly examine the head, ear, nose, throat, face, and neck of patients. When there is no underlying etiology, it is referred to as classical NIN. Some secondary reasons have been reported: herpes zoster, temporomandibular joint dysfunction, nasopharyngeal carcinoma, petrous bone osteoma, and neuroborreliosis.

Bottom Line Statement

Similar to trigeminal neuralgia, the genesis of n. intermedius neuralgia is a mystery. It is presumed that the etiology of n. intermedius neuralgia is analogous to that of trigeminal neuralgia. Calvin and colleagues concluded that both peripheral and central mechanisms are required for the production of trigeminal neuralgia. Fromm and associates proposed that a peripheral nerve lesion (in the trigeminal root or distal) is the first event in a process that leads to central synaptic changes. The response of the central synapses to altered peripheral events leads to the development of the trigeminal neuralgia.

Medico-Legal Traps

Misdiagnosis or Delayed Diagnosis

- Nervus intermedius neuralgia (NIN) is extremely rare and may be confused with more common causes of otalgia, such as trigeminal neuralgia or temporomandibular disorders. Delayed or incorrect diagnosis can lead to ineffective treatments or worsened patient outcomes. This increases the risk of legal claims related to mismanagement or inappropriate procedures.
- **Thumb Rule Consideration:** Always consider NIN in patients with paroxysmal otalgia that radiates to the parieto-occipital region, particularly if pain is triggered by auditory canal stimulation. Apply the ICHD-3 diagnostic criteria and exclude other common causes through a thorough clinical evaluation.

Failure to Exclude Secondary Causes

- Many conditions, such as herpes zoster, nasopharyngeal carcinoma, or temporomandibular joint dysfunction, can present with similar symptoms to NIN. Failing to investigate these potential secondary causes can result in missed diagnoses and legal ramifications, especially if untreated conditions progress.
- **Thumb Rule Consideration:** Always conduct imaging and further investigations to exclude secondary causes of neuralgia. Consider MRI, especially in cases where there is concern for malignancy, structural abnormalities, or infection like neuroborreliosis.

Inadequate Pain Management

- Patients with NIN suffer from severe, paroxysmal pain that can drastically impact their quality of life. Inadequate pain management may lead to patient dissatisfaction and potential legal complaints.
- **Thumb Rule Consideration:** Develop a comprehensive pain management plan that includes medications like anticonvulsants (e.g., carbamazepine) and possible interventions such as nerve blocks, tailored to the patient's needs.

Surgical Risk in Treating Intractable Cases

- For patients who do not respond to conservative treatment, surgical intervention such as microvascular decompression may be considered. However, there are risks of complications like hearing loss or facial nerve damage, leading to medico-legal concerns if informed consent is inadequate.
- **Thumb Rule Consideration:** Ensure that patients fully understand the risks and benefits of surgical intervention, including potential complications. Document detailed informed consent discussions before proceeding with invasive treatments.

Neglecting Psychological Impact

- The chronic and severe nature of NIN can result in secondary psychological effects such as anxiety, depression, or diminished quality of life. Failure to recognize and address these mental health issues may result in claims of incomplete care.
- **Thumb Rule Consideration:** Regularly assess the psychological impact of chronic pain on patients and incorporate mental health support, such as counseling or psychiatric referrals, into the management plan to provide holistic care.

REFERENCES

- Alcaraz N, King WA, Wackym PA: Endoscopy during neurotomy of the nervus intermedius for geniculate neuralgia, Otolaryngol Head Neck Surg 121:334–336, 1999.
- Bhagra A, Stead LG: Nervus intermedius neuralgia: a rare entity, Ann Emerg Med 47:579, 584, 2006.
- Gantz BJ, Redleaf MI, Perry BP, Gubbels SP: Management of Bell's palsy and nervus intermedius neuralgia. In Brackmann DE, Shelton C, Arriaga MA, editors:Otologic surgery, ed 3, Philadelphia, 2010, Elsevier, pp 335–346.
- Persson A, Bergström T, Lindh M, Namvar L, Studahl M: Varicella-zoster virus CNS disease: viral load, clinical manifestations and sequels, J Clin Virol 46:249–253, 2009.
- Taguchi T, Ueda S, Kudo T, et al: Ramsay-Hunt syndrome, J Infect 62:180–181, 2011.
- Ulusoy Ş, Özkan G, Bektaş D, et al: Nervus intermedius neuralgia in renal transplantation recipient: a case report, Transplant Proc 42:1986–1988, 2010.
- Once-Daily Gastroretentive Gabapentin for Postherpetic Neuralgia: Integrated Efficacy, Time to Onset of Pain Relief and Safety Analyses of Data From Two Phase 3, Multicenter, Randomized, Double-Blind, Placebo-Controlled Studies. Rauck et al. Journal of Pain and Symptom ManagementNovember 12, 2012.
- Tang IP, Freeman SR, Kontorinis G, Tang MY, Rutherford SA, King AT, Lloyd SK. Geniculate neuralgia: A systematic review. J Laryngol Otol. 2014;128:394–399.

NUMMULAR HEADACHE

The International Classification of Headache Disorders has broadly classified headache disorders into primary and secondary based on their origin. Primary headache disorders include migraine, trigeminal autonomic cephalgia, tension-type headache, and other primary headache disorders. Nummular headache categorizes under other primary headache disorders. It may be continuous or with intermittent exacerbations. The involved area is sharply contoured, fixed in size and shape, round or elliptical and about 1 to 6 cm in diameter, which has led to the name "coin-shaped headache." Unlike migraine headache, nummular headache is not accompanied by nausea, vomiting, rhinorrhea, lacrimation, conjunctival injection, light or sound sensitivity or focal neurologic symptoms.

Cuadrado ML, López-Ruiz P, Guerrero ÁL. Nummular headache: an update and future prospects. Expert Rev Neurother. 2018 Jan;18(1):9-19.

Clinical Description

Nummular headache is an uncommon chronic headache syndrome characterized by constant localized pain with superimposed paroxysms of stabbing jabs and jolts of mild to moderate intensity that occur in a coin-shaped localized area of the scalp. The pain remains confined to the same symptomatic area which does not change in shape or size with time. The pain is continuous but lancinating exacerbations lasting for several seconds or gradually increasing from 10 mins to 2 h may superimpose the baseline pain. The temporal pattern is either chronic or remitting.

Most commonly located in the parietal region, the pain of nummular headache is unilateral and localized to a single area. It rarely if ever switches sides. The scalp overlying the area may be tender to touch and stimulation of the area; for example, the brushing of hair may exacerbate the pain. Nummular headache occurs slightly more commonly in women and is generally not seen before the fourth decade of life, but rare reports of children suffering from nummular headache sporadically appear in the literature. Nummular headache is also known as coin-shaped headache.

Pearls & Oysters

Nummular headache is not associated with any psychiatric disorders, anxiety, and depression. Migraine and tension headaches may be concurrently present with a nummular headache but are not related. This evidence proves once again that the central origin of nummular headache is unlikely. Because of the above evidence, nummular headaches have a provisional classification as epicrania. Epicrania include headaches that arise from epicranial tissue such as internal and external layers of the skull, all the layers of the scalp including epicranial nerves and arteries.

Nummular headache is a relatively new diagnosis, and there is limited evidence of any complications that may arise in longstanding cases. However, treatment with neuromodulators can cause excessive drowsiness; hence patients should be cautioned about operating heavy machinery and driving.

Bottom Line Statement

Although nummular headache is a primary headache disorder, the possibility of a secondary cause mimicking the symptoms require rigorous exclusion through neurologic exams, laboratory tests, and neuroimaging. The nurse practitioner, primary care provider, emergency department physician, neurologist, and an internist should inform the patient about the benign nature of this disorder. However, any focal neurologic symptoms, new-onset headache, persistent or morning headaches apart from the nummular headache, should prompt a physician consultation.

Nummular headaches, along with all headaches disorders, are best addressed in a collaborative, interprofessional team approach regarding both diagnosis and treatment. This healthcare team includes physicians and specialists, neuroscience specialty trained nursing staff, and pharmacists, working collaboratively to bring about optimal patient care and results. Often the pharmacist will need to assist in medication management and assist in educating the patient regarding compliance. A coordinated interprofessional approach will result in the best outcomes. [Level V]

Medico-Legal Traps

Misdiagnosis as Migraine or Tension Headache

- Due to its chronic nature and episodic exacerbations, nummular headache can easily be confused with more common headache disorders such as migraine or tension-type headache. Misdiagnosis can lead to inappropriate treatment plans, including unnecessary medications or invasive procedures, exposing clinicians to legal risks.
- **Thumb Rule Consideration:** Always differentiate NH from other headache disorders by identifying its hallmark "coin-shaped" area of pain, absence of associated symptoms like nausea, and fixed size of the affected scalp area.

Failure to Rule Out Secondary Causes

- Although NH is a primary headache disorder, secondary causes such as neuralgia, scalp lesions, or intracranial pathology may mimic its symptoms. Failure to exclude these causes can result in legal issues, especially if a serious condition like a tumor is overlooked.
- **Thumb Rule Consideration:** Conduct thorough neurologic exams, neuroimaging (MRI/CT), and laboratory tests to rule out secondary causes before concluding a diagnosis of NH.

Neglecting Patient Education on Benign Nature

- NH can be alarming to patients due to its chronic and localized pain, leading to anxiety. If healthcare providers fail to communicate the benign nature of NH and its non-life-threatening aspects, this could lead to patient dissatisfaction and medico-legal consequences.•
- **Thumb Rule Consideration:** Clearly explain the benign nature of NH to patients, reassure them of the prognosis, and encourage follow-up for any new or unusual symptoms.

Inappropriate Use of Neuromodulators

- Neuromodulators like gabapentin or amitriptyline are often used for NH, but improper dosing or failure to warn patients about potential side effects (e.g., excessive drowsiness) can lead to accidents or complications, triggering legal claims.
- **Thumb Rule Consideration:** Prescribe neuromodulators carefully, monitor side effects, and ensure patients are cautioned about operating heavy machinery or driving while under treatment.

Delayed Diagnosis Due to Rare Condition

- NH is a rare condition and often goes undiagnosed for long periods. Delayed diagnosis may lead to prolonged patient suffering and potential legal consequences, especially if the delay results in worsened symptoms or mismanagement of other coexisting conditions like neuralgias.
- **Thumb Rule Consideration:** Maintain a high index of suspicion for NH in patients with localized scalp pain that does not fit into typical headache patterns and ensure prompt referral to specialists if needed.

REFERENCES

- Grosberg BM, Solomon S, Lipton RB. Nummular headache. Curr Pain Headache Rep. 2007 Aug;11(4):310-2.
- Chen WH, Chen YT, Lin CS, Li TH, Lee LH, Chen CJ. A high prevalence of autoimmune indices and disorders in primary nummular headache. J Neurol Sci. 2012 Sep 15;320(1-2):127-30.
- Maniam R, Kaye AD, Vadivelu N, Urman RD. Facial Pain Update: Advances in Neurostimulation for the

Treatment of Facial Pain. Curr Pain Headache Rep. 2016 Apr;20(4):24.

- Magis D, Schoenen J. Advances and challenges in neurostimulation for headaches. Lancet Neurol. 2012 Aug;11(8):708-19.
- Cohen GL: Nummular headache: what denomination? Headache 10:1417–1418, 2005.
- Evens RW, Pareja JA: Nummular headache, Headache 45:164–165, 2005.

OBTURATOR NEURALGIA

Obturator neuropathy is a difficult clinical problem to evaluate. One possible cause of pain is due to fascial entrapment of the nerve. Symptoms include medial thigh or groin pain, weakness with leg adduction, and sensory loss in the medial thigh of the affected side. Radiographic imaging provides limited diagnostic help. MRI may detect atrophy in the adductors of the leg. However, it is unable to detect any abnormality of the nerve or in the fibro-osseus tunnel. The best test for diagnosis is by electromyography (EMG) and can be confirmed by a local nerve block. Pharmacologic management of pain and physical therapy can be helpful in the acute phase of injury. Surgical decompression of the nerve should be considered for lesions documented by EMG or local nerve block, for those with predisposing risk factors (prior surgery, pelvic trauma, or hematoma) and with prolonged or severe lesions.

Curr Rev Musculoskelet Med. 2008 Dec; 1(3-4): 234–237.

Clinical Description

Persistent pain in the groin and thigh area is a difficult clinical problem to evaluate. There are many entities that produce groin pain including tendonitis, bursitis, osteitis pubis, stress fracture, sports hernias or athletic pubalgia, nerve entrapment. In some instances, a report of obturator nerve compression, specifically its anterior division, is one possible cause of pain in the adductor region. Entrapment of the obturator nerve has been documented by nerve conduction studies. Subsequent surgical decompression of the anterior division of the obturator nerve has produced favorable results.

The most common presenting symptom is sensory alteration in the medial thigh. These symptoms can include paresthesias, sensory loss, or pain. The most frequent reported symptom in one study was medial thigh or groin pain. A deep ache may be described in the adductor origin region at the pubic bone and may extend to the medial aspect of the thigh to the knee. Exacerbation of pain may be caused by maneuvers that stretch the nerve either by extension or lateral leg movement [9]. There is also possibly diminished sensation along the medial thigh. In some instances, these sensory complaints may extend to the medial calf. However, the obturator nerve very rarely provides sensation distal to the knee.

Despite the fact that many muscles used in thigh adduction are intervated by nerves other than the obturator n. adduction on the affected side is usually weak. Sometimes medial thigh wasting can be observed. With severe injuries, loss of adduction and internal rotation occur. During ambulation, the hip is externally rotated and abnormally abducted, which results in a circumducting, wide based gait. Ipsilateral loss of the hip adductor tendon reflex can be present, but is only suggestive, not pathognomonic of obturator neuropathy. Because this reflex does not always occur in healthy individuals, presence of this reflex on the contralateral, asymptomatic leg must occur for the finding to be useful.

Pearls & Oysters

There may be a temporal relationship between nerve injury, therapy, and recovery. Therefore athletes with diagnosed obturator neuropathy should try only a limited course of conservative therapy. Sorenson et al. stated that patients with acute onset of obturator neuropathy had good recovery with conservative management. Conversely, those with chronic neuropathy have less chance for improvement and, thus, result in a poorer outcome.

Bottom Line Statement

Mononeuropathies of the obturator nerve are rare. Athletes will present with pain, weakness in leg adduction, and sensory loss over a small area in the medial thigh sometimes just with exercise or exacerbated after exercise. Often, obturator neuropathy is caused by pelvic trauma or surgery so athletes should be questioned regarding previous surgery. Definitive diagnosis is made with electrophysiologic studies and can be confirmed by obturator nerve block with local anesthesia. Conservative therapy can be helpful in athletes with acute symptoms. Surgical exploration should be considered for lesions documented by EMG or local nerve block, for those with predisposing risk factors (prior surgery, pelvic trauma, or hematoma) and with prolonged or severe lesions.

Medico-Legal Traps

Misdiagnosis of Groin and Thigh Pain

- Obturator neuralgia presents with symptoms such as groin and medial thigh pain, which can be mistaken for more common conditions like tendonitis, bursitis, or sports hernias. Misdiagnosis can lead to prolonged patient suffering, inappropriate treatments, and potential legal implications for healthcare providers.•
- **Thumb Rule Consideration:** Always consider obturator neuralgia in cases of persistent groin pain, especially in athletes, and confirm the diagnosis with electromyography (EMG) or nerve block before ruling it out.

Failure to Investigate Pelvic Trauma History

- Obturator neuralgia is often associated with previous pelvic trauma, surgery, or hematoma. Failure to inquire about a detailed surgical or trauma history may lead to delayed diagnosis and ineffective treatment, creating liability risks for physicians.•
- **Thumb Rule Consideration:** Take a thorough medical history, specifically asking about prior pelvic trauma or surgeries, when assessing patients with symptoms of obturator neuralgia.

Overlooking Electrophysiological Studies

- Diagnosis of obturator neuralgia cannot be reliably made with imaging alone, as MRI and other scans may not show abnormalities. Relying solely on these methods and neglecting to perform electrophysiological studies like EMG may result in missed diagnoses and delayed treatment.•
- **Thumb Rule Consideration:** Use EMG and nerve blocks to confirm obturator neuropathy when clinical symptoms are present but imaging is inconclusive.

Delayed Surgical Intervention

- Conservative treatment, such as physical therapy, may benefit patients with acute obturator neuralgia, but continuing conservative management in chronic cases with no improvement increases the risk of prolonged pain and legal action.•
- **Thumb Rule Consideration:** If symptoms persist despite conservative management, especially in chronic cases, consider timely surgical exploration or decompression to prevent further deterioration.

Inadequate Pain Management

- Obturator neuralgia can cause significant pain, but failing to properly manage pain with appropriate medications or procedures, such as nerve blocks, can lead to patient dissatisfaction and legal claims of inadequate care.•
- **Thumb Rule Consideration:** Implement a comprehensive pain management plan, including pharmacologic treatments and nerve blocks, especially in severe or persistent cases, to ensure proper symptom relief.

REFERENCES

- Ashby EC. Chronic obscure groin pain is commonly caused by enthesopathy: 'Tennis elbow' of the groin. Br J Surg. 1994;81:1632–4. doi: 10.1002/bjs.1800811123.
- Martens MA, Hansen L, Mulier JC. Adductor tendonitis and musculus rectus abdominis tendonopathy. Am J Sports Med. 1987;15:353–6. doi: 10.1177/036354658701500410.

- Zimmerman G. Groin pain in athletes. Aust Fam Physician. 1988;17:1046–52.
- Bradshaw C, McCrory P, Bell S, Brukner P. Obturator neuropathy: a cause of chronic groin pain in athletes. Am J Sports Med. 1997;25:402–8. doi: 10.1177/036354659702500322.
- Stewart JD. Focal peripheral neuropathies. 2. New York: Raven Press; 1993.
- Sunderland S. Nerves and nerve injuries. 2. Edinburgh: Churchill Livingstone; 1978.
- Dawson DM, Hallet M, Wilbourn AJ. Miscellaneous uncommon syndromes of the lower extremity. In: Entrapment neuropathies. 3rd ed. Philadelphia: Lippincott-Raven; 1988, p. 369–79.
- Sorenson EJ, Chen JJ, Daube JR. Obturator neuropathy: causes and outcome. Muscle Nerve. 2002;25(4):605–7. doi: 10.1002/mus.10065.
- Busis NA. Entrapment and other focal neuropathies. Neurol Clin. 1999;17(3):633–53. doi: 10.1016/S0733-8619(05)70156-0.
- Mumenthaler M, Schliack H. Lesions of individual nerves of the lower limb plexus and the lower extremity. In: Peripheral nerve lesions. Diagnosis and therapy. New York: Thieme Medical Publishers; 1991, p. 297–343.
- Pavlov H, Nelson TL, Warren RF, Torg JS, Burstein AH. Stress fractures of the pubic ramus. A report of twelve cases. J Bone Joint Surg Am. 1982;64A:1020–5.

OMOHYOID SYNDROME

Omohyoid muscle syndrome (OMS) is a condition that causes a X-shaped lateral neck lump on swallowing, caused by the failure of the central tendon of the omohyoid muscle to restrict movement of the muscle during swallowing.

Ann Otol Rhinol Laryngol. 2021 Oct;130(10):1181-1189

Clinical Description

OMS could be genetic as all cases were Asian in ethnicity. The deep cervical fascia which usually envelopes the omohyoid muscle may be weakened by stress as 20% of cases had a preceding traumatic event. Real-time ultrasonography establishes the diagnosis, demonstrating the anterolateral displacement of the sternocleidomastoid muscle by a thickened omohyoid muscle during swallowing. Surgical transection can achieve cure, but due to limited studies available, they should be reserved for patients who are extremely bothered. Intramuscular injection of botulinum toxin is an effective alternative, but recurrence is expected. Omohyoid muscle syndrome is a rare condition that presents as a characteristic X-shaped lateral protruding neck mass that occurs on swallowing. This dynamic bulging neck mass is usually painless and is caused by the omohyoid muscle displacing the overlying SCM.

Pearls & Oysters

Omohyoid muscle syndrome is a rare clinical condition that shows unmistakable signs of an X-shaped lateral neck mass caused by displacement of the sternocleidomastoid muscle superficially due to aberrant movement of the omohyoid muscle. There have been several hypotheses about the mechanism responsible for this syndrome. The first proposed mechanism is that it is caused by failure of omohyoid muscle to lengthen due to muscle fiber degeneration. A recent anatomical study regarding morphologies of the superior belly of omohyoid muscle reported that four types of intermediate morphologies were observed in 18 of 67 samples, and four of them were considered to be caused by the poor development of the myofibers. The other hypothesis regarding omohyoid muscle is that it is caused by a failure of the fascial-retaining mechanism of the omohyoid muscle. The major complication in the treatment of patients thought to have omohyoid syndrome is wrong diagnosis. Occult cervical spine fractures or instability after trauma remain an ever-present possibility. Failure to diagnose such injuries can put the patient at significant risk for permanent neurological sequelae.

Bottom Line Statement

Omohyoid muscle syndrome is a rare condition that might occur after trauma such as chokehold to the neck. Imaging on this syndrome quite challenging especially when there were no other symptoms experienced. If it is proven to be strictly cosmetic, most patients will choose to have a conservative therapy.

Medico-Legal Traps

Misdiagnosis and Overlooking of Serious Underlying Conditions

- Omohyoid syndrome presents with an X-shaped neck mass during swallowing, which can easily be misdiagnosed as other neck conditions, such as cervical spine trauma, occult fractures, or malignancies. Failing to correctly diagnose the condition or overlooking potential coexisting conditions like cervical instability can lead to serious consequences, including neurological damage.
- **Thumb Rule Consideration:** Always conduct a thorough diagnostic evaluation using imaging and real-time ultrasonography to exclude more serious conditions before diagnosing omohyoid syndrome.

Underestimating the Genetic and Trauma Factors

- Omohyoid muscle syndrome is more commonly reported in individuals of Asian descent, with trauma playing a role in some cases. Failure to take a comprehensive history regarding ethnic background or recent neck trauma could lead to delayed or incorrect diagnosis, especially when dealing with populations less prone to this condition.
- **Thumb Rule Consideration:** Always take a detailed patient history, including ethnic background and any recent traumatic events, when evaluating a neck mass, even if the symptoms seem primarily cosmetic.

Failure to Consider Conservative and Reversible Treatments First

- Surgery can cure omohyoid syndrome, but it carries risks and should not be a first-line treatment for a cosmetic condition. Rushing to surgery without first attempting conservative measures like botulinum toxin injections could expose providers to legal risk if complications arise.
- **Thumb Rule Consideration:** Recommend conservative treatments like botulinum toxin injections before considering surgical intervention, especially when the primary concern is cosmetic.

Complications from Surgery Due to Inadequate Preoperative Planning

- Surgical transection of the omohyoid muscle carries risks, including damage to surrounding neurovascular structures, and improper preoperative planning could lead to complications. Failing to inform the patient about the risks of recurrence or complications from surgery can lead to malpractice claims.
- **Thumb Rule Consideration:** Ensure that patients are fully informed about all treatment options, including risks and the likelihood of recurrence, and make surgical interventions only after careful preoperative planning.

Failure to Document Cosmetic Nature and Patient Consent

- Given that many patients with omohyoid syndrome seek treatment for cosmetic reasons, providers must ensure that this is clearly documented. Failure to obtain informed consent that acknowledges the cosmetic nature of the condition and treatment could result in legal claims if the outcome does not meet the patient's expectations.
- **Thumb Rule Consideration:** Clearly document the cosmetic nature of the syndrome and ensure thorough informed consent discussions with the patient regarding expected outcomes and risks.

REFERENCES

- Buntine JA. The omohyoid muscle and fascia: morphology and anomalies. Aust N Z J Surg. 1970;40:86-88.
- Gurgel F. Brazilian Jiu-Jitsu Advanced Techniques. Tel Aviv, Israel: Dekel Publishing House; 2007.
- Caswell HT., Jr. The omohyoid syndrome. Lancet. 1969;2:319.
- Kim L, Kwon H, Pyun S-B. Pseudodysphagia due to omohyoid muscle syndrome. Dysphagia. 2009;24:357-361.
- Standring S. Gray's Anatomy: The Anatomical Basis of Clinical Practice. 40th ed. Edinburgh, UK: Churchill Livingstone/Elsevier; 2008.
- Zachary RB, Young A, Hammond JD. The omohyoid syndrome. Lancet. 1969 Jul;2(7611):104-5.

ORCHIALGIA

Chronic orchialgia is defined as 3 months of intermittent or constant testicular pain that is significantly bothersome to the patient. It is the cause of about 2.5% to 5% of all urology consultations and currently affects about 100000 men in the United States each year. When it cannot be directly be attributed to any specific, identifiable source, the condition is called idiopathic chronic orchialgia.

Polackwich AS, Arora HC, Li J, Levine L, Tojuola B, Parekattil S, Shoskes DA. Development of a clinically relevant symptom index to assess patients with chronic orchialgia/chronic scrotal content pain. Transl Androl Urol. 2018 May;7(Suppl 2):S163-S168.

Clinical Description

Evaluation can be confusing as the underlying cause is often idiopathic and conservative therapy is often unsuccessful making this a challenging condition to diagnose and treat. Conservative therapy is usually tried first, but more invasive treatments are used when first-line options fail. Surgical options include spermatic cord blocks, varicocelectomy, epididymectomy, vasovasostomy (if the patient has had a vasectomy), microsurgical denervation of the spermatic cord (MDSC), botulinum toxin injections, and orchiectomy.

Possible identifiable organic causes include structural disorders such as spermatoceles, varicoceles, infection, trauma, fibrosis, tumors, intermittent torsion, torsion of a testicular appendage, chronic epididymitis, low back strain, vasculitis (such as Henoch-Schonlein purpura), post-vasectomy pain syndrome, nerve entrapment from hernia surgery or perineural fibrosis, pelvic floor dysfunction, or referred pain from another site such as a ureteral stone. Less common causes include diabetic neuropathy, retroperitoneal tumors, interstitial cystitis, abdominal aortic aneurysms, peritonitis, amiodarone-induced epididymal inflammation, pelvic musculoskeletal disorders, osteitis pubis, and polyarteritis nodosa. Chronic orchialgia may also be associated with chronic pelvic pain syndrome (CPPS), possibly through intraprostatic reflux, or the 2 may sometimes be describing the same entity. Up to 50% of men with chronic pelvic pain syndrome or chronic prostatitis will also claim to have chronic orchialgia.

There is often a psychological component in chronic orchialgia including such problems as somatization disorder, major depression, chronic pain other than in the genitals and chemical dependency. When no specific etiology can be identified, which happens in about 25% to 50% of all cases, it is called idiopathic chronic orchialgia and is thought to be due to neurogenic inflammation or nerve sensitization possibly from prolonged overstimulation.

Pearls & Oysters

Buspirone, an anxiolytic drug, shows some promise for chronic orchialgia but there are no published studies on it yet.

Sacral nerve stimulation has been used anecdotally for intractable, neuropathic testicular pain with some success. This may prove to be useful in selected patients prior to more invasive surgical options.

Pulsed radiofrequency therapy to denervate the spermatic cord has been tried with encouraging early results, although its final efficacy and duration is still uncertain.

Ultrasound-guided targeted micro-cryoablation of the peri-spermatic cord is an alternative therapy when MDSC has failed. Spermatic cord nerves, like other nerves, are sensitive to freezing injuries. When exposed to temperatures of -15 C to -20 C, the nerves become completely desensitized. Men who have failed MDSC might have some residual, functioning nerve fibers in the spermatic cord that could contribute to persistent pain. Freezing these nerves is a reasonable alternative to an orchiectomy. Early results suggest successful pain relief in up to 74% of patients.

Botulinum toxin injections can inhibit neurogenic inflammation and reduce chronic pain by blocking the release of neuropeptides. Neurogenic inflammation and Wallerian degeneration of nerve fibers in the spermatic cord are thought to be one possible etiology of idiopathic chronic orchialgia. As such, it is reasonable to expect an inhibitory effect from botulinum toxin on this process by providing an anti-nociceptive effect. Early results suggest significant relief of pain in 70% of patients when botulinum toxin is injected medial and lateral to the spermatic cord at the external ring.

AminoFix is an injectable, dehydrated amniotic/chorionic membrane allograft derived from human amniotic tissues. It has been shown to have a beneficial effect on slowing scar tissue formation, promoting healing and reducing inflammation. Experimentally, it has been injected similar to botulinum toxin with about 50% of patients indicating significant reductions in their pain after treatment.

Bottom Line Statement

Chronic orchialgia is likely to remain a challenging condition for an interprofessional team of nurses, nurse practitioners, physician assistants, and physicians to evaluate and treat due to multiple possible etiologies, limited tools for diagnostic evaluation and the multitude of treatment options. Conservative therapies are often unsuccessful, and diagnostic methods frequently fail to identify a specific etiology. Psychological factors appear to play an important role in this painful syndrome. Physical therapy and pelvic floor trigger point dry needling can be useful and effective non-surgical treatments. Scrotal ultrasound and spermatic cord blocks are the most useful diagnostic tools currently available. an interprofessional approach to this difficult problem is recommended.

When conservative and alternative means are unsuccessful in relieving the pain, surgical intervention is justified. Microsurgical denervation of the spermatic cord appears to be a highly successful surgical means of dealing with idiopathic chronic orchialgia without resorting to more aggressive surgical resections. Orchiectomy remains as the surgical treatment of last resort, but even this drastic procedure is not always successful in relieving chronic testicular pain. Further studies are needed to identify better treatment options and improve long-term patient outcomes.

Medico-Legal Traps

1. Failure to Diagnose the Underlying Cause

- Chronic orchialgia has multiple potential etiologies ranging from infections, tumors, and nerve entrapments to idiopathic causes. If clinicians fail to properly investigate and identify the underlying condition through imaging, ultrasound, or nerve conduction studies, it can lead to mismanagement, delayed treatment, and poor outcomes for the patient, increasing the risk of legal consequences.
- **Thumb Rule Consideration:** Conduct thorough diagnostic evaluations, including imaging and nerve studies, to rule out identifiable causes before considering the condition as idiopathic.

2. Ignoring Psychological Components

- Chronic orchialgia is frequently associated with psychological issues, including somatization disorder, depression, or chronic pain syndromes. Failure to recognize and address the psychological aspects of chronic orchialgia can lead to inadequate treatment and prolonged suffering, increasing the potential for litigation.
- **Thumb Rule Consideration:** Include a mental health assessment in the diagnostic process, and offer psychological support or therapy as part of the treatment plan.

3. Inappropriate Use of Surgical Interventions

- Surgical options such as microsurgical denervation of the spermatic cord (MDSC) or orchiectomy should only be considered after conservative and less invasive treatments fail. Rushing to surgery without exhausting non-surgical alternatives may expose healthcare providers to legal risks, especially if complications arise or the surgery does not relieve the pain.
- **Thumb Rule Consideration:** Exhaust conservative options (e.g., physical therapy, nerve blocks, or botulinum toxin injections) before recommending surgical interventions.

4. Failure to Obtain Informed Consent for Treatment Options

- Given the variety of treatment options available for chronic orchialgia, including nerve blocks, surgery, and cryoablation, patients may not fully understand the risks and benefits of each approach. Failure to provide thorough informed consent regarding the expected outcomes, potential complications, and the possibility of pain persistence post-surgery can result in legal action.
- **Thumb Rule Consideration:** Provide detailed explanations of all treatment options, including success rates, risks, and the possibility of persistent pain, and obtain thorough informed consent from the patient.

5. Overlooking Recurrence Risk After Non-Surgical Treatments

- Non-surgical treatments, such as botulinum toxin injections and nerve blocks, may provide temporary relief but often lead to recurrence of pain. Failure to prepare patients for the possibility of recurrence or incomplete relief could lead to dissatisfaction and potential legal claims.
- **Thumb Rule Consideration:** Educate patients about the likelihood of recurrence or incomplete relief after non-surgical treatments and set realistic expectations regarding long-term outcomes.

REFERENCES

- Polackwich AS, Arora HC, Li J, Levine L, Tojuola B, Parekattil S, Shoskes DA. Development of a clinically relevant symptom index to assess patients with chronic orchialgia/chronic scrotal content pain. Transl Androl Urol. 2018 May;7(Suppl 2):S163-S168.
- Shoskes DA, Calixte N, Tadros N, Li J, Parekattil S. Validation of the Chronic Orchialgia Symptom Index for Men With Chronic Orchialgia/Chronic Scrotal Contents Pain. Urology. 2018 Sep;119:39-43.
- Calixte N, Brahmbhatt J, Parekattil S. Chronic Testicular and Groin Pain: Pathway to Relief. Curr Urol Rep. 2017 Sep 02;18(10):83.
- Grayson CT, Criman ET, Cefalu LM, Roedel EQ, Hong SS, Yheulon CG. Litigation Patterns in Inguinal Hernia Surgery: A 25 Year Review. J Surg Res. 2018 Dec;232:266-270.
- Redmond EJ, Mac Namara FT, Giri SK, Flood HD. Blunt testicular trauma - is surgical exploration necessary? Ir J Med Sci. 2018 Nov;187(4):1109-1113.
- Moore JR, Pathak RA, Snowden C, Bolan CW, Young PR, Broderick GA. Multispecialty retrospective review of

the clinical utility of pelvic magnetic resonance imaging in the setting of pelvic pain. Transl Androl Urol. 2017 Dec;6(6):1155-1158.

- Calixte N, Tojuola B, Kartal I, Gudeloglu A, Hirsch M, Etafy M, Mendelson R, Djokic B, Sherba S, Shah K, Brahmbhatt J, Parekattil S. Targeted Robotic Assisted Microsurgical Denervation of the Spermatic Cord for the Treatment of Chronic Orchialgia or Groin Pain: A Single Center, Large Series Review. J Urol. 2018 Apr;199(4):1015-1022.
- Ching CB, Hays SR, Kaffenberger SD, Stephany HA, Luckett TR, Clayton DB, Tanaka ST, Thomas JC, Adams MC, Brock JW, Pope JC. Pediatric chronic orchialgia: patient population and patterns of care. J Pediatr Urol. 2014 Oct;10(5):799-803.
- Parekattil SJ, Cohen MS. Robotic surgery in male infertility and chronic orchialgia. Curr Opin Urol. 2010 Jan;20(1):75-9.

OS ACROMIALE PAIN SYNDROME

Os acromiale is from Ancient Greek, "os" is bone, and "acromiale" is a possessive form of "acromion", a compound word: akros, "highest", ōmos, "shoulder". Os acromiale is an uncommon cause of shoulder pain with symptoms often resulting from an unstable meso-acromion. The associated pain may be due to impingement from the unfused fragment, a concomitant rotator cuff tear, or gross motion at the os acromiale site. Currently, initial treatment includes physical therapy, nonsteroidal anti-inflammatory agents, and subacromial corticosteroid injections. Surgical intervention is reserved for patients who do not respond to nonoperative treatment.

J Shoulder Elbow Surg. 2002 Sep-Oct;11(5):521-8.

Clinical Description

Os acromiale represents an unfused accessory center of ossification of the acromion of the scapula. It is regarded as one of the reasons for rotator cuff tears and shoulder impingement, which is generally asymptomatic and discovered accidentally. This anatomic deformity occurs more frequently in persons of Black ancestry than in persons of White, Native American and Middle Eastern ancestries. Treatment for symptomatic patients is primarily non-operative, like nonsteroidal anti-inflammatory drug, physical therapy or corticosteroid injection. Surgical procedures are typically recommended only after non-operative treatments have failed. Common procedures include arthroscopic subacromial decompression with acromioplasty, open or arthroscopically assisted reduction and internal fixation with or without bone grafting7, 8, and open or arthroscopic excision of the os fragment.

Pearls & Oysters

Hardware-sourced problems were often occurred after tension band fixation. Depending on the fixation technique, the incidence of nonunion after internal fixation was from 0% to 100%. In addition, Boehm et al. showed the postoperative infection rate with two superficial infections (6%) and four deep infections (13%). One of the deep infection cases was following ORIF (5%, 1/22), one case was following open excision (17%, 1/6), and two cases were following open acromioplasty (40%, 2/5) as well. Two cases of superficial infection followed ORIF (9%, 2/22).

Bottom Line Statement

An Os Acromiale is an unfused secondary ossification center of the acromion that can be associated with shoulder impingement and rotator cuff tendonitis. Diagnosis is made with axillary lateral radiographs of the shoulder. Treatment is observation in the majority of cases with operative management reserved for patients who have persistent shoulder impingement or rotator cuff disease that have failed nonoperative management.

Medico-Legal Traps

1. Failure to Diagnose Os Acromiale

- Os acromiale is often asymptomatic and may go undiagnosed in patients with shoulder pain. Failure to recognize it as a cause of shoulder impingement, rotator cuff pathology, or subacromial pain may result in prolonged suffering for the patient and a delay in appropriate treatment, potentially leading to malpractice claims.
- **Thumb Rule Consideration:** Always include os acromiale in the differential diagnosis for patients presenting with shoulder pain, especially if there are signs of impingement or rotator cuff dysfunction, and confirm diagnosis with proper imaging.

2. Inadequate Imaging and Misinterpretation

- Reliance on standard imaging techniques such as AP (anteroposterior) radiographs may miss the diagnosis of os acromiale, which requires more specific imaging (e.g., axillary lateral radiographs or MRI). Misinterpreting imaging or failing to order appropriate views can lead to misdiagnosis, unnecessary treatments, and potential legal ramifications.
- **Thumb Rule Consideration:** Use axillary lateral radiographs and MRI to confirm os acromiale diagnosis and rule out associated pathologies such as rotator cuff tears.

3. Improper Surgical Indication and Technique

- Surgery for os acromiale should only be considered after nonoperative treatment options fail. Rushing into surgery without exhausting conservative treatments (physical therapy, NSAIDs, corticosteroid injections) may increase the risk of poor outcomes and potential lawsuits. Furthermore, improper surgical techniques (e.g., suboptimal fixation or excision) can result in complications like nonunion or infection.
- **Thumb Rule Consideration:** Reserve surgery for cases that fail nonoperative management, and ensure that surgical fixation or excision is

performed by an experienced orthopedic surgeon to minimize risks.

4. Neglecting Postoperative Complications

- Surgical treatment for os acromiale, particularly open or arthroscopic procedures, carries risks such as infection, nonunion, hardware failure, or incomplete resolution of symptoms. Failure to monitor and address these complications promptly can lead to malpractice claims, especially if patients suffer long-term dysfunction.
- **Thumb Rule Consideration:** Closely monitor postoperative patients for complications such as infections, nonunion, and hardware failure, and address them immediately to prevent further deterioration.

5. Inadequate Patient Education and Informed Consent

- Patients with os acromiale must be fully informed about the nature of the condition, the likelihood of complications, and the expected outcomes of both nonoperative and operative treatments. Failing to provide comprehensive informed consent, particularly regarding the risks of surgery and potential complications, can lead to legal action if the patient is dissatisfied with the outcome.
- **Thumb Rule Consideration:** Ensure thorough patient education about all treatment options, the potential for complications, and realistic expectations regarding outcomes, especially before proceeding with surgical interventions.

REFERENCES

- Acar B, Kose O. Shoulder pain after falling from bicycle. Turk J Emerg Med, 2016, 16: 91–92.
- Familiari F, Huri G, Gonzalez-Zapata A, McFarland EG. Scapula fracture and os acromiale after reverse total shoulder arthroplasty. Orthopedics, 2014, 37: 434, 492–495.
- Harris JD, Griesser MJ, Jones GL. Systematic review of the surgical treatment for symptomatic os acromiale. Int J Shoulder Surg, 2011, 5: 9–16.
- Sahajpal D, Strauss EJ, Ishak C, Keyes JM, Joseph G, Jazrawi LM. Surgical management of os acromiale: a case report and review of the literature. Bull NYU Hosp Jt Dis, 2007, 65: 312–316
- Kaplan P. Musculoskeletal MRI. W B Saunders Co. (2001) ISBN:0721690270.
- Papatheodorou A, Ellinas P, Takis F et-al. US of the shoulder: rotator cuff and non-rotator cuff disorders. Radiographics. 26 (1): e23.
- Haaga JR, Boll D. CT and MRI of the whole body. Mosby. (2009) ISBN:0323053750.
- Butler P, Mitchell A, Healy JC. Applied Radiological Anatomy. Cambridge University Press. (2012) ISBN:0521766664.
- Zlatkin MB. MRI of the shoulder. Lippincott Williams & Wilkins. ISBN:0781715903.
- Smith J, Dahm DL, Newcomer-Aney KL. Role of sonography in the evaluation of unstable os acromiale. J Ultrasound Med. 2009;27 (10): 1521-6. Kaplan P. Musculoskeletal MRI. W B Saunders Co. (2001) ISBN:0721690270.
- Ryu RK, Fan RS, Dunbar WH. The treatment of symptomatic os acromiale. Orthopedics, 1999, 22: 325–328.
- Maffulli N, Longo UG, Berton A, Loppini M, Denaro V. Biological factors in the pathogenesis of rotator cuff tears. Sports Med Arthrosc Rev, 2011, 19: 194–201.

OS SUPRATROCHLEARE-RELATED ELBOW PAIN

Elbow Arthritis represents a difficult therapeutic challenge. The complaints are classically characterized by pain, weakness, and loss of motion. Functional range of motion required for activities of daily living is considered to be an arc of motion of 100° (30° of extension to 130° of flexion) and a 100°arc of forearm rotation (50° of pronation to 50° of supination). Elbow arthritis can result from rheumatoid arthritis, sequelae of joint infection, crystalline arthropathy, hemophilia, primary osteoarthritis, and, most commonly, trauma to the elbow. Treatment options should include non operative and operative techniques, all attempting to provide pain relief and restoration of function.

J Hand Surg 2009;34A:761–768.

Clinical Description

Elbow pain secondary to os supratrochleare is being seen with increasing frequency in clinical practice owing to the increased interest in physical fitness and the use of exercise machines. Os supratrochleare is the name given to an accessory ossicle occasionally found in the posterior elbow. This accessory ossicle often is found adjacent to the proximal aspect of the olecranon process. It is thought that accessory ossicles such as os supratrochleare bones serve to decrease the friction and pressure of tendons as they pass in proximity to a joint. Similar accessory ossicles are found in the feet, hands, and wrists. Elbow pain secondary to os supratrochleare is characterized by tenderness and pain over the posterior elbow. Patients often describe a feeling of having gravel in their elbow and may report a grating sensation with flexion and extension of the elbow. The pain of os supratrochleare worsens with activities that require repeated flexion and extension of the elbow or with forceful overhead throwing. Os supratrochleare is often associated with loose bodies in the elbow joint and may coexist with olecranon bursitis.

Pearls & Oysters

The major complication of injection of os supratrochleare is infection. This complication should be exceedingly rare if strict aseptic technique is followed. Approximately 25% of patients report a transient increase in pain after injection of the os supratrochleare and should be warned of this possibility. Another potential risk of this injection technique is trauma to the extensor tendons from the injection itself.

Pain emanating from the elbow is a common problem encountered in clinical practice. Os supratrochleare must be distinguished from fractures of the elbow, fractures of the os supratrochleare itself, entrapment neuropathies of the ulnar nerve, bursitis, tendinitis, and epicondylitis. Less common causes of posterior elbow pain are osteochondritis dissecans, Panner disease, and synovial chondromatosis.

Bottom Line Statement

Pain emanating from the elbow is a common problem encountered in clinical practice. Os supratrochleare must be distinguished from fractures of the elbow, fractures of the os supratrochleare itself, entrapment neuropathies of the ulnar nerve, bursitis, tendinitis, and epicondylitis. Less common causes of posterior elbow pain are osteochondritis dissecans, Panner's disease, and synovial chondromatosis.

Medico-Legal Traps

1. Failure to Diagnose Os Supratrochleare

- Os supratrochleare-related elbow pain may be misdiagnosed as more common elbow pathologies such as fractures, tendinitis, or epicondylitis. Delayed or incorrect diagnosis can result in inappropriate treatment and prolonged patient suffering, potentially leading to malpractice claims.
- **Thumb Rule Consideration:** Always consider os supratrochleare in the differential diagnosis for persistent posterior elbow pain, especially in patients with a history of repetitive motion activities, and confirm the diagnosis with imaging studies like X-ray or MRI.

2. Inadequate Imaging

- Relying solely on standard radiographs may miss os supratrochleare or its associated conditions such as loose bodies. Failing to use advanced imaging (e.g., MRI or CT scan) when clinical suspicion persists can lead to misdiagnosis or delayed treatment, increasing the likelihood of legal consequences.

- **Thumb Rule Consideration:** Use appropriate imaging modalities like MRI or CT to accurately diagnose os supratrochleare-related elbow pain and assess for associated conditions such as loose bodies or olecranon bursitis.

---

3. Improper Injection Technique

- Injections for pain relief, such as corticosteroid or anesthetic injections, can lead to complications like infection, tissue damage, or extensor tendon trauma if not performed correctly. Improper aseptic technique or incorrect needle placement can worsen the patient's condition and expose the clinician to liability.
- **Thumb Rule Consideration:** Ensure strict aseptic technique and proper anatomical knowledge when administering injections for os supratrochleare pain, and fully inform the patient about potential risks such as transient pain or infection.

---

4. Overlooking Associated Pathologies

- Os supratrochleare is often associated with other elbow conditions like loose bodies, olecranon bursitis, or ulnar nerve entrapment. Focusing solely on the os supratrochleare without evaluating for these coexisting pathologies can lead to incomplete treatment, poor outcomes, and potential legal repercussions.
- **Thumb Rule Consideration:** Conduct a comprehensive evaluation of the elbow, including assessment for loose bodies, bursitis, and nerve entrapment, to provide a holistic treatment approach and avoid missing associated conditions.

---

5. Inadequate Patient Education and Informed Consent

- Patients may not fully understand the nature of os supratrochleare-related elbow pain, its treatment options, and the potential risks of procedures. Failing to provide detailed explanations about conservative versus surgical treatments or the risks associated with injections can lead to dissatisfaction and legal challenges.
- **Thumb Rule Consideration:** Ensure comprehensive patient education about the condition, treatment options, and risks, especially prior to invasive procedures like injections or surgery, and obtain informed consent with thorough documentation.

REFERENCES

- Rettig LA, Hastings H II, Feinberg JR. Primary osteoarthritis of the elbow: lack of radiographic evidence for morphologic predisposition, results of operative debridement at intermediate follow-up, and basis for a new radiographic classification system. J Shoulder Elbow Surg 2008;17:97–105.
- Brasington R. TNF-alpha antagonists and other recombinant proteins for the treatment of rheumatoid arthritis. J Hand Surg 2009;34A:349 –350.
- van Brakel RW, Eygendaal D. Intra-articular injection of hyaluronicacid is not effective for the treatment of post-traumatic osteoarthritisof the elbow. Arthroscopy 2006;22:1199 –1203.
- Fuerst M, Fink B, Rüther W. Survival analysis and longterm results of elbow synovectomy in rheumatoid arthritis. J Rheumatol 2006;33:892– 896.
- Tanaka N, Sakahashi H, Hirose K, Ishima T, Ishii S. Arthroscopicand open synovectomy of the elbow in rheumatoid arthritis. J BoneJoint Surg 2006;88A:521–525.
- Gudmundsen E, Østensen H: Accessory ossicles in the elbow, Acta Orthop Scand 58:130–132, 1987.
- McFarland EG, Gill HS, Laporte DM, Streiff M: Miscellaneous conditions about the elbow in athletes [review], Clin Sports Med 23:743–763, 2004.
- Waldman SD: Functional anatomy of the elbow. In Waldman SD, editor: Pain review, Philadelphia, 2009, Saunders, pp 76–77.
- Wood VE, Campbell GS: The supratrochleare dorsale accessory ossicle in the elbow, J Shoulder Elbow Surg 3:395–398, 1994.

OS TRIGONUM PAIN SYNDROME

Os trigonum syndrome is a recognized cause of pain in the posterior aspect of the foot and ankle. The symptoms and physical findings, however, are often nonspecific and difficult to differentiate from other causes of posterior ankle pain.

Iowa Orthop J. 1999; 19: 122–126.

Clinical Description

The os trigonum is a small bone on the posterolateral aspect of the talus formed from a separate ossification center which fails to unite with the talus itself. The incidence of the os trigonum has been reported to be 3-15% and it is more often bilateral than unilateral3. The os trigonum syndrome is characterized by pain, and sometimes swelling, in the posterolateral aspect of the ankle. The two mechanisms of injury originally described by McDougal involve either micro trauma from repetitive hyperplantar flexion or an episode of acute forced hyperplantarflexion. These mechanisms make it easy to understand why this syndrome has been most frequently described in ballet dancers1, and soccer players. Much less frequently, forced dorsiflexion causing avulsion of the os trigonum by the posterior talofibular ligament or direct trauma to the posterior aspect of the ankle may cause a painful os trigonum.

The diagnosis can be difficult to make as symptoms and physical exam findings mimic those that occur with problems related to an accessory soleus muscle, flexor hallucis longus, posterior tibialis, or peroneal tendons; or arthritis involving the posterior tibiotalar or subtalar joints. Radiographs typically reveal an os trigonum less than one centimeter in size and, in chronic cases, the margins may appear irregular with cystic and sclerotic changes along either the talus or the ossicle. Tomograms, CT scans, and MRI have all been described with subtle, nonspecific findings. Bone scintigraphy which shows increased uptake in the posterior aspect of the talus has been recommended by several authors to aid in the diagnosis.

Pearls & Oysters

With os trigonum syndrome, technetium bone scanning may demonstrate increased uptake in the posterior aspect of the talus. However, positive scans are sometimes bilateral and have unclear predictive value. MRI may show only fluid between the synchondrosis and can be helpful with excluding other causes of posterior ankle pain10. Injection of local anesthesia under fluoroscopic guidance into the area of the trigonal synchondrosis has been suggested as a method of confirming the diagnosis in isolated cases.

Bottom Line Statement

The differential diagnosis of posterior ankle pain includes Achilles tendon problems, flexor hallucis longus tenosynovitis, inflammation of the retrocalcaneal bursa, subluxation of the peroneal tendons, painful accessory soleus muscle, tarsal tunnel syndrome, fracture of the dome or posterior process of the talus, focal posterior tibiotalar or subtalar arthritis or osteonecrosis of the talus. Most of these conditions can be diagnosed with a careful physical and radiographic examination. The diagnosis of the os trigonum syndrome is usually a diagnosis of exclusion based solely upon the presence of posterior ankle pain and an os trigonum. The mean duration of symptoms prior to diagnosis in our series was over one year and most patients had seen an average of three physicians prior to referral to the senior author. The problem with making the diagnosis is well described in the literature and a higher degree of suspicion in dancers and soccer players may lead to a quicker diagnosis. It is particularly important to rule out associated tenosynovitis of the flexor hallucis longus by assuring pain free active and passive flexion of the FHL tendon and absence of medial sided tenderness.

Medico-Legal Traps

Failure to Diagnose or Misdiagnosis

- Os trigonum syndrome is frequently misdiagnosed as other posterior ankle conditions like Achilles tendinitis, flexor hallucis longus tenosynovitis, or subtalar arthritis. Misdiagnosis can lead to improper treatments and delayed recovery, potentially resulting in malpractice claims.
- **Thumb Rule Consideration:** Always consider os trigonum syndrome in athletes with posterior ankle pain, especially those involved in repetitive plantarflexion. Utilize diagnostic tools like bone scintigraphy and MRI to confirm the condition.

Overlooking Differential Diagnoses

- Os trigonum syndrome presents similarly to other conditions such as retrocalcaneal bursitis, tarsal tunnel syndrome, and peroneal tendon subluxation. Failure to differentiate can lead to incorrect treatment, dissatisfaction, and legal repercussions.
- **Thumb Rule Consideration:** Perform a thorough differential diagnosis with physical examination and imaging studies to rule out other causes of posterior ankle pain before confirming os trigonum syndrome.

Improper Use of Diagnostic Imaging

- Imaging techniques like X-rays and MRIs may not always clearly identify os trigonum syndrome, leading to delayed diagnosis or misattribution to other conditions. This can cause unnecessary treatments and worsen patient outcomes, increasing the risk of legal consequences.
- **Thumb Rule Consideration:** Use MRI, CT, and bone scintigraphy appropriately, and consider diagnostic injections under fluoroscopic guidance when imaging findings are subtle or inconclusive.

Ineffective Non-Surgical Treatment

- If non-surgical interventions like NSAIDs, physical therapy, or corticosteroid injections fail but no further action is taken, this may prolong suffering and lead to legal action. Clinicians who do not escalate treatment risk being accused of negligence.
- **Thumb Rule Consideration:** Transition to surgical options promptly if conservative measures fail to improve symptoms after a reasonable period, especially in cases affecting athletic performance or daily activities.

Complications from Surgery or Delayed Referral

- Surgical treatments, such as excision of the os trigonum, carry risks like infection or nonunion. Delayed referrals to specialists or not providing surgical options when indicated can prolong disability, raising the possibility of malpractice claims.
- **Thumb Rule Consideration:** Refer patients to an orthopedic or foot specialist when conservative treatment fails, and ensure patients are fully informed of the surgical risks and benefits.

REFERENCES

- Hamilton WG, Geppert MJ, Thompson FM. Pain in the posterior aspect of the ankle in dancers. J Bone Joint Surg. 1996;78A:1491–1500.
- Johnson RP, Collier BD, Carrera GF. The os trigonum syndrome: Use of bone scan in the diagnosis. J Trauma. 1984;24:761–764.
- Grogan DP, Walling AK, Odgen JA. Anatomy of the os trigonum. J Pediatr Orthop. 1990;10:618–622.
- Wenig JA. Os trigonum syndrome. J Amer Podiatric Med Assoc. 1990;80:278–282.
- McDougall A. The os trigonum. J Bone Joint Surg. 1955;37B:257–265.

- Brodsky AE, Khalil MA. Talar compression syndrome. Amer J Sports Med. 1986;6:472–476.
- Marotta JJ, Micheli LJ. Os trigonum impingement in dancers. Amer J Sports Med. 1992;20:533–536.
- Quirk R. Talar compression syndrome in dancers. Foot and Ankle. 1982;3:65–68.
- Wredmark T, Carlstedt DA, Bauer H, Saartok T. Os trigonum syndrome: A clinical entity in ballet dancers. Foot and Ankle. 1991;11:404–406.
- Karasick D, Schweitzer ME. The Os trigonum syndrome: Imaging features. Amer J Rad. 1996;166:125–129.
- Hedrick MR, McBryde AM. Posterior ankle impingement. Foot and Ankle. 1994;15:2–8.
- Veazey BL, Heckman JD, Galindo MJ, McGanity PLJ. Excision of ununited fractures of the posterior process of the talus: A treatment for chronic posterior ankle pain. Foot and Ankle. 1992;13:453–457.

OSTEONECROSIS OF THE ELBOW JOINT

Avascular necrosis is the death of bone tissue due to a lack of blood supply. Also called osteonecrosis, it can lead to tiny breaks in the bone and cause the bone to collapse. The process usually takes months to years.A broken bone or dislocated joint can stop the blood flow to a section of bone. Avascular necrosis is also associated with long-term use of high-dose steroid medications and too much alcohol. Avascular necrosis (AVN) may be asymptomatic and is occasionally discovered incidentally on radiographs. Symptoms depend on the affected joint. Medullary infarcts are usually silent, and infarcts of the small bones of the hands and feet are often symptomatic.

Clin Orthop Relat Res. 2000 Apr;(373):141-5.

Clinical Description

Osteonecrosis of the elbow joint is a diagnosis that is often missed, leading to considerable unnecessary pain and disability. Osteonecrosis is a disease that leads to joint destruction and often involves large joints, such as the hips, knees, and shoulders. In contrast to the pediatric population, osteonecrosis of the adult elbow potentially can lead to end stage arthritis. If the osteonecrosis is diagnosed early, nonoperative treatment may be effective in relieving pain, although the long-term results of these treatments remain unknown. Osteonecrosis occurs when part of the bone does not get blood flow and dies. After a while, the bone can collapse. If osteonecrosis is not treated, the joint deteriorates, leading to severe arthritis. Osteonecrosis can be caused by disease or by severe trauma, such as a fracture or dislocation, that affects the blood supply to the bone. Osteonecrosis can also occur without trauma or disease. This is called idiopathic -- meaning it occurs without any known cause. When osteonecrosis occurs in the shoulder joint, it is usually due to long-term treatment with steroids, a history of trauma to the shoulder, or the person has sickle cell disease.

Pearls & Oysters

Advanced osteonecrosis can lead to osteoarthritis and permanent decreased mobility. Failure to surgically treat significant osteonecrosis of the elbow joint usually will result in continued pain and disability and in most patients will lead to ongoing damage to the elbow joint Severe cases may require joint replacement. Use the minimum effective dose of systemic corticosteroids; when possible, use steroid-sparing agents. Early diagnosis and treatment are important; the earlier AVN is detected, the more treatment (and less invasive) options available to the patient. Provide patient education for high-risk patients

Bottom Line Statement

Osteonecrosis of the adult elbow is a relatively rare disease and represents approximately 0.7% of all the patatients. As is true in osteonecrosis, the adult capitellum and the lateral epicondyle appeared to be involved most often. This condition may happen in any bone. It most commonly happens in the ends of a long bone. It may affect one bone, several bones at one time, or different bones at different times. AVN usually involves the epiphysis (end part of a long bone), such as the femoral and humeral heads and the femoral condyles, but small bones can also be affected. In clinical practice, AVN is most commonly encountered in the hip.

Medico-Legal Traps

Delayed or Missed Diagnosis

- Osteonecrosis of the elbow is often missed or diagnosed late due to non-specific symptoms and its rarity, leading to prolonged patient suffering, joint destruction, and avoidable disability. Missing early signs can result in legal repercussions for failing to provide timely diagnosis and treatment.
- **Thumb Rule Consideration:** Maintain a high index of suspicion in patients with risk factors such as steroid use, alcohol abuse, or trauma history, and use advanced imaging like MRI for early detection.

Failure to Provide Timely Surgical Intervention

- Failure to escalate treatment when nonoperative management is ineffective can result in worsening joint damage, arthritis, and increased disability. Surgical options like joint preservation procedures or replacement are necessary in advanced cases, and delays may lead to lawsuits for inadequate care.
- **Thumb Rule Consideration:** If conservative treatments fail or disease progression is evident, promptly refer for orthopedic evaluation to explore surgical options before significant joint damage occurs.

Inadequate Management of Risk Factors

- Patients on long-term corticosteroids, with alcohol dependency, or with underlying conditions like sickle cell disease, are at high risk for osteonecrosis. Failing to manage or minimize these risk factors (e.g., steroid-sparing treatments) can increase the likelihood of osteonecrosis and expose healthcare providers to medico-legal risks.

- **Thumb Rule Consideration:** Educate patients on risk mitigation, minimize steroid use, and monitor high-risk patients regularly with imaging to detect osteonecrosis early.

Overlooking Secondary Causes of Elbow Pain

- The symptoms of osteonecrosis can mimic other conditions like lateral epicondylitis or radial head fractures. Misdiagnosis or incomplete workups leading to ineffective treatments (such as corticosteroid injections, which may exacerbate osteonecrosis) can result in poor outcomes and legal consequences.
- **Thumb Rule Consideration:** Ensure a comprehensive diagnostic approach, using clinical history, physical examination, and imaging to differentiate osteonecrosis from other common elbow pathologies.

Failure to Inform Patients About Prognosis and Treatment Options

- Inadequate communication about the potential for progression to severe arthritis or joint collapse can lead to patient dissatisfaction and claims of uninformed consent. Patients must understand the chronic nature of osteonecrosis and the possible need for surgery in advanced stages.
- **Thumb Rule Consideration:** Provide clear, thorough information on the prognosis, risks, and treatment options, including non-surgical and surgical approaches, and document patient consent after discussing potential outcomes.

REFERENCES

- Matthews AH, Davis DD, Fish MJ, Stitson D. Avascular Necrosis. 2022 Jan.
- Bose VC, Baruah BD. Resurfacing arthroplasty of the hip for avascular necrosis of the femoral head: a minimum follow-up of four years. J Bone Joint Surg Br. 2010 Jul. 92(7):922-8.
- McAlindon T, Ward RJ. Osteonecrosis. In: Hochberg MC, Gravallese EM, Silman AJ, Smolen JS, Weinblatt ME, Weisman MH, eds. Rheumatology. 7th ed. Philadelphia, PA: Elsevier; 2019:chap 206.
- Whyte MP. Osteonecrosis, osteosclerosis/hyperostosis, and other disorders of the bone. In: Goldman L, Schafer AI, eds. Goldman-Cecil Medicine. 26th ed. Philadelphia, PA: Elsevier; 2020:chap 234.
- Collaborative Osteonecrosis Group: Multifocal os- teonecrosis. A multicenter study. Clin Orthop 3691312-326, 1999.
- Cui Q, Wang GJ, Su CC, Balian G: Lovastatin prevents steroid induced adipogenesis and osteonecrosis. Clin Orthop 344:8-19, 1997.
- Delanois RE, Mont MA, Yoon TR, Mizel M, Hungerford DS: Atraumatic osteonecrosis of the talus. J Bone Joint Surg 80A:529-536, 1998.
- Ficat RP, Arlet J: Coxopathies ischemiques. Rev Chir Orthop 58543-561, 1972.

PAGET'S DISEASE

Paget's disease is an uncommon cause of back pain that is frequently diagnosed on plain radiographs obtained for other purposes or when the patient notices swelling of a long bone. Paget's disease is also known as osteitis deformans, and its cause is unknown. The incidence of Paget's disease is approximately 2%, with the disease occurring much less commonly in India, Japan, the Middle East, and Scandinavia.

Ralston SH: Pathogenesis of Paget's disease of bone, Bone 43:819–825, 2008.

Clinical Description

Neurologic complications of PDB have been reviewed [Schmidek, 1977; Poncelet, 1999; McCloskey and Kanis, 2002; Rubin and Levin, 2009]. Some symptoms and neurologic complications may be related to skull involvement. Patients with skull involvement may have headaches [Siris and Roodman, 2008]. Cranial nerve deficits have been reported but appear to be rare. Optic atrophy, ophthalmoplegia, anosmia, trigeminal neuralgia, and facial palsy have been reported [Rubin and Levin, 2009]. Hearing loss may occur when the temporal bone is involved. Presbycusis and PDB affect similar populations and it may be difficult to differentiate presbycusis from pagetic hearing loss [Bone, 2006]. Pagetic hearing loss is sensori-neural which is greater at high pitches and characteristically accompanied by low-frequency 'air-bone gap' [Monsell, 2004]. The hearing loss appears to be caused by loss of bone density in the cochlear capsule [Monsell et al. 1999; Monsell, 2004]. Some patients may have tinnitus. Another neurologic complication resulting from skull involvement is basilar invagi-nation from softening of the skull base which may cause cause hydrocephalus with headache and dizziness. This basilar invagination can result in syringomyelia and compression of the brainstem. This neurologic syndrome is usually slowly progressive and symptoms may include ataxia, vertigo, tinnitus, dysphagia, and dysarthria [Rubin and Levin, 2009].

Spinal involvement may cause pain, neurologic symptoms, and even paralysis. These may be caused by a compression of the spinal cord or nerve roots as well as ischemia due to 'vascular steal' [Herzberg and Bayliss, 1980]. Peripheral neuropathies such as ulnar, median, sciatic, and posterior tibial have been reported [Rubin and Levin, 2009]. Neurologic symptoms may improve with calcitonin [Chen et al. 1979; Herzberg and Bayliss, 1980] or bisphosphonate [Wallace et al. 1995; Pane, 2007] therapy.

Pearls & Oysters

PDB is often asymptomatic and is frequently discovered incidentally when an elevated serum alkaline phosphatase (SAP) is found on routine laboratory testing, or radiographically on x-rays performed for unrelated reasons. A recent population-based study from Olmsted County, Minnesota, USA [Wermers et al. 2008] found that 58% of the patients had symptoms at diagnosis. Seventy-two percent of these patients had polyostotic disease. Skeletal complications included bowing deformity in 7.6%, fracture of pagetic bone in 9.7%, and osteosarcoma in 0.4%. Osteoarthritis was present in 73%. Hearing loss was present in the 61%. Neurologic symptoms were uncommon. Overall survival was slightly better than predicted. PDB appears to have an adverse effect on some domains of quality of life [Gold et al. 1996; Langston et al. 2007].

Bottom Line Statement

PDB is a common condition, particularly in older persons of Northern European extraction. The incidence and severity of this condition may be decreasing. PDB is caused by accelerated osteoclastic bone resorption followed by increased bone formation in one or more bones resulting in skeletal lesions which can be osteolytic, mixed osteolytic/osteosclerotic, or osteosclerotic. Recently the SQSTM1 gene has been found to be one important cause of familial PDB. Symptoms and complications related to PDB can include bone pain, fracture, bone deformity, osteoarthri-tis, hearing loss, neurologic symptoms, cardiovascular complications, and, rarely, malignant transformation. Very effective medical therapy with potent aminobisphosphonates is available for patients requiring specific antipagetic treatment. Surgery is occasionally needed on pagetic bone and when possible should only be undertaken following effective medical therapy and by surgeons with significant experience treating this condition.

Medico-Legal Traps

Failure to Diagnose Early Due to Asymptomatic Nature

- Paget's disease is frequently asymptomatic and may go unnoticed until radiographs or blood tests for other reasons reveal abnormalities. Delayed diagnosis can result in irreversible complications such as fractures, bone deformities, or neurological deficits. Patients may claim negligence if symptoms are overlooked in routine evaluations.
- **Thumb Rule Consideration:** Always investigate elevated serum

alkaline phosphatase levels or incidental radiographic findings in older patients, especially those of Northern European ancestry, to rule out Paget's disease.

Misattributing Neurological Symptoms to Other Conditions

- Neurological symptoms from PDB, such as hearing loss, headaches, or cranial nerve involvement, may be misattributed to age-related conditions like presbycusis or degenerative diseases. Misdiagnosis can result in worsening symptoms, including paralysis or brainstem compression.
- **Thumb Rule Consideration:** Consider Paget's disease in patients with unexplained neurological symptoms, especially those with skull or spinal involvement, and perform imaging to rule out bone-related causes.

Failure to Administer Timely Bisphosphonate Therapy

- Early medical treatment with bisphosphonates can significantly improve outcomes, but failure to initiate treatment promptly could result in unnecessary pain, fractures, or other skeletal complications. Legal consequences may arise from delayed treatment that could have been prevented.
- **Thumb Rule Consideration:** Initiate bisphosphonate therapy as soon as Paget's disease is diagnosed in symptomatic patients or those at high risk for complications, and monitor treatment response.

Surgical Intervention Without Adequate Pre-Treatment

- Performing surgery on pagetic bone without proper medical management, such as bisphosphonate therapy, increases the risk of complications like delayed healing, infections, or fractures. Surgeons may face legal issues for poor outcomes in untreated bones.
- **Thumb Rule Consideration:** Ensure patients undergo effective medical therapy prior to any surgical intervention on pagetic bone, and refer complex cases to surgeons experienced with Paget's disease.

Overlooking Secondary Complications Like Osteosarcoma

- Paget's disease has a rare but serious association with osteosarcoma. Failure to monitor or detect malignant transformation could result in claims of mismanagement, especially in cases of unexplained bone pain or swelling.
- **Thumb Rule Consideration:** Closely monitor for signs of malignant transformation in Paget's disease, particularly in patients with new or worsening symptoms, and ensure regular follow-up with imaging when indicated.

REFERENCES

- Rousière M, Michou L, Cornélis F, Orcel P: Paget's disease of bone, Best Pract Res Clin Rheumatol 17:1019–1041, 2003.
- Rousière M, Michou L, Cornélis F, Orcel P: Paget's disease of bone, Best Pract Res Clin Rheumatol 17:1019–1041, 2003.
- Rousière M, Michou L, Cornélis F, Orcel P: Paget's disease. In Waldman SD, Campbell RSD, editors: Imaging of pain, Philadelphia, 2010, Saunders.
- Walsh JP, Attewell R, Stuckey BGA, et al: Eisman treatment of Paget's disease of bone: a survey of clinical practice in Australia, Bone 42:1219–1225, 2008.
- Abrahamsen B., Eiken P., Eastell R. (2009a) Subtrochanteric and diaphyseal femur fractures in patients treated with alendronate: A register-based national cohort study. J Bone Miner Res 24: 1095–1102 [
- Abrahamsen B., Eiken P., Eastell R. (2009b) More on reports of esophageal cancer with oral bisphosphonate use. N Engl J Med 360: 1789.
- Altman R.D. (1999) Arthritis in Paget's disease of bone. J Bone Miner Res 14(supplement 2): 85–87.
- Altman R.D. (2002) Epidemiology of Paget's disease of bone. Clin Rev Bone Miner Metab 1: 99–102
- Altman R.D., Collins B. (1980) Musculoskeletal manifestations of Paget's disease of bone. Arthritis Rheum 23: 1121–1127
- Alvarez L., Guanabens N., Peris P., Monegal A., Bedini J.L., Deulofeu R., et al. (1995) Discriminative value of biochemical markers of bone turnover in assessing the activity of Paget's disease. J Bone Miner Res 10: 458–465.
- Alvarez L., Guanabens N., Peris P., Vidal S., Ros I., Monegal A., et al. (2001) Usefulness of biochemical markers of bone turnover in assessing response to treatment of Paget's disease. Bone 29: 447–452.

PARSONAGE-TURNER SYNDROME

Idiopathic brachial plexopathy was reported in the Lancet in 1948 by Parsonage and Turner. Parsonage-Turner Syndrome (PTS), also referred to as idiopathic brachial plexopathy or neuralgic amyotrophy, is a rare disorder consisting of a complex constellation of symptoms with abrupt onset of shoulder pain, usually unilaterally, followed by progressive neurologic deficits of motor weakness, dysesthesias, and numbness. Although the etiology of the syndrome is unclear, it is reported in various clinical situations, including postoperatively, postinfectious, posttraumatic, and postvaccination. The identification of the syndrome in the postoperative patient remains a challenge as symptoms may easily be attributed to sequelae of surgical positioning, postoperative recovery, or postanesthetic block pain.

Parsonage MJ, Turner JWA. The shoulder girdle syndrome. Lancet. 1948;1:973–978. doi: 10.1016/S0140-6736(48)90611-4.

Clinical Description

Parsonage-Turner Syndrome (PTS) is a rare syndrome that may occur in otherwise normal healthy individuals with sudden, rather abrupt, unilateral shoulder pain that may begin rather insidiously but quickly amplifies in severity and intensity. The acute period of pain is subsequently replaced over a course of a few days to weeks with progressive weakness, reflex changes, and sensory abnormalities in varying presentations that typically involve the shoulder girdle musculature and proximal upper limb muscles. The condition, also known as neuralgic amyotrophy or brachial neuritis, has been reported in numerous clinical situations that involve some sort of antecedent impact on the patient, whether it be surgical, infectious, traumatic, or even therapeutic, such as cases involving vaccinations or antibiotic treatments. The postsurgical patient who develops PTS poses a specific diagnostic dilemma. In these individuals, the patient has undergone a rather traumatic experience to the body considering perioperative administration of antibiotics, intraoperative anesthesia, operative manipulation of tissue, and various positioning techniques used to facilitate surgical techniques. It is no mystery that, when this cohort of patients develops PTS, it is often attributed to intraoperative positioning or even part of the rehabilitative process manifested as shoulder strain with therapy.

Pearls & Oysters

The pain of Parsonage-Turner syndrome is difficult to treat. It responds poorly to opioid analgesics and may respond poorly to the previously mentioned medications. The uncontrolled pain of Parsonage-Turner syndrome has led to suicide, and hospitalization of such patients should be strongly considered. Researchers are studying the use of intravenous immune globulin (IVIG) therapy to treat individuals with PTS. Immune globulins are specialized proteins known as antibodies that are found in blood and other bodily fluids of animals. Antibodies are used by the immune system to fight foreign substances like bacteria and viruses. More research is necessary to determine the long-term safety and effectiveness of IVIG therapy for individuals with PTS.

Bottom Line Statement

PTS is a condition that usually presents suddenly with disabling pain and is often difficult to diagnose in its acute state. The pain is generally self-limiting, and the natural history of PTS leads to a generally favorable functional recovery. Early diagnosis with a good clinical evaluation, electrodiagnostics, and relevant imaging can allow for aggressive short-term pain management, help outline proper therapy, and provide comfort to both patient and physician in establishing a diagnosis. Proper diagnosis can also avoid unnecessary additional testing or surgical exploration. Limited follow-up EMG testing can be useful in demonstrating early electrodiagnostic signs of recovery which can precede clinical evidence of recovery. This finding can help alleviate the patient's psychological concerns about their disability and functional recovery and also provide the treating medical team with information regarding the patient's prognosis and, ultimately, recovery.

Medico-Legal Traps

Misdiagnosis Due to Postoperative Presentation

- Parsonage-Turner Syndrome (PTS) can easily be mistaken for complications related to surgical positioning, anesthesia, or normal postoperative recovery due to its presentation with severe shoulder pain and weakness following surgery. Misdiagnosing it as a surgical complication may delay appropriate treatment, leading to prolonged disability.
- **Thumb Rule Consideration:** Always consider PTS as a differential diagnosis in postoperative patients presenting with severe shoulder pain and neurological deficits, especially when symptoms do not correlate with typical surgical complications.

Failure to Recognize Vaccine or Infection-Related Onset

- PTS can be triggered by vaccinations, infections, or even minor trauma, yet this is often overlooked. Failure to link these antecedent events to the onset of PTS can result in delayed diagnosis and treatment, increasing the risk of prolonged suffering.
- **Thumb Rule Consideration:** In patients presenting with acute shoulder

pain and weakness, always review recent medical history, including vaccinations, infections, and minor injuries, to rule out PTS as a potential diagnosis.

Inadequate Pain Management

- The pain of PTS can be severe and unresponsive to typical analgesics like opioids. Failure to properly manage the intense pain may lead to unnecessary suffering, psychological distress, and even suicide. Legal issues may arise if pain is inadequately treated or if the patient is not hospitalized when necessary.
- **Thumb Rule Consideration:** Aggressively manage PTS pain with a multidisciplinary approach, including non-opioid analgesics, nerve blocks, or advanced therapies like IVIG, and consider hospitalization for severe cases.

Overuse of Unnecessary Surgical or Diagnostic Procedures

- Misdiagnosis of PTS as a structural or mechanical issue can lead to unnecessary imaging, exploratory surgeries, or invasive diagnostic procedures, which may cause further harm to the patient. This mismanagement can result in legal claims of medical malpractice.
- **Thumb Rule Consideration:** Utilize a thorough clinical evaluation, electromyography (EMG), and focused imaging early to establish a diagnosis of PTS, avoiding unnecessary surgeries or tests.

Failure to Reassure and Manage Expectations

- PTS often leads to prolonged functional impairment, and patients may experience anxiety about their prognosis. Failure to provide clear communication about the natural course of the condition and expected recovery can result in dissatisfaction and potential litigation.
- **Thumb Rule Consideration:** Regularly update patients on their prognosis and recovery expectations, and use follow-up EMG testing to monitor progress, providing psychological reassurance and reducing unnecessary anxiety.

REFERENCES

- Allan SG, Towla HMA, Smith CC, Downie AW. Painful brachial plexopathy: an unusual presentation of polyarteritis nodosa. Postgrad Med J. 1982;58:311–313.
- Allen IM. The neurological complication of serum treatment. Lancet. 1931;2:1128–1131. doi: 10.1016/S0140-6736(00)78218-3.
- Anderton JM, Schady W, Markham DE. An unusual case of postoperative brachial palsy. B J Anaesth. 1994;72:605.
- Cape CA, Fincham RW. Paralytic brachial neuritis with diaphragmatic paralysis; contralateral recurrence.

Neurology. 1965;15:191–193.

- Dubinsky RM, Kabbani H, El-Chami Z, et al. Practice parameter: treatment of postherpetic neuralgia: an evidence-based report of the Quality Standards Subcommittee of the American Academy of Neurology. Neurology. 2004;63:959–965.
- Mileto A, Gaeta M: Calcific tendonitis of supraspinatus simulating acute brachial neuritis (Parsonage-Turner syndrome), Clin Radiol 66:578–581, 2011.
- Schreiber AL, Abramov R, Fried GW, Herbison GJ. Expanding the differential of shoulder pain: Parsonage-Turner syndrome. J Am Osteopath Assoc. 2009;109:415-422.

PECTORALIS MAJOR TEAR SYNDROME

Injuries of the pectoralis major muscle are rare. Although the injury typically occurs while lifting weights, specifically while performing a bench press, it has also been known to occur in several other sports. Several factors, including delay in care and recognition of the injury, can delay appropriate treatment and result in worse outcomes for the patient. Specific treatment of this injury depends on the severity of the injury, the patient's activity level, and daily living needs.

ElMaraghy AW, Devereaux MW. A systematic review and comprehensive classification of pectoralis major tears. J Shoulder Elbow Surg. 2012 Mar;21(3):412-22.

Clinical Description

Tears and/or ruptures of the pectoralis major muscle are rare, with only 400 noted cases in the literature. They are becoming increasingly more common and almost exclusively occur in otherwise healthy males between the ages of 20 and 40 years old. This increase is potentially a result of greater participation in bodybuilding and weightlifting training. The majority of injuries take place at the musculotendinous junction, with only a small percentage occurring in the muscle belly. Injuries occur with excessive tension on a maximally eccentrically contracted muscle. The muscle is typically extended, abducted, and externally rotated during the downward deceleration phase of the bench press exercise. The inferior fibers of the sternal head are maximally stretched during the final 30 degrees of humeral extension and thus the most vulnerable to rupture in this position (i.e. final stage of bench press). Tears/ruptures occur in four locations: humeral insertion musculotendinous junction (muscle belly muscle tearing off the sternum (very rare). Patients will describe a "sharp tearing sensation" or an audible snap/pop during resisted adduction and internal rotation.

There has been some association between increased risk of rupture and anabolic steroid use, with the weakening of tendons becoming a contributing factor. However, this injury can occur in individuals who do not use anabolic steroids.

Iatrogenic injury to the pectoralis major tendon can also occur during rotator cuff repair.

Pearls & Oysters

Presentation to a healthcare provider often gets delayed as patients treat the injury like a typical strain or sprain. A pectoralis major tear can be more difficult to detect after the initial pain and swelling have subsided. Persistent weakness and asymmetry after the resolution of the initial symptoms usually suggest a more severe injury. In contrast, an acute pectoralis major tear may be more challenging to detect due to swelling, an intact fascial covering, or the overlying and uninjured clavicular head obstructing a palpable or visible defect.

Bottom Line Statement

Pectoralis major tears are rare injuries, and there may be a delay in the presentation to the emergency department or primary care provider. To improve the morbidity of the disorder, an interprofessional team approach is a recommendation. Healthcare practitioners should order an MRI if a pectoralis major tear is suspected. The patient should obtain a referral to a sports physician, orthopedic surgeon, or rehabilitation specialist. Early diagnosis and treatment are important as chronic injuries may lead to more technically difficult surgery and suboptimal outcomes. The pain may need to be managed by the practitioner. Patients need to be educated on the adverse effects of analgesics and should opt for non-pharmacological measures like ice, massage, and acupressure. For those who are young, active, and want a faster recovery, referral to an orthopedic surgeon is the proper course. The recovery after conservative treatment is often long; after surgery, the recovery is faster, but there is always the risk of complications. Irrespective of the approach, the patient should be encouraged to seek physical therapy. The outcomes in most patients are good. Orthopedic specialty-trained nurses can assist with either surgical or conservative care, and act as a bridge between physical therapists and rehabilitation specialists and the surgeon. All members of the interprofessional healthcare team must communicate and have access to the same level of information regarding the case to drive optimal patient outcomes.

Medico-Legal Traps

Delay in Diagnosis and Initial Treatment

- Pectoralis major tears often present late, as patients may mistake the injury for a strain or sprain. Missing the diagnosis early can result in worse outcomes, especially in athletes. The delay may complicate surgical repairs and lead to suboptimal results.
- **Thumb Rule Consideration:** Always consider a pectoralis major tear in patients with acute shoulder pain, particularly those involved in weightlifting or other high-tension activities. Use MRI promptly to confirm the diagnosis.

Failure to Educate on Non-Pharmacological Pain Management

- Focusing solely on pharmacological interventions, particularly opioids, without adequate patient education on alternative pain management can lead to unnecessary medication use, increased risk of addiction, or complications.
- **Thumb Rule Consideration:** Emphasize non-pharmacological pain relief measures such as ice, physical therapy, massage, and acupressure in managing pectoralis major tear pain. Only prescribe analgesics when necessary and monitor their use closely.

Inadequate Postoperative Rehabilitation

- Failing to implement proper rehabilitation following surgical or non-surgical treatment can delay recovery and impact long-term outcomes. This can also lead to legal claims if patients perceive a lack of care coordination.
- **Thumb Rule Consideration:** Ensure that patients are referred to physical therapy early and receive a structured rehabilitation plan, with close follow-up from both physical therapists and orthopedic surgeons.

Overlooking Risks Associated with Anabolic Steroid Use

- Patients using anabolic steroids are at higher risk for tendon injuries. Ignoring this factor during the evaluation or failure to counsel patients on the dangers of steroids can result in recurrent injuries and potential legal issues.
- **Thumb Rule Consideration:** Screen all patients for anabolic steroid use during the initial evaluation and educate them on the associated risks, including increased tendon fragility.

Inadequate Informed Consent Regarding Surgical Risks

- Failure to properly inform patients about the risks associated with surgical repair, such as complications, possible nonunion, or long-term functional limitations, can result in medico-legal repercussions if outcomes are poor.
- **Thumb Rule Consideration:** Provide detailed informed consent that outlines all potential risks of surgery, including complications and the possibility of incomplete recovery, ensuring patients have realistic expectations.

REFERENCES

- ElMaraghy AW, Devereaux MW. A systematic review and comprehensive classification of pectoralis major tears. J Shoulder Elbow Surg. 2012 Mar;21(3):412-22.
- Wolfe SW, Wickiewicz TL, Cavanaugh JT. Ruptures of the pectoralis major muscle. An anatomic and clinical analysis. Am J Sports Med. 1992 Sep-Oct;20(5):587-93.
- de Castro Pochini A, Andreoli CV, Belangero PS, Figueiredo EA, Terra BB, Cohen C, Andrade Mdos S, Cohen M, Ejnisman B. Clinical considerations for the surgical treatment of pectoralis major muscle ruptures based on 60 cases: a prospective study and literature review. Am J Sports Med. 2014 Jan;42(1):95-102.

- Haley CA, Zacchilli MA. Pectoralis major injuries: evaluation and treatment. Clin Sports Med. 2014 Oct;33(4):739-56.
- Petilon J, Carr DR, Sekiya JK, Unger DV. Pectoralis major muscle injuries: evaluation and management. J Am Acad Orthop Surg. 2005 Jan-Feb;13(1):59-68.
- Zeman SC, Rosenfeld RT, Lipscomb PR. Tears of the pectoralis major muscle. Am J Sports Med. 1979 Nov-Dec;7(6):343-7.
- Kircher J, Ziskoven C, Patzer T, Zaps D, Bittersohl B, Krauspe R. Surgical and nonsurgical treatment of total rupture of the pectoralis major muscle in athletes: update and critical appraisal. Open Access J Sports Med. 2010 Oct 11;1:201-5.
- Schepsis AA, Grafe MW, Jones HP, Lemos MJ. Rupture of the pectoralis major muscle. Outcome after repair of acute and chronic injuries. Am J Sports Med. 2000 Jan-Feb;28(1):9-15.
- Äärimaa V, Rantanen J, Heikkilä J, Helttula I, Orava S. Rupture of the pectoralis major muscle. Am J Sports Med. 2004 Jul-Aug;32(5):1256-62.

PES ANSERINE BURSITIS

The pes anserine describes a region where tendinous structures of the semitendinosus, gracilis, and sartorius muscles join to insert at the medial knee. The pes anserine bursa is sandwiched between the proximal medial tibia and the insertion point of the 3 tendons. Pes anserine bursitis is a clinical entity associated with pain at the medial knee and upper tibial region.

Alvarez-Nemegyei J, Canoso JJ. Evidence-Based Soft Tissue Rheumatology IV: Anserine Bursitis. J Clin Rheumatol. 2004 Aug;10(4):205-6.

Clinical Description

Bursitis is the general term used to describe inflammation of any bursa. The bursae are cavitary structures lined with synovial tissue that cushions and assists during the motion of joints and muscles. Bursitis is usually accompanied by tenderness; however, swelling and redness may also be present.

Pes anserine bursitis is a clinical entity associated with pain at the medial knee and the proximal medial tibial region. A more generic term, pes anserine pain syndrome, has been applied to refer to medial knee pain, which may or may not include inflammation of the bursal sac.

Sartorius, gracilis, and semitendinous tendons insert roughly 5 cm distal to the medial knee joint line forming a structure that mimics the natatory membrane of the goose and hence is called "goosefoot" or pes anserinus in Latin. The 3 muscles are primary knee flexors and play a secondary role in tibial internal rotation with a resultant protective effect against rotation and valgus stress. There are thirteen bursae around the knee, one of them is the pes anserinus bursa. The pes anserinus bursa is situated immediately beneath the pes anserinus separating it from the upper medial tibia. Usually, there is no communication between the pes anserinus bursa and the knee joint.

In 1937, Moschcowitz was the first to describe pes anserinus bursitis changes when he reported the complaint of knee pain almost exclusively in females with pain complaint with ascending or descending stairs or rising from a seated position or difficulty with knee flexion. It is challenging to differentiate between pes anserine bursitis and tendinitis as both the tendons and bursa are anatomically close to each other. However, management is the same.

Pearls & Oysters

Complications of pes anserine bursitis are rare but usually result from a lack of treatment. These can include increased pain and inflammation, with a subsequent weakening of the muscles and tendons around the knee joint.

Pes anserine bursitis refers specifically to the inflammatory condition of the bursal sac located between the muscular tendons (sartorius, gracilis, and semitendinosus) and their insertion at the proximal medial tibia. These three muscles act to help in the "cross-legged" position. Thus, any repetitive activity that requires this form of motion may exacerbate the symptoms of the condition.

Underlying osteoarthritis, obesity, and the female gender are risk factors for developing this syndrome.

Treatment of pes anserine bursitis is generally supportive with steroid injections reserved for refractory cases.

Bottom Line Statement

Patients with pes anserine bursitis may be seen in all practice settings from outpatient offices, urgent care centers, and emergency departments. Referral to a specialist is not often needed unless the patient has another underlying condition that may be causing this syndrome or if there is unrelenting discomfort despite supportive measures.

Most data on diagnosis and treatment of pes anserine is derived from case series, relying heavily on expert opinions for direction and care goals. An interprofessional team approach will result in the best outcomes.

Medico-Legal Traps

Failure to Differentiate Between Bursitis and Tendinitis

- Pes anserine bursitis and tendinitis are anatomically close and share similar symptoms, making diagnosis challenging. Misdiagnosis can lead to ineffective treatment or prolonged patient suffering.
- **Thumb Rule Consideration:** Perform a thorough clinical evaluation, considering imaging or diagnostic ultrasound if necessary, to distinguish between tendinitis and bursitis for appropriate management.

Inadequate Attention to Underlying Risk Factors

- Obesity, osteoarthritis, and the female gender are common risk factors for pes anserine bursitis. Ignoring these underlying conditions may result in incomplete treatment and recurrence of symptoms.
- **Thumb Rule Consideration:** Always assess for and address contributing factors such as obesity and underlying osteoarthritis, using a multidisciplinary approach for comprehensive management.

Overuse of Steroid Injections Without Conservative Therapy

- While steroid injections may provide relief, over-reliance on this treatment without trying conservative measures first can lead to complications such as weakening of tendons. This can also expose healthcare providers to liability if complications arise from repeated injections.
- **Thumb Rule Consideration:** Reserve steroid injections for refractory cases and prioritize conservative therapies like rest, ice, physical therapy, and NSAIDs in the initial treatment plan.

Delay in Diagnosis Due to Overlapping Symptoms with Other Knee Conditions

- The symptoms of pes anserine bursitis may mimic other conditions such as medial meniscus tears, osteoarthritis, or patellofemoral pain syndrome. Misattributing pain to these conditions can delay the correct diagnosis and treatment.
- **Thumb Rule Consideration:** Maintain a broad differential diagnosis for medial knee pain and use diagnostic tests like ultrasound or MRI if necessary to confirm pes anserine bursitis.

Lack of Patient Education and Prevention Strategies

- Failing to educate patients on the role of repetitive activities, poor posture, or improper exercise techniques in exacerbating the condition may lead to recurrent episodes of pain.
- **Thumb Rule Consideration:** Educate patients on proper body mechanics, weight loss, and activity modifications to prevent recurrence, and ensure they understand the importance of completing physical therapy for long-term recovery.

REFERENCES

- Alvarez-Nemegyei J, Canoso JJ. Evidence-Based Soft Tissue Rheumatology IV: Anserine Bursitis. J Clin Rheumatol. 2004 Aug;10(4):205-6.
- Hubbard MJ, Hildebrand BA, Battafarano MM, Battafarano DF. Common Soft Tissue Musculoskeletal Pain Disorders. Prim Care. 2018 Jun;45(2):289-303.
- Cohen SE, Mahul O, Meir R, Rubinow A. Anserine bursitis and non-insulin dependent diabetes mellitus. J Rheumatol. 1997 Nov;24(11):2162-5.
- Sapp GH, Herman DC. Pay Attention to the Pes Anserine in Knee Osteoarthritis. Curr Sports Med Rep. 2018 Feb;17(2):41.
- Safran MR, Fu FH. Uncommon causes of knee pain in the athlete. Orthop Clin North Am. 1995 Jul;26(3):547-59.
- Huang TW, Wang CJ, Huang SC. Polyethylene-induced pes anserinus bursitis mimicking an infected total knee arthroplasty: a case report and review of the literature. J Arthroplasty. 2003 Apr;18(3):383-6.
- Larsson LG, Baum J. The syndrome of anserina bursitis: an overlooked diagnosis. Arthritis Rheum. 1985 Sep;28(9):1062-5.

- Brookler MI, Mongan ES. Anserina bursitis. A treatable cause of knee pain in patients with degenerative arthritis. Calif Med. 1973 Jul;119(1):8-10.
- Alvarez-Nemegyei J, Peláez-Ballestas I, Goñi M, Julián-Santiago F, García-García C, Quintana R, Silvestre AM, García-Olivera I, Mathern NA, Loyola-Sanchez A, Conti S, Sanabria AJ, Pons-Estel BA. Prevalence of rheumatic regional pain syndromes in Latin-American indigenous groups: a census study based on COPCORD methodology and syndrome-specific diagnostic criteria. Clin Rheumatol. 2016 Jul;35 Suppl 1(Suppl 1):63-70.
- Gnanadesigan N, Smith RL. Knee pain: osteoarthritis or anserine bursitis? J Am Med Dir Assoc. 2003 May-Jun;4(3):164-6.
- Handy JR. Anserine bursitis: a brief review. South Med J. 1997 Apr;90(4):376-7.
- Larsson LG, Baum J. The syndromes of bursitis. Bull Rheum Dis. 1986;36(1):1-8.
- Helfenstein M, Kuromoto J. Anserine syndrome. Rev Bras Reumatol. 2010 May-Jun;50(3):313-27.
- Pompan DC. Pes Anserine Bursitis: An Underdiagnosed Cause of Knee Pain in Overweight Women. Am Fam Physician. 2016 Feb 01;93(3):170.
- Hemler DE, Ward WK, Karstetter KW, Bryant PM. Saphenous nerve entrapment caused by pes anserine bursitis mimicking stress fracture of the tibia. Arch Phys Med Rehabil. 1991 Apr;72(5):336-7.

POST–DURAL PUNCTURE HEADACHE

Postdural puncture headache is a potential complication of a lumbar puncture, with symptoms caused by traction on pain-sensitive structures from low cerebrospinal fluid pressure (intracranial hypotension) following a leak of cerebrospinal fluid at the puncture site. Symptoms of this condition include a bilateral frontal or occipital headache that is worse in the upright position, along with nausea, neck pain, dizziness, visual changes, tinnitius, hearing loss, or radicular symptoms in the arms.

Tubben RE, Jain S, Murphy PB. StatPearls [Internet]. StatPearls Publishing; Treasure Island (FL): Jul 4, 2022. Epidural Blood Patch.

Clinical Description

Postdural puncture headache (PDPH) is a potential expected complication of a lumbar puncture, with symptoms related to traction on pain-sensitive structures from low cerebrospinal fluid (CSF) pressure (intracranial hypotension) following a leak of CSF at the puncture site.

The symptoms of post–dural puncture headache begin almost immediately after the patient moves from a horizontal to an upright position. The intensity peaks within 1 or 2 minutes and abates within several minutes of the patient again assuming the horizontal position. The headache is pounding in character, and its intensity is severe, with the intensity increasing the longer the patient remains upright. The headache is almost always bilateral and located in the frontal, temporal, and occipital regions. Nausea and vomiting and dizziness frequently accompany the headache pain, especially if the patient remains upright for long periods. If cranial nerve palsy occurs, visual disturbance may occur.

Rarely, prolonged or severe cases can result in cerebral venous thrombosis, subdural hematoma from traction on dural veins, seizures, hypopituitarism, syringomyelia, herniation, coma, and death.

Pearls & Oysters

PDPH needs to be evaluated and diagnosed when symptomatic Mild symptoms may be managed conservatively whereas with severe symptoms, an EBP should be offered. A second EBP may be offered if the clinical history is clearly UDP related; other causes of HA need to be considered in the differential diagnosis. Post discharge, a telephone follow-up is essential with appropriate documentation in the medical record PDPH education should be provided to the parturient along with long-term follow-up for those with persistent headache.

Failure to recognize, diagnose, and treat post–dural puncture headache promptly may result in considerable pain and suffering for the patient. If the low cerebrospinal fluid pressure is allowed to persist, cranial nerve deficits may occur. In most instances, the cranial nerve deficits are temporary, but in rare instances, these deficits may become permanent, especially in patients with vulnerable nerves, such as those with diabetes. MRI of the brain is indicated in all patients thought to be suffering from headaches associated with dural puncture. Failure to diagnose central nervous system infection correctly can result in significant mortality and morbidity.

Bottom Line Statement

The most important consideration in preventing PDPH is the use of a small gauge, pencil-tipped, non-cutting spinal needle. There is no evidence to support supplemental fluid or bedrest following procedure to prevent PDPH. Intravenous aminophylline, adrenocorticotrophic hormone (ACTH), or epidural morphine may reduce the incidence of PDPH, but further investigation is needed to prove efficacy.

PDPH can lead to longer hospitilizations and higher healthcare costs. Many measures have been suggested to help prevent the disorder but, thus far, none have been shown to be effective in randomized, controlled trials. The use of ultrasound does show promise as it can accurately predict the depth of the epidural space but until randomized studies are done, the utility of ultrasound remains academic.

Many pharmaceutical agents have been investigated for prevention of PDPH but, so far, most have not lowered the risk of the condition. There even remains controversy about prophylactic bed rest and hydration prior to the procedure.

Medico-Legal Traps

Failure to Diagnose Early and Properly

- PDPH can be misdiagnosed as tension headaches, migraines, or other neurological conditions due to overlapping symptoms. A delay in proper diagnosis can result in prolonged patient suffering and increase the risk of complications such as cranial nerve deficits.
- **Thumb Rule Consideration:** Always suspect PDPH in patients presenting with positional headaches following lumbar puncture or epidural anesthesia, and promptly investigate.

Inappropriate Needle Selection During Lumbar Puncture

- The use of larger, cutting needles increases the risk of dural puncture and subsequent CSF leakage, leading to PDPH. Inadequate precautions during the procedure can be grounds for negligence.
- **Thumb Rule Consideration:** Use small-gauge, pencil-point needles to minimize the risk of dural puncture and subsequent PDPH, and follow best practices for technique.

Failure to Recognize or Treat Severe Cases Promptly

- Severe, untreated PDPH can lead to complications like cerebral venous thrombosis, subdural hematoma, or cranial nerve palsies, which could have been avoided with timely intervention.
- **Thumb Rule Consideration:** Offer an epidural blood patch (EBP) as soon as conservative measures fail in moderate to severe cases, and monitor for complications such as nerve palsy or subdural hematoma.

Inadequate Patient Education Post-Procedure

- Failure to inform patients about the possibility of PDPH and its symptoms could result in delayed care-seeking behavior, worsening the condition. This could expose healthcare providers to claims of poor informed consent.
- **Thumb Rule Consideration:** Thoroughly educate patients post-procedure about the signs of PDPH, emphasizing the importance of reporting symptoms early for appropriate management.

Lack of Documentation and Follow-Up

- Inadequate documentation of the procedure, patient complaints, and follow-up care can result in medico-legal complications, especially if the patient develops long-term issues.•
- **Thumb Rule Consideration:** Document every step of the procedure, including needle type, patient education, follow-up calls, and any interventions made for PDPH. Ensure robust follow-up protocols to monitor patient recovery.

REFERENCES

- Goldszmidt E, Kern R, Chaput A, Macarthur A. The incidence and etiology of postpartum headaches: a prospective cohort study. Can J Anaesth. Nov 2005;52(9):971-7.
- Vincent RD, Jr., Chestnut DH. Epidural analgesia during labor. Am Fam Physician. Nov 15 1998;58(8):1785-92.
- Ranganathan P, Golfeiz C, Phelps AL, et al. Chronic headache and backache are long-term sequelae of unintentional dural puncture in the obstetric population. J Clin Anesth. May 2015;27(3):201-6. doi:10.1016/j.jclinane.2014.
- Wu C, Lian Y, Guan D, Wang L, Miao Y, Xie N, Chen Y, Zheng Y. A Multicenter Clinical Study on Treating

Post-Dural Puncture Headache with an Intravenous Injection of Aminophylline. Pain Physician. 2016 Jul;19(5):E761-5.

- Basurto Ona X, Osorio D, Bonfill Cosp X. Drug therapy for treating post-dural puncture headache. Cochrane Database Syst Rev. 2015 Jul 15;(7):CD007887.

POSTERIOR TIBIAL TENDINITIS

Posterior tibial tendon dysfunction is the most common cause of adult acquired flatfoot. Degenerative changes in this tendon, lead to pain and weakness and if not identified and treated will progress to deformity of the foot and degenerative changes in the surrounding joints. Patients will complain of medial foot pain, weakness, and a slowly progressive foot deformity. A "too many toes" sign may be present and patients will be unable to perform a single heal raise test. Investigations such X-ray, ultrasound and magnetic resonance imaging will help stage the disease and decide on management. The optimal manage may change based on the progression of deformity and stage of disease. Early identification and prompt initiation of treatment can halt progression of the disease.

J Family Med Prim Care. 2015 Jan-Mar; 4(1): 26–29.

Clinical Description

Posterior tibial tendon dysfunction is the most common cause of adult acquired flatfoot disease. The changes of advanced disease are obvious and have significant morbidity associated with it. Tendon degeneration, however, begins far before clinical disease is apparent. By detecting early posterior tibial tendon disease, progression may be halted with nonoperative means; if left to progress, surgical reconstruction with osteotomy and arthrodesis becomes necessary. The purpose of this article is to review the pathphysiology, clinical stages, investigations and treatment options for posterior tibial tendon dysfunction, so that general practitioners can easily identify early disease and initiate treatment before deformity sets.

Tibialis posterior originates from the posterolateral tibia, posteromedial fibula and interosseous membrane. It runs through the deep posterior compartment of the leg and its tendon passes behind the medial malleolus. Blood supply to the tendon is poorest in this area and is the most common site for rupture. Close to its insertion site the tendon splits into a main, plantar and recurrent components, with the main component inserting onto the navicular tuberosity, the plantar portion onto the second, third, fourth metatarsals, second and third cuneiforms and cuboid. The recurrent component attaches to the sustentaculum tali of the calcaneus.

Tibialis posterior acts as the primary dynamic stabilizer of the medial longitudinal arch and main inverter of the midfoot.[5,6] Its contraction also elevates the medial longitudinal arch, causing the hind foot and midfoot to become a rigid structure. This allows the gastrocnemius to act with greater efficiency during the gait cycle.

Johnson and Strom developed a classification scheme in 1989 to describe the stages of posterior tibial tendon dysfunction. Originally three stages were described, with Stage I having an intact tendon with inflammation, but no clinical deformity. Treatment at this stage is conservative, with tenosynovectomy and debridement for severe cases. In Stage II the tendon is ruptured or otherwise nonfunctional, resulting in a planovalgus deformity which is passively correctable. In Stage III the foot deformity is no longer correctable and osteoarthritis is seen in the subtalar joint. A fourth stage, added by Myerson, describes patients with a valgus tilt of the talus in the ankle joint with tibiotalar degeneration. Surgical correction of Stage III and IV involves fusion of one or more joints, including the subtalar, calcaneocuboid, talonavicular and ankle joints.

Pearls & Oysters

Weight bearing anteroposterior and lateral views of both feet, in addition to bilateral weight bearing ankle views, should be obtained. Changes may not be apparent on X-ray in the early stages but as the disease progresses, collapse of the medial longitudinal arch and joint degeneration may become evident.

Ultrasound is a quick, readily available, low-cost investigation which gives information about tendon size, degeneration and presence of fluid. Quality of results, however, can be ultrasonographer dependent.

Magnetic resonance imaging (MRI) is useful in detecting early changes within the tendon and for assessing joint degeneration in later disease.[25,28,29,30] Detecting early tendon changes and prompt initiation of nonoperative treatment may avert the need for surgery. MRI is also useful in more advanced stages of the disease, where precise delineation of joint degeneration plays a part in preoperative planning.

Bottom Line Statement

Posterior tibial tendon dysfunction characteristically is a slow onset condition mainly affecting middle-aged, obese women. Risk factors include obesity, hypertension, diabetes, steroid use and seronegative arthropathies. Patients may complain of pain and swelling around the medial ankle, difficulty mobilizing or exacerbation of an existing limp. Examination may show tenderness along the course of the tendon, difficulty performing a single heel raise or "too many toes" when feet are viewed standing from behind. X-ray and MRI can confirm diagnosis, help stage disease and assist in preoperative planning. The disease as an entity is under-recognized, and early stages of the disease can be misdiagnosed, but prompt treatment can prevent deformity and need for surgery.

Medico-Legal Traps

Failure to Diagnose Early Stage Disease

- Early-stage posterior tibial tendon dysfunction (Stage I) may be subtle and often missed, leading to progression to irreversible deformity and joint degeneration. Misdiagnosis or delayed diagnosis can result in worsened patient outcomes and potential legal claims.
- **Thumb Rule Consideration:** Suspect PTTD in middle-aged or older patients, especially women, presenting with medial ankle pain and difficulty mobilizing. Perform a thorough clinical exam and consider early imaging like ultrasound or MRI to catch early tendon degeneration.

Inadequate Use of Imaging

- Relying solely on standard X-rays may miss early-stage disease, as changes are often not visible until more advanced stages. Missing these early changes can lead to progression of the condition without timely intervention.
- **Thumb Rule Consideration:** Always include advanced imaging techniques such as MRI or ultrasound in cases of suspected PTTD, especially if early-stage disease is suspected and X-rays are normal.

Overlooking Nonoperative Treatment Options in Early Stages

- Early detection and prompt nonoperative treatment (e.g., orthotics, physical therapy, weight loss) can prevent progression of PTTD. Missing the window for conservative treatment may lead to legal issues for unnecessary progression to surgery.
- **Thumb Rule Consideration:** Prioritize conservative treatment in Stage I and early Stage II patients with tendon inflammation or rupture, before resorting to surgical interventions.

Failure to Consider Patient Risk Factors

- Not assessing risk factors like obesity, hypertension, diabetes, or steroid use may result in inappropriate treatment plans or complications. These conditions can exacerbate PTTD and influence the treatment approach.
- **Thumb Rule Consideration:** Always evaluate for systemic risk factors and address modifiable ones (e.g., obesity) alongside PTTD management to reduce progression and complication risks.

Inappropriate Surgical Decision-Making

- Premature surgical intervention or failure to provide surgery in severe cases (Stage III or IV) can result in either unnecessary morbidity or long-term deformity and disability. Misjudgment in surgical timing or choice may lead to patient harm and legal consequences.
- **Thumb Rule Consideration:** Reserve surgery for patients with advanced deformity (Stage III/IV) or failure of conservative management. Preoperative imaging is crucial for planning, particularly to assess joint degeneration and choose appropriate procedures.

REFERENCES

- GJohnson KA. Tibialis posterior tendon rupture. Clin Orthop Relat Res. 1983:140–7.
- Arangio GA, Salathe EP. A biomechanical analysis of posterior tibial tendon dysfunction, medial displacement calcaneal osteotomy and flexor digitorum longus transfer in adult acquired flat foot. Clin Biomech. 2009;24:385–90.
- Deland JT, de Asla RJ, Sung IH, Ernberg LA, Potter HG. Posterior tibial tendon insufficiency: Which ligaments are involved? Foot Ankle Int. 2005;26:427–35.
- Kohls-Gatzoulis J, Angel JC, Singh D, Haddad F, Livingstone J, Berry G. Tibialis posterior dysfunction: A common and treatable cause of adult acquired flatfoot. BMJ. 2004;329:1328–33.
- Myerson MS. Adult acquired flat foot deformity. J Bone Joint Surg. 1996;78A:780–92.
- Khazen G, Khazen C. Tendoscopy in stage I posterior tibial tendon dysfunction. Foot Ankle Clin. 2012;17:399–406.
- Myerson M, Solomon G, Shereff M. Posterior tibial tendon dysfunction: Its association with seronegative inflammatory disease. Foot Ankle. 1989;9:219–25.
- Geideman WM, Johnson JE. Posterior tibial tendon dysfunction. J Orthop Sports Phys Ther. 2000;30:68–77.
- Shereff MJ. Treatment of ruptured posterior tibial tendon with direct repair and FDL tenodesis. Foot Ankle Clin. 1997;2:281–96.
- Kong A, Van Der Vliet A. Imaging of tibialis posterior dysfunction. Br J Radiol. 2008;81:826–36.
- Miller SD, Van Holsbeeck M, Boruta PM, Wu KK, Katcherian DA. Ultrasound in the diagnosis of posterior tibial tendon pathology. Foot Ankle Int. 1996;17:555–8.

PRIMARY THUNDERCLAP HEADACHE

The term' thunderclap headache' (TCH) was coined by Day and Raskin in 1986. They discovered it in a patient suffering from an unruptured cerebral aneurysm who presented with multiple episodes of an abrupt onset of a severe form of headache, later labeled as a thunderclap headache. Thunderclap headache is defined as a severe form of headache that occurs abruptly, like a "clap of thunder," as suggested by the name, peaks within 30 seconds to 1 minute of the onset, and usually fades in the next few hours. The sufferers often describe it as the worst headache of their life.

Ravishankar K. Looking at "thunderclap headache" differently? Circa 2016. Ann Indian Acad Neurol. 2016 Jul-Sep;19(3):295-301.

Clinical Description

Thunderclap headache is an uncommon type of headache that may be the result of an underlying vascular or nonvascular intracranial abnormality or may represent a primary headache syndrome of unknown cause. The more benign, though no less painful, primary thunderclap headache occurs over three times more frequently than the serious secondary thunderclap headache. Because of the often-threatening causes of the less common secondary thunderclap headache (e.g., subarachnoid hemorrhage, cerebral venous thrombosis), urgent evaluation including computed tomography (CT) and/or magnetic resonance imaging of the brain and cerebrospinal fluid analysis are indicated in all patients suspected of having thunderclap headache.

One of the most severe headaches encountered in clinical practice, thunderclap headache is characterized by a very rapid onset to peak of less than 1 minute. The headache may last from 1 to 10 days and, because of its intensity, almost always provokes an urgent trip to the emergency department, where the headache is invariably initially misdiagnosed as the sentinel headache of acute subarachnoid hemorrhage or other potentially catastrophic headache syndromes. This is not surprising in that primary thunderclap headache is virtually indistinguishable clinically from subarachnoid hemorrhage, one of the most neurologically devastating forms of cerebrovascular accident. Thus, because of the serious consequences of misdiagnosis, by necessity primary thunderclap headache is a diagnosis of exclusion..

Pearls & Oysters

Complications and pitfalls in the diagnosis and treatment of primary thunderclap headache generally fall into three categories. The first category involves the failure to recognize a sentinel bleed associated with subarachnoid hemorrhage and evaluate and treat the patient before significant morbidity or mortality occurs. The second category involves misdiagnosis that results in unnecessary testing, in particular, cerebral angiography, which itself is associated with significant morbidity and rarely death. The third category involves iatrogenic morbidity and rarely mortality from the use of medications to treat primary thunderclap headache (e.g., triptans, ergots) that not only do not treat this primary headache syndrome but also have significant side effects.

Bottom Line Statement

Primary thunderclap headache is a diagnosis of exclusion. It is frequently misdiagnosed as the sentinel headache of subarachnoid hemorrhage, causing the treating physician to order urgent diagnostic testing, which is associated with its own significant mortality and morbidity. The lack of focal neurological findings in a patient with acute headache should point the clinician toward the diagnosis of benign primary headaches including primary thunderclap headache, cough headache, exertional headache atypical migraine, and headache associated with sexual activity. This does not mean that urgent computerized scanning of the brain and analysis of the patient's cerebrospinal fluid are not indicated.

Medico-Legal Traps

Failure to Differentiate Between Primary and Secondary Causes

- Thunderclap headaches can be caused by life-threatening conditions such as subarachnoid hemorrhage. Failure to differentiate between primary benign thunderclap headaches and secondary serious causes can lead to devastating outcomes, including untreated intracranial hemorrhage or aneurysm rupture.
- **Thumb Rule Consideration:** Always treat thunderclap headaches as potentially life-threatening until proven otherwise. Conduct urgent imaging and cerebrospinal fluid analysis to rule out secondary causes.

Misdiagnosis and Unnecessary Testing

- Primary thunderclap headache often mimics serious conditions, leading to unnecessary diagnostic procedures such as cerebral angiography, which carries risks of morbidity and mortality. Misdiagnosis can also result in a cascade of unnecessary testing and associated costs.
- **Thumb Rule Consideration:** If initial imaging (CT scan) and cerebrospinal fluid analysis are normal, and there are no focal neurological

signs, reconsider the need for more invasive testing like angiography. Proceed conservatively after excluding critical conditions.

Use of Inappropriate Medications

- Medications like triptans and ergots, often used to treat migraines, are ineffective for thunderclap headaches and can cause significant side effects such as vasoconstriction, which could exacerbate an underlying vascular condition.
- **Thumb Rule Consideration:** Avoid using triptans, ergots, or vasoconstrictive agents for treating primary thunderclap headaches until life-threatening vascular conditions have been excluded.

Delayed Diagnosis Leading to Patient Harm

- Delays in diagnosis can occur when patients presenting with thunderclap headache are not evaluated immediately with appropriate imaging or neurological assessment. This can result in missed diagnoses of critical conditions like subarachnoid hemorrhage, increasing the risk of severe morbidity or mortality.
- **Thumb Rule Consideration:** Rapid assessment and imaging (CT and lumbar puncture) should be initiated in all patients with sudden, severe headache, especially when described as the "worst headache of their life."

Overlooking Underlying Risk Factors

- Patients with thunderclap headaches may have underlying risk factors like aneurysms or vascular malformations that could complicate diagnosis. Failure to consider and investigate these risk factors appropriately can lead to serious legal consequences.
- **Thumb Rule Consideration:** Always investigate patient history for potential risk factors like aneurysms, vascular malformations, or prior history of headaches. Conduct thorough imaging and follow-up evaluations as necessary.

REFERENCES

- Anderson T: Current and evolving management of subarachnoid hemorrhage, Crit Care Nurs Clin North Am 21:529–539, 2009.
- Chih-Ming H, Ya-Ju L, Yang-Kai F, Shih-Pin C, Tzu-Hsien L: Isolated thunderclap headache during sex: orgasmic headache or reversible cerebral vasoconstriction syndrome? J Clin Neurosci 17:1349–1351, 2010.
- de Bruijn SFTM, Stam J, Kappelle LJ: CVST Study Group: Thunderclap headache as first symptom of cerebral venous sinus thrombosis, Lancet 348:1623–1625, 1996.
- Janardhan V, Biondi A, Riina HA, et al: Vasospasm in aneurysmal subarachnoid hemorrhage: diagnosis, prevention, and management, Neuroimaging Clin N Am 6:483–496, 2006.
- Linn FHH: Primary thunderclap headache. In: Aminoff MJ, editor: Handbook of clinical neurology, vol 97, New York, 2010, Elsevier, pp 473–481.

- Manno EM: Subarachnoid hemorrhage, Neurol Clin 22:347–366, 2004.
- Newfield P: Intracranial aneurysms: vasospasm and other issues. In Atlee JL, editor: Complications in anesthesia, ed 2, Philadelphia, 2007, Saunders, pp 719–723.
- Palestrant D, Connolly ES: Subarachnoid hemorrhage, Neurobiol Dis 265–270, 2007.

POSTMASTECTOMY PAIN

After having breast cancer surgery, some women have problems with nerve (neuropathic) pain in the chest wall, armpit, and/or arm that doesn't go away over time. This is called post-mastectomy pain syndrome (PMPS) because it was first noticed in women who had mastectomies, but it can also happen after other types of breast-conserving surgery (such as a lumpectomy).

Grossman SA, Nesbit S. Cancer-related Pain. In: Niederhuber JE, Armitage JO, Doroshow JH, Kastan MB, Tepper JE, eds. Abeloff's Clinical Oncology. 5th ed. Philadelphia: Elsevier, 2014:608-619.

Clinical Description

Postmastectomy pain syndrome (PMPS) is a type of neuropathic pain, a complex chronic pain state that is typically associated with nerve fiber injury. The pain is typically localized to the anterior/lateral chest wall, axilla, and/or medial upper arm and persists more than three months after surgery when all other causes of pain, such as infection or recurrence, have been eliminated. The characteristics include classic features of neuropathic pain such as burning, tingling, shooting, stinging, or stabbing pains and hyperesthesia.

The definition of PMPS has not been standardized. The current definition for PMPS used by the International Association for Study of Pain is "chronic pain in the anterior aspect of the thorax, axilla, and/or upper half of the arm beginning after mastectomy or quadrantectomy and persisting for more than three months after surgery". While some studies define PMPS as pain persisting for more than three months, and others define it as pain persisting for more than 18 months, the author of this topic defines PMPS as pain persisting for more than six months after breast surgery.

Studies have shown that between 20% and 30% of women develop symptoms of PMPS after surgery. It's most common after operations that remove tissue in the upper outside portion of the breast or the underarm area.

PMPS is thought to be linked to damage done to the nerves in the armpit and chest during surgery. But the causes are not known for sure. Women who are younger, who have had a full axillary lymph node dissection (ALND) and not just a sentinel lymph node biopsy, or who were treated with radiation after surgery are more likely to have problems with PMPS. Because ALND is done less often now, PMPS is less common than it once was.

Pearls & Oysters

Reliable diagnosis and identification of neuropathic pain, defined by the International Association for the Study of Pain as pain caused by lesioned or dysfunctional nerves, remains challenging. Four types of pain after breast cancer surgery were identified by a recent review of neuropathic pain in this population: Intercostabrachial neuralgia, neuroma pain, phantom pain and pain caused by other neuronal damage. Intercostabrachial neuralgia pain accompanies sensorial changes in the region of intercostabrachial nerve distribution. Neuroma pain stems from scar tissue in the breast, chest, or arm that is triggered by percussion.

Bottom Line Statement

PMPS is a common complication of breast cancer surgery that significantly affects daily life activities. Its prevalence becomes especially high (87.6%) if patients experiencing PMPS-like symptoms are included. The main risk factors for PMPS in this population were tumor localization in the upper lateral quadrant and secondary treatment with radiotherapy. Our survey strategy was modified to fit our study population, combining multiple surveys and accounting for education levels of by allowing verbal completion of surveys. Confirming these risk factors and identifying alterations in treatment strategies that reduce the incidence of PMPS will require prospective randomized controlled studies.

Medico-Legal Traps

Failure to Diagnose PMPS in a Timely Manner

- Postmastectomy pain is often underreported or mistaken for typical post-surgical discomfort, leading to delayed diagnosis and treatment. This delay can result in chronic pain and suffering for patients, with the potential for claims of negligence due to inadequate post-operative care.
- **Thumb Rule Consideration:** Always evaluate any pain persisting beyond three months after surgery for possible PMPS. Early identification is crucial to managing symptoms and improving outcomes.

Inadequate Informed Consent

- Patients may not be adequately informed about the risk of developing PMPS during discussions about breast cancer surgery. Failing to inform patients about this potential complication can result in legal claims of lack of informed consent.
- **Thumb Rule Consideration:** Ensure comprehensive pre-surgical

counseling includes a clear explanation of the potential risks of developing PMPS, especially in patients undergoing axillary lymph node dissection or radiation.

Mismanagement of Post-Operative Pain

- Chronic pain management in PMPS may be improperly handled if general practitioners are unfamiliar with the neuropathic nature of the condition, leading to the inappropriate use of pain management techniques like opioids, which are often ineffective for neuropathic pain.
- **Thumb Rule Consideration:** Utilize appropriate neuropathic pain treatments, such as gabapentin or tricyclic antidepressants, and refer patients to pain management specialists when necessary.

Failure to Document or Monitor Pain Symptoms

- A lack of thorough documentation or failure to monitor ongoing pain complaints can expose healthcare providers to medico-legal claims, especially if PMPS is not diagnosed early and leads to long-term complications.
- **Thumb Rule Consideration:** Maintain detailed records of all patient complaints related to post-surgical pain, and ensure regular follow-ups to assess for the development of PMPS.

Neglecting Psychological Impact

- PMPS is associated with significant psychological distress, yet this is often overlooked by healthcare providers. Ignoring the emotional and psychological aspects of chronic pain can result in claims of inadequate care.
- **Thumb Rule Consideration:** Always consider psychological support as part of the comprehensive treatment plan for PMPS, including referrals to mental health professionals when necessary to address anxiety, depression, or quality of life concerns.

REFERENCES

- Johannsen M, Christensen S, Zachariae R, Jensen AB. Socio-demographic, treatment-related, and health behavioral predictors of persistent pain 15 months and 7-9 years after surgery: a nationwide prospective study of women treated for primary breast cancer. Breast Cancer Res Treat. 2015;152(3):645-658.
- Leysen L, Beckwée D, Nijs J, et al. Risk factors of pain in breast cancer survivors: a systematic review and meta-analysis. Support Care Cancer. 2017;25(12):3607-3643.
- Wolff AC, Domcheck SM, Davidson ND, Sacchini V, McCormick B. Cancer of the Breast. In: Niederhuber JE, Armitage JO, Doroshow JH, Kastan MB, Tepper JE, eds. Abeloff's Clinical Oncology. 5th ed. Philadelphia: Elsevier, 2014:1630-1692.
- Gärtner R, Jensen MB, Nielsen J, et al. Prevalence of and factors associated with persistent pain following breast cancer surgery. JAMA 2009; 302:1985.

- Caviggioli F, Maione L, Forcellini D, et al. Autologous fat graft in postmastectomy pain syndrome. Plast Reconstr Surg 2011; 128:349.
- Stubblefield MD, Custodio CM. Upper-extremity pain disorders in breast cancer. Arch Phys Med Rehabil 2006; 87:S96.
- Smith WC, Bourne D, Squair J, et al. A retrospective cohort study of post mastectomy pain syndrome. Pain 1999; 83:91.
- Miguel R, Kuhn AM, Shons AR, et al. The effect of sentinel node selective axillary lymphadenectomy on the incidence of postmastectomy pain syndrome. Cancer Control 2001; 8:427.
- Caffo O, Amichetti M, Ferro A, et al. Pain and quality of life after surgery for breast cancer. Breast Cancer Res Treat 2003; 80:39.
- Tasmuth T, von Smitten K, Hietanen P, et al. Pain and other symptoms after different treatment modalities of breast cancer. Ann Oncol 1995; 6:453.
- Bokhari F, Sawatzky JA. Chronic neuropathic pain in women after breast cancer treatment. Pain Manag Nurs 2009; 10:197.

PROCTALGIA FUGAX

Proctalgia fugax or functional recurrent anorectal pain is part of a spectrum of functional gastrointestinal disorders defined by the Rome III diagnostic criteria as episodes of sharp fleeting pain that recur over weeks, are localized to the anus or lower rectum, and last from seconds to several minutes with no pain between episodes. There is no diurnal variation. There are numerous precipitants including sexual activity, stress, constipation, defecation and menstruation, although the condition can occur without a trigger. It should be differentiated from chronic proctalgia, a functional anorectal pain disorder with a vague, dull ache or pressure sensation high in the rectum, often worse when sitting than when standing or lying down, and lasts at least 20 minutes.

Bharucha AE, Wald A, Enck P, et al. Functional anorectal disorders. Gastroenterology 2006;130: 1510–8.

Clinical Description

The prevalence of proctalgia fugax in the general population may be as high as 8%–18%. Many patients present to primary health care physicians and often do not require further consultation because the symptoms are fleeting. This condition is more common among women than among men, and usually affects patients between 30 and 60 years of age. Although the cause of proctalgia fugax is unclear, spasm of the anal sphincter is commonly implicated. The condition may be more likely to occur after sclerotherapy for hemorrhoids and vaginal hysterectomy. There are also associations with other functional pathologies, such as irritable bowel syndrome and anxiety. Other causes of anorectal pain (e.g., hemorrhoids, cryptitis, ischemia, abscess, fissure, rectocele and malignant disease) must be excluded before the diagnosis can be made. Proctalgia fugax is estimated to affect 4 to 18 percent of the general population. However, only 17 to 20 percent of patients report their symptoms to a physician. Although proctalgia has been reported in adult patients ranging from 18 to 87 years of age, it usually affects individuals between 30 and 60 years of age. Proctalgia fugax is more common among female patients as compared with males.

Pearls & Oysters

The patient will complain of episodes of localized pain at the lower rectum and anus, the episode lasts for a second to minutes (20 minutes maximum) with no pain between episodes. Symptoms may occur once per month, with no factors that trigger symptoms, however, anxiety and stress may induce symptoms. Symptoms like; nausea, vomiting, sweating, and dizziness are rare. Episodes occur at irregular intervals and are unpredicted. In a study the intervals range from 1-180 times/ year, another study demonstrated the recurrence of proctalgia fugax less than 5 times/ year in 51% of patients.

Bottom Line Statement

It is a transitory disorder that usually does not need further investigations and can be treated by a primary health care physician. It is difficult to detect its prevalence as the patient does not seek a doctor's help unless the symptoms become severe it represents about 8- 18% and is more common among women than men between 30 and 60 years most affected age.

Abnormal smooth muscle contraction and the increase in anal pressure were suggested to be the cause of pain sensation, because the intermittent, infrequent, and the short duration of the pain associated with proctalgia fugax make identifying its mechanism difficult. The definite causes of proctalgia are still unclear but first, exclusion of any pelvic or anorectal pathophysiology is important. Proctalgia fugax is common after vaginal hysterectomy, sclerotherapy for hemorrhoids, and intramuscular abscess. Anxiety, stressful conditions, and irritable bowel syndrome in addition to an abscess, anal fissure, or hypertrophy of the internal anal sphincter.

Medico-Legal Traps

Failure to Rule Out Other Serious Anorectal Pathologies

- Proctalgia fugax can mimic other serious conditions like anal fissures, hemorrhoids, or malignancies. If these are not ruled out through appropriate investigation, there is a risk of misdiagnosis, leading to delayed treatment of more serious conditions.
- **Thumb Rule Consideration:** Always perform a thorough anorectal examination and consider further investigation to exclude other potential pathologies before diagnosing proctalgia fugax.

Mismanagement Due to Lack of Diagnosis

- Because proctalgia fugax presents with fleeting symptoms, healthcare providers may dismiss or overlook the condition, leading to inadequate management. This could result in patient dissatisfaction and potential claims of negligence.
- **Thumb Rule Consideration:** Take patient complaints of episodic anorectal pain seriously and document symptom patterns, even if the pain is brief, to ensure appropriate follow-up and management.

Inadequate Patient Education and Communication

- Patients may be alarmed by the sudden, severe pain associated with proctalgia fugax. Failure to adequately educate patients about the benign nature of the condition can lead to anxiety, unnecessary visits to the emergency department, and potential claims of insufficient communication.
- **Thumb Rule Consideration:** Provide clear and thorough explanations to patients about the episodic and benign nature of proctalgia fugax, and reassure them while outlining management strategies.

Failure to Address Triggering Factors

- Stress, anxiety, and other functional gastrointestinal disorders like irritable bowel syndrome (IBS) may exacerbate symptoms of proctalgia fugax. Ignoring these potential triggers can worsen patient outcomes and result in dissatisfaction with treatment.
- **Thumb Rule Consideration:** Identify and address potential triggers such as stress or concurrent gastrointestinal issues, and consider a multidisciplinary approach involving stress management techniques if appropriate.

Over-Treatment or Unnecessary Investigations

- Since proctalgia fugax symptoms are usually self-limited and benign, unnecessary imaging or invasive procedures may be performed if the condition is misinterpreted, increasing patient costs and procedural risks.•
- **Thumb Rule Consideration:** Avoid over-investigating mild cases of proctalgia fugax unless symptoms are severe or atypical, and focus on reassurance and conservative management.

REFERENCES

- Whitehead WE, Wald A, Diamant NE, et al. Functional disorders of the anus and rectum. Gut 1999; 45(Suppl 2):II55–9
- Boyce PM, Talley NJ, Burke C, et al. Epidemiology of the functional gastrointestinal disorders diagnosed according to Rome II criteria: an Australian population-based study. Intern Med J 2006; 36:28–36 [
- Bharucha AE, Trabuco E. Functional and chronic anorectal and pelvic pain disorders. Gastroenterol Clin North Am 2008;37:685–96
- Jeyarajah S, Chow A, Ziprin P, et al. Proctalgia fugax, an evidence-based management pathway. Int J Colorectal Dis 2010;25:1037–46.
- Drossman DA, Li Z, Andruzzi E, Temple RD, Talley NJ, Thompson WG, et al. U.S. householder survey of functional gastrointestinal disorders. Prevalence, sociodemography, and health impact. Dig Dis Sci. 1993;38(9):1569–80.
- Celik AF, Katsinelos P, Read NW, Khan MI, Donnelly TC. Hereditary proctalgia fugax and constipation: report of a second family. Gut. 1995 Apr 1;36(4):581-4.
- de Parades V, Etienney I, Bauer P, Taouk M, Atienza P. Proctalgia fugax: demographic and clinical characteristics. What every doctor should know from a prospective study of 54 patients. Diseases of the colon & rectum. 2007 Jun;50(6):893-8.

PRONATOR TERES SYNDROME

Pronator teres syndrome (PTS), first described by Henrik Seyffarth in 1951, is caused by a compression of the median nerve (MN) by the pronator teres (PT) muscle in the forearm. The PT muscle is named because of its action and shape; it is a rounded muscle that pronates. In the majority of cases (66%), it arises from unequal two heads: the larger humeral head from the upper part of the medial epicondyle and the smaller ulnar head from the coronoid process of the ulna. They pass down to the forearm, form a common flexor tendon, and insert into the radial shaft. Before the two heads unite, the median nerve passes between them in 74% to 82% of the cases, innervating both heads from C6-7 roots. The absence of the ulnar head is rare (14%) and may reduce the risk of median nerve entrapment.

Lacey SH, Soldatis JJ. Bilateral pronator syndrome associated with anomalous heads of the pronator teres muscle: a case report. J Hand Surg Am. 1993 Mar;18(2):349-51.

Clinical Description

Pronator teres syndrome (PTS), first described by Henrik Seyffarth in 1951, is caused by a compression of the median nerve (MN) by the pronator teres (PT) muscle in the forearm. The PT muscle is named because of its action and shape; it is a rounded muscle that pronates the forearm. In the majority of cases (66%), it arises from unequal two heads: the larger humeral head from the upper part of the medial epicondyle and the smaller ulnar head from the coronoid process of the ulna. They pass down to the forearm, form a common flexor tendon, and insert into the radial shaft. Before the two heads unite, the median nerve passes between them in 74% to 82% of the cases, innervating both heads from C6-7 roots. The absence of the ulnar head is rare (14%) and may reduce the risk of median nerve entrapment. Many individuals have additional fibrous brands within the two heads of the PT muscle. The anterior interosseous nerve (AIN) then branches from the MN about 5 to 8 cm distal to the medial epicondyle.

Pearls & Oysters

Complications of surgical treatment are rare. In one study of 72 patients treated with pronator teres syndrome, no complications were recorded during the operations with an overall postoperative satisfaction rate (very satisfied and satisfied) of 59%. Theoretical complications from surgery include: Infection; Seroma/hematoma formation; Nerve injury; Scar formation.

When considering conservative treatment, patients should be advised on minimizing their engagement of activities that involve frequent forearm pronation. These activities include: Hammering; Ladling food; Cleaning dishes; Playing tennis; Pouring drinks (an activity frequently performed by waitresses/bartenders); Carrying books (an activity frequently performed by librarians); Twisting of clothes.

Bottom Line Statement

Pronator teres syndrome can be often misdiagnosed as it shares symptoms with more common carpal tunnel syndrome. The etiology may vary, and it may affect various people ranging from a patient with multiple comorbidities (e.g., hemodialysis) to healthy individuals who are involved in sports or other physical activities requiring repetitive pronation movements of the forearm as well as people with specific anatomic variations of the elbow region. Different specialists may encounter patients with pronator teres syndrome including urgent care medical professionals, primary care physicians, sports physicians, and others. The role of a physiatrist or a neurologist who specializes in neuromuscular conditions and performs NCV/EMG studies is crucial in the diagnosis and treatment of this condition. The radiologist also plays a role in diagnosing pronator teres syndrome, but he/she will need proper guidance from the referring specialist. Physical and occupational therapists manage conservative treatment, but if it fails, the surgeon gets involved. Thus it takes an interprofessional group of specialists to manage patients with pronator teres syndrome. Existing evidence regarding pronator teres syndrome is inadequate.

Medico-Legal Traps

Failure to Differentiate from Carpal Tunnel Syndrome

- PTS shares several symptoms with the more common carpal tunnel syndrome, often leading to misdiagnosis. This can delay appropriate treatment and increase the risk of chronic pain or disability.
- **Thumb Rule Consideration:** Always differentiate PTS from carpal tunnel syndrome by evaluating forearm pain during pronation, weakness, and lack of nighttime symptoms, and consider EMG/NCV studies for precise diagnosis.

Inadequate Pre-Surgical Evaluation

- Surgical intervention in PTS may be recommended prematurely without fully exploring conservative management options, such as physical therapy and lifestyle modifications. This can lead to avoidable complications and legal implications if surgery fails or causes harm.

- **Thumb Rule Consideration:** Exhaust conservative treatment options, including physical therapy and activity modification, before considering surgical intervention.

Complications from Surgery

- Surgical treatment for PTS, while rare, can lead to complications such as infection, nerve injury, or scar formation, especially if postoperative care is inadequate.
- **Thumb Rule Consideration:** Ensure comprehensive preoperative counseling, informing patients about potential risks, and meticulously follow postoperative protocols to prevent complications.

Delayed Diagnosis Due to Subtle Symptoms

- Pronator teres syndrome often presents with vague symptoms, leading to a delay in diagnosis and treatment. This may result in worsening of the condition or mismanagement, increasing legal liability.
- **Thumb Rule Consideration:** Maintain a high index of suspicion in patients with repetitive forearm pronation activities and persistent pain, and promptly refer for diagnostic studies like EMG/NCV when symptoms persist.

Overlooking Anatomical Variations

- Variations such as an absent ulnar head of the pronator teres or additional fibrous bands can influence the severity of nerve entrapment, but these are often overlooked in treatment planning. This oversight can lead to suboptimal outcomes in both conservative and surgical treatment.
- **Thumb Rule Consideration:** Always account for anatomical variations when diagnosing and planning treatment for PTS, using imaging studies like MRI or ultrasound if necessary.

REFERENCES

- SEYFFARTH H. Primary myoses in the M. pronator teres as cause of lesion of the N. medianus (the pronator syndrome). Acta Psychiatr Neurol Scand Suppl. 1951;74:251-4.
- Olewnik Ł, Podgórski M, Polguj M, Wysiadecki G, Topol M. Anatomical variations of the pronator teres muscle in a Central European population and its clinical significance. Anat Sci Int. 2018 Mar;93(2):299-306.
- Vymazalová K, Vargová L, Joukal M. Variability of the pronator teres muscle and its clinical significance. Rom J Morphol Embryol. 2015;56(3):1127-35.
- Nebot-Cegarra J, Perez-Berruezo J, Reina de la Torre F. Variations of the pronator teres muscle: predispositional role to median nerve entrapment. 1991-1992Arch Anat Histol Embryol. 74:35-45.
- Hsiao CW, Shih JT, Hung ST. Concurrent carpal tunnel syndrome and pronator syndrome: A retrospective study of 21 cases. Orthop Traumatol Surg Res. 2017 Feb;103(1):101-103.
- Hartz CR, Linscheid RL, Gramse RR, Daube JR. The pronator teres syndrome: compressive neuropathy of the median nerve. J Bone Joint Surg Am. 1981 Jul;63(6):885-90.
- Afshar A. Pronator Syndrome Due to Schwannoma. J Hand Microsurg. 2015 Jun;7(1):119-22.

PROSTATODYNIA

Prostatodynia is a clinical entity associated with voiding symptoms and pelvic pain suggestive of prostatitis but with a normal prostate examination and without evidence of inflammation or infection in expressed prostatic secretions. The problem tends to be chronic and is vexing in its management. Although thought to be a common condition, prevalence data are generally lacking.

Mil Med. 1997 Jun;162(6):380-3.

Clinical Description

The term chronic pelvic pain syndrome (CPPS) is used to designate unexplained chronic pelvic pain in men. This pain is associated with irritative voiding symptoms and/or pain in the groin, genitalia, or perineum in the absence of pyuria and bacteriuria (no pus cells or bacteria seen on microscopic analysis of the urine). However, excess white blood cells (WBCs) or bacteria seen on Gram stain and culture of expressed prostatic secretions (EPS) may be found.

CPPS has also been termed prostatodynia; however, the use of this term is not encouraged in current practice, as it carries the negative historical connotation of being a "wastebasket" designation for a melange of psychosomatic symptoms and suggests that the source of the patient's symptoms invariably lies within the prostate gland itself. Current research has provided evidence of numerous extraprostatic considerations, including neuropathic and other systemic pathologies.

The pain of prostatodynia is characterized by dull, aching, or or burning pain of the perineum and underlying structures. The intensity of pain is mild to moderate and may worsen with urination or sexual activity. The pain may be referred to the penis, testicles, scrotum, or inner thigh. Irritative urinary outflow symptoms and sexual dysfunction often coexist with the pain of prostatodynia. The history of all patients with chronic prostatodynia should include specific questioning regarding a history of sexual abuse.

Pearls & Oysters

Symptoms parallel those experienced by persons with chronic bacterial and nonbacterial prostatitis. The typical patient is a young to middle-aged man with variable symptoms of chronic, irritative, and/or obstructive voiding accompanied by moderate to severe pain in the pelvis, lower back, perineum, and/or genitalia.

Erectile dysfunction is the symptom that initially brings many men to seek medical attention; however, the patient often waits until the end of the interview to mention the problem or he may avoid mentioning it at all unless the physician specifically inquires.

Bottom Line Statement

In 2015, Prostate Cancer UK released consensus guidelines for the diagnosis and management of chronic bacterial prostatitis (CBP) and chronic prostatitis/ chronic pelvic pain syndrome (CP/CPPS). The guidelines define early-stage disease as persistent, recurrent symptoms for <6 months in antibiotic□naïve men. In later-stage disease, patients experience persistent, recurrent symptoms for >6 months that are refractory to initial lines of pharmacotherapy. The recommendations for evaluation include the following :

Use of reliable instruments, such as the National Institutes of Health Chronic Prostatitis Symptom Index (NIH□CPSI), International Prostate Symptom Score (IPSS), and UPOINT system, should be considered to assess initial symptom severity, evaluate phenotypic differences, and monitor patients' response to therapeutic intervention.

Patients should be screened for psychosocial symptoms (eg, anxiety or stress).

Referral to a mental health specialist (eg, psychiatrist, clinical psychologist) should be considered if clinically relevant levels of psychosocial symptoms are present.

Other concerns or differential diagnoses, including urological cancers and infertility, should be discussed with the patient to establish a full patient history.

Patients should be informed of the underlying causes of CBP and CP/CPPS to help improve their understanding. This may include an explanation of basic pelvic anatomy, the chronic pain cycle, and potential routes for pain (neuropathic vs nociceptive).

Medico-Legal Traps

Misdiagnosis as Prostatitis or Infection

- Prostatodynia presents with symptoms similar to bacterial prostatitis, such as pelvic pain and voiding issues, which often leads to misdiagnosis. Incorrectly prescribing antibiotics when no infection is present can result in prolonged patient discomfort and unnecessary treatment costs.
- **Thumb Rule Consideration:** Ensure thorough diagnostic evaluation with urine analysis, cultures, and prostatic secretion studies before initiating antibiotics. Confirm the absence of infection or inflammation.

Failure to Recognize Extraprostatic Causes

- Prostatodynia is frequently associated with neuropathic, muscular, or psychological causes, but these are often overlooked due to the focus on prostate-related issues. Mismanaging the condition as solely prostate-based leads to incomplete care.
- **Thumb Rule Consideration:** Evaluate for extraprostatic causes such as neuropathy, pelvic floor dysfunction, and psychological factors. Use multidisciplinary approaches, including pain management and mental health consultation, as needed.

Inadequate Attention to Psychosomatic Components

- Historically dismissed as psychosomatic, prostatodynia may have significant psychological components, including anxiety, depression, or trauma. Ignoring these factors can lead to ineffective treatment and patient dissatisfaction.
- **Thumb Rule Consideration:** Screen all patients with chronic prostatodynia for psychosocial symptoms, such as anxiety or past trauma, and consider referring to mental health specialists when necessary.

Delayed or Incomplete Sexual Dysfunction Inquiry

- Erectile dysfunction and sexual dysfunction are common in patients with prostatodynia, but these issues are often not fully addressed during initial consultations. This oversight may worsen the patient's quality of life and contribute to legal challenges.
- **Thumb Rule Consideration:** Always ask direct questions about sexual health and dysfunction, and address these issues as part of comprehensive management to avoid delayed diagnoses and patient distress.

Neglecting Long-Term Management and Multidisciplinary Care

- Prostatodynia can be chronic and refractory to initial treatments. Failing to offer long-term management options or involve a multidisciplinary team can result in prolonged suffering and dissatisfaction.
- **Thumb Rule Consideration:** Create a long-term management plan involving urologists, physiotherapists, and pain specialists, ensuring follow-up and adjustment of therapies based on symptom progression and patient response.

REFERENCES

- [Guideline] Rees J, Abrahams M, Doble A, Cooper A, Prostatitis Expert Reference Group (PERG). Diagnosis and treatment of chronic bacterial prostatitis and chronic prostatitis/chronic pelvic pain syndrome: a consensus guideline. BJU Int. 2015 Oct. 116 (4):509-25. [Full Text].

- Pontari MA, Ruggieri MR. Mechanisms in prostatitis/chronic pelvic pain syndrome. J Urol. 2004 Sep. 172(3):839-45.
- Jain P, Ghosh A, Jana D, Pal DK. Chronic pelvic pain syndrome/chronic prostatitis: Is it related to human papillomavirus infection? A case-control study from Eastern India. Urologia. 2020 Jan 16. 391560319899848.
- Krieger JN, Riley DE. Chronic prostatitis: Charlottesville to Seattle. J Urol. 2004 Dec. 172(6 Pt 2):2557-60.
- Cohen RJ, Shannon BA, McNeal JE, Shannon T, Garrett KL. Propionibacterium acnes associated with inflammation in radical prostatectomy specimens: a possible link to cancer evolution?. J Urol. 2005 Jun. 173(6):1969-74.
- Rudick CN, Berry RE, Johnson JR, et al. Uropathogenic Escherichia coli induces chronic pelvic pain. Infect Immun. 2011 Feb. 79(2):628-35. [Full Text].
- Soto SM, Smithson A, Martinez JA, Horcajada JP, Mensa J, Vila J. Biofilm formation in uropathogenic Escherichia coli strains: relationship with prostatitis, urovirulence factors and antimicrobial resistance. J Urol. 2007 Jan. 177(1):365-8.
- Westesson KE, Shoskes DA. Chronic prostatitis/chronic pelvic pain syndrome and pelvic floor spasm: can we diagnose and treat?. Curr Urol Rep. 2010 Jul. 11 (4):261-4.

PSOAS BURSITIS

Psoas bursitis is a condition in which the bursa, a small fluid-filled sac that helps reduce friction between tissues, becomes inflamed in the area just below the crease of the groin, resulting in pain in the hip and groin region. It is often misdiagnosed as an inguinal hernia or attributed to a primary hip pathological process. Psoas bursitis can be caused by acute trauma, such as a seat belt injury, or by repeated microtrauma from activities such as running up stairs or overuse of exercise equipment. It is important to distinguish psoas bursitis from lumbar radiculopathy, as the latter involves back pain associated with reflex, motor, and sensory changes, while psoas bursitis only results in secondary back pain due to altered gait and no neurological changes. Radiographs of the hip and electromyography can help differentiate between the two conditions. Treatment of psoas bursitis may include rest, physical therapy, and injection of the bursa with a corticosteroid medication.

Johnston CA, Wiley JP, Lindsay DM, Wiseman DA. Iliopsoas bursitis and tendinitis. Sports Medicine 1998;25(4):271-83.

Clinical Description

Psoas bursitis is a condition characterized by inflammation of the psoas bursa, a fluid-filled sac located between the psoas muscle and the front of the neck of the femur. This condition can cause pain in the groin and hip region, as well as difficulty sleeping on the affected side and a sharp, catching sensation during range of motion of the hip. It can be caused by acute trauma or repeated microtrauma, such as running up stairs or overuse of exercise equipment, and may be more common in athletes and other physically active individuals. Treatment options for psoas bursitis may include rest, physical therapy, and anti-inflammatory medications. In some cases, corticosteroid injections may be used to reduce inflammation and pain. If the condition becomes chronic, calcification of the bursa may occur.

Pearls & Oysters

It is essential that injections of the psoas bursa be performed by clinicians who have a thorough understanding of the regional anatomy and are experienced in performing injection techniques. This is due to the close proximity of the femoral nerve to the bursa. It is not uncommon for patients to report an increase in pain temporarily following the injection of the bursa. It is important for clinicians to be aware of this potential side effect and to properly advise patients beforehand.

Bottom Line Statement

It is important to consider other potential causes of groin pain, such as inguinal hernia and entrapment neuropathies of the ilioinguinal, genitofemoral, and femoral nerves, before proceeding with injection of the psoas bursa. While injection of the bursa can be an effective treatment for psoas bursitis, it is crucial to take precautions to avoid trauma to the femoral nerve.

After the injection procedure, physical modalities such as local heat and gentle stretching exercises can be introduced several days later to aid in recovery. However, it is important to avoid vigorous exercises, as they may exacerbate symptoms. In addition, simple analgesics, non-steroidal anti-inflammatory drugs (NSAIDs), and antimyotonic agents such as tizanidine may be used in conjunction with injection of the bursa to manage pain and muscle spasms.

Medico-Legal Traps

Misdiagnosis as Inguinal Hernia or Hip Pathology

- Psoas bursitis is frequently misdiagnosed as an inguinal hernia or primary hip condition, which can lead to delayed or inappropriate treatment. Missing the correct diagnosis can result in prolonged patient suffering and potential legal challenges.
- **Thumb Rule Consideration:** Always include psoas bursitis in the differential diagnosis of groin pain, particularly when the patient lacks clear signs of hernia or hip pathology. Confirm the diagnosis with imaging and clinical tests before proceeding with treatments.

Failure to Differentiate from Lumbar Radiculopathy

- Psoas bursitis can be mistaken for lumbar radiculopathy due to similar presenting symptoms, particularly lower back pain. However, radiculopathy involves neurological deficits, which are absent in psoas bursitis. Incorrectly treating for radiculopathy may lead to worsening symptoms.
- **Thumb Rule Consideration:** Conduct a thorough neurological examination, including reflex, motor, and sensory tests, to rule out lumbar radiculopathy. Use electromyography and hip radiographs to clarify the diagnosis.

Inadequate Precision During Corticosteroid Injections

- Due to the proximity of the femoral nerve to the psoas bursa, injections into the bursa can inadvertently damage the nerve, leading to complications such as femoral nerve palsy. Inexperienced clinicians are at a higher risk of causing such iatrogenic injuries.

- **Thumb Rule Consideration:** Ensure that the practitioner performing the injection has a detailed understanding of the regional anatomy and significant experience with such procedures. Utilize imaging guidance, such as ultrasound, to improve injection accuracy.

Neglecting to Rule Out Entrapment Neuropathies

- Groin pain can also be caused by entrapment neuropathies of the ilioinguinal, genitofemoral, or femoral nerves. Failing to exclude these conditions before initiating treatment for psoas bursitis can result in ineffective management and legal risks due to misdiagnosis.
- **Thumb Rule Consideration:** Thoroughly assess and rule out nerve entrapment syndromes when evaluating patients with groin pain. Use targeted diagnostic techniques, such as nerve conduction studies, to ensure accurate diagnosis.

Lack of Patient Education About Post-Injection Pain

- Temporary worsening of pain following corticosteroid injection into the psoas bursa is common, but failure to inform patients of this possibility beforehand can lead to dissatisfaction, complaints, and potential legal actions.
- **Thumb Rule Consideration:** Clearly inform patients about the potential for increased pain following the injection and provide detailed instructions on post-procedure care, including rest, use of analgesics, and gradual reintroduction of physical therapy.

REFERENCES

- Van de Perre S, Vanwambeke K, Vanhoenacker FM, De Schepper AM. Posttraumatic iliopsoas bursitis. JBR BTR 2005;88(3):154.
- Matsumoto T, Juji T, Mori T. Enlarged psoas muscle and iliopsoas bursitis associated with a rapidly destructive hip in a patient with rheumatoid arthritis. Modern rheumatology 2006;16(1):52-4.
- Arromdee E, Matteson EL. Bursitis: common condition, uncommon challenge. The Journal of Musculoskeletal Medicine. 2001;18(4):213-224.
- Tibor LM, Sekiya JK. Differential diagnosis of pain around the hip joint. Arthroscopy: The Journal of Arthroscopic & Related Surgery 2008;24(12):1407-21.
- Skiadas V, Koutoulidis V, Plotas A. An atypical case of noninfected iliopsoas bursitis-MRI findings. Journal of radiology case reports 2009;3(10):15.
- Wyss J, Patel A. Therapeutic programs for musculoskeletal disorders.New York, NY: Demos Medical Publishing; 2013.
- Noesberger B, Eichenberger AR. Overuse injuries of the hip and snapping hip syndrome. Operative Techniques in Sports Medicine. 1997;5(3):138-42.
- Gilliland WR, Murphey MD, Papadoupolos PJ, Zembrzuska H. Iliopsoas bursitis. J Musculoskelet Med 2012;3:53-4.
- Rowbotham EL, Grainger AJ. Ultrasound-guided intervention around the hip joint. American Journal of Roentgenology. 201;197(1):W122-7.
- Johnston CA, Lindsay DM, Wiley JP. Treatment of iliopsoas syndrome with a hip rotation strengthening

program: a retrospective case series. Journal of Orthopaedic & Sports Physical Therapy 1999 Apr;29(4):218-24.

- O'Sullivan, K., Smith, S.M., & Sainsbury, D. (2010). Electromyographic analysis of the three subdivisions of gluteus medius during weight-bearing exercises. BMC Sports Science, Medicine & Rehabilitation. doi:10.1186/1758-2555-2-17 (Level of evidence: 2C)
- Quinn A. Hip and groin pain: physiotherapy and rehabilitation issues. The open sports medicine journal. 2010;4(1).

QUADRICEPS EXPANSION SYNDROME

The intraarticular fat pad is a mass of intracapsular but extrasynovial adipose tissue that occupies the potential spaces within the knee joint. They act as a protective cushion between the quadriceps and patellar tendon, patella, and distal femur, prevent friction, and improve patellofemoral engagement during deep knee flexion and extension.

Grando H, Chang EY, Chen KC, Chung CB (2014) MR imaging of extrasynovial inflammation and impingement about the knee. Magn Reson Imaging Clin N Am 22:725–741.

Clinical Description

Several types of quadriceps injuries can occur, the most common being the quadriceps contusion, which is painful and disabling. The usual cause of the quadriceps contusion is a direct blow to the anterior thigh from an object or another person (eg, helmet, knee). Very rarely, this injury can be severe enough to progress to an acute compartment syndrome.

Because the quadriceps is in contact with the femur throughout its length, it is susceptible to compression forces. The rectus femoris is the most commonly injured portion of the muscle because of its anterior location. Minimally, impact causes cellular edema of the muscle, but complete capillary disruption with localized hemorrhage leading to a tense anterior compartment can occur. The muscle is more resistant to injury if it is struck while in a contracted nonfatigued state. Other quadriceps injuries range from simple strains to more complex and disabling muscle ruptures.

Other types of quadriceps injuries include strains of the quadriceps tendon, complete and partial tears of the quadriceps tendon, and fascial rupture of the quadriceps muscle. Specific areas of the quadriceps are affected for each of these diagnoses. The classic quadriceps strain occurs at the conjoined muscle tendon junction (jumper's knee). The partial tear of the quadriceps most commonly affects the indirect (distal) head of the rectus femoris. Fascial rupture usually occurs anteriorly at the mid thigh and causes a muscle hernia.

Causes of quadriceps injury are as follows:

Quadriceps contusion or compartment syndrome - Direct blow to anterior aspect of thigh

Quadriceps strain or rupture - Acute stretch or repeated eccentric muscle contractions with immediate or delayed (1-3 d) presentation of pain, stiffness, and decreased function

Pearls & Oysters

In one study, only one third of patients with acute quadriceps tendon rupture were accurately diagnosed at the first visit. Therefore, if complete rupture is suspected but the diagnosis cannot be confirmed clinically, MRI is the study of choice. Late diagnosis of a complete tear of the quadriceps tendon can lead to retraction of the muscle proximally with scarring. The consequence of this is that the surgical repair is more difficult and the clinical results are not as good.

Bottom Line Statement

Most people are able to return to their previous occupations and activities after recovering from a quadriceps tendon tear. Slightly over half of people have thigh weakness and soreness at the site of the tear. People who require surgery do better if the repair is performed early after the injury.

If you are a competitive athlete, the surgeon will do very thorough assessment before giving a go-ahead to return to your sport. Your surgeon will compare your leg strength using some functional knee testing (like hopping). The goal is for your injured leg to be at least 85-90% as strong as your uninjured leg. In addition to leg strength, your surgeon will assess your leg's endurance, your balance, and if you have any swelling.

Medico-Legal Traps

Delayed or Missed Diagnosis of Quadriceps Tendon Rupture

- Misdiagnosing or delaying the diagnosis of a complete quadriceps tendon rupture is common, with studies showing only one-third of cases accurately diagnosed during the first visit. Delayed diagnosis can result in retraction of the muscle and make surgical repair more difficult with poorer outcomes.
- **Thumb Rule Consideration:** If a complete rupture is suspected but not confirmed clinically, always order an MRI. Early diagnosis is crucial to avoid complications and ensure better surgical outcomes.

Failure to Differentiate Between Strain and Compartment Syndrome

- Quadriceps injuries can range from mild strains to severe compartment syndromes. Misinterpreting a quadriceps contusion for a simple strain can be dangerous if compartment syndrome is present, leading to increased risk of permanent damage due to delayed decompression.

- **Thumb Rule Consideration:** Always assess for signs of compartment syndrome after a direct blow to the anterior thigh, especially when swelling, pain out of proportion, or paresthesia is present. Consider pressure measurement or MRI in ambiguous cases.

Improper Post-Surgical Assessment for Return to Sport

- Athletes recovering from quadriceps tendon tears often rush back to high-impact sports, risking re-injury or improper healing. Inadequate post-surgical functional assessments increase the legal liability for physicians and can cause lasting damage to the athlete's ability to perform.
- **Thumb Rule Consideration:** Conduct thorough functional testing (strength, endurance, and balance) before clearing an athlete to return to sport. Injured leg strength should be at least 85-90% of the uninjured leg, with no signs of swelling or imbalance.

Overlooking Potential Complications from Contusions

- Complications like myositis ossificans can arise from untreated or poorly managed quadriceps contusions. Physicians who fail to educate patients about proper rest, icing, and follow-up imaging may face legal action if complications develop later.
- **Thumb Rule Consideration:** Educate patients about the risk of complications, including myositis ossificans, and emphasize the importance of following prescribed rest, icing, and therapy protocols. Schedule follow-ups to monitor progress.

Failure to Address Long-Term Weakness After Recovery

- Even after surgical repair and recovery, patients may experience residual weakness or soreness in the affected thigh. Failure to inform patients about these possible long-term issues can lead to dissatisfaction and potential legal claims.
- **Thumb Rule Consideration:** Set realistic expectations with patients regarding long-term outcomes after quadriceps injury recovery. Inform them that some weakness and soreness are common, but ensure that rehabilitation and strengthening exercises are tailored to minimize these effects.

REFERENCES

- Ryan JB, Wheeler JH, Hopkinson WJ, Arciero RA, Kolakowski KR. Quadriceps contusions. West Point update. Am J Sports Med. 1991 May-Jun. 19(3):299-304.
- Eckard TG, Kerr ZY, Padua DA, Djoko A, Dompier TP. Epidemiology of Quadriceps Strains in National Collegiate Athletic Association Athletes, 2009-2010 Through 2014-2015. J Athl Train. 2017 May. 52 (5):474-481.

- Arnold EP, Sedgewick JA, Wortman RJ, Stamm MA, Mulcahey MK. Acute Quadriceps Tendon Rupture: Presentation, Diagnosis, and Management. JBJS Rev. 2022 Feb 7. 10 (2):
- Falkowski AL, Jacobson JA, Hirschmann MT, Kalia V. MR imaging of the quadriceps femoris tendon: distal tear characterization and clinical significance of rupture types. Eur Radiol. 2021 Oct. 31 (10):7674-83.
- Langenhan R, Baumann M, Ricart P, Hak D, Probst A, Badke A. Postoperative functional rehabilitation after repair of quadriceps tendon ruptures: a comparison of two different protocols. Knee Surg Sports Traumatol Arthrosc. 2012 Feb 4.
- Almekinders LC. Anti-inflammatory treatment of muscular injuries in sport. An update of recent studies. Sports Med. 1999 Dec. 28(6):383-8.

QUADRILATERAL SPACE SYNDROME

Quadrilateral space syndrome (QSS) is a rare disorder characterized by axillary nerve and posterior humeral circumflex artery (PHCA) compression within the quadrilateral space. Impingement is most frequently due to trauma, fibrous bands, or hypertrophy of one of the muscular borders. Diagnosis can be complicated by the presence of concurrent traumatic injuries, particularly in athletes. Since many other conditions can mimic QSS, it is often a diagnosis of exclusion.

Chen D., Cai P., Lao G., Gu Y. Quadrilateral space syndrome. Chin. Med. J. 1995;108:109–112.

Clinical Description

Quadrilateral space syndrome (QSS) is a rare disorder characterized by axillary nerve and posterior humeral circumflex artery (PHCA) compression within the quadrilateral space, first described by Cahill and Palmer in 1983.

Cahill originally described four distinct features of QSS:

(1) diffuse pain around the shoulder;

(2) paresthesia in a nondermatomal distribution;

(3) point tenderness above the quadrilateral space; and•

(4) positive angiogram finding in provocative positioning.

The condition is commonly attributed to repeated overhead activity (such as baseball or volleyball athletes), but a variety of other pathologies including lipomas, hematomas, and labral cysts may cause compression in the quadrilateral space.

While neurovascular compression does account for the acute findings in QSS including pain, paraesthesia, and atrophy, it is debated whether this is primarily a problem of neural entrapment or vascular compression. Compression may occur at rest or with movement and QSS should be considered for all patients with a chief complaint of neck pain, shoulder pain, lateral arm paraesthesia, and/or quadrilateral space tenderness.

Pearls & Oysters

Shoulder pain and weakness are common presenting symptoms and common entities like rotator cuff pathology and degenerative changes may be present in patients who have QSS. It is important for providers to be aware that various common pathologies such as presence of rotator cuff tendinopathy do not mean QSS is excluded. The clinical exam should be directed towards identifying the specific muscle or muscles involved. A finding of atrophy of deltoid or teres minor should raise suspicion of QSS even in patients with known tendinopathy or shoulder or acromioclavicular joint pathologies. MRI is indicated in all patients thought to have quadrilateral space syndrome, and aggressive treatment of surgically correctable causes is generally indicated sooner rather than later to avoid ongoing irreversible shoulder damage.

Bottom Line Statement

QSS is a rare disorder with signficant morbidity. Because many symptoms of QSS are nonspecific, there may be a delay in diagnosis and subsequent delay in care. In one study, it was shown that the mean interval from the commencement of symptoms to surgical decompression was 14.5 months, with a range from 6–24 months. Practitioner awareness of QSS as a differential diagnosis, particularly in at-risk populations such as athletes, is also critical for timely and accurate diagnosis. Careful analysis of imaging studies is necessary to exclude differential diagnoses, understand etiology, and to devise the best treatment strategy for QSS. Future investigations could include studies on the prevalence of QSS and a more thorough analysis on the barriers of diagnosis, including limited practitioner awareness of the condition, nonspecific presentation, and the absence of a gold standard workup.

Medico-Legal Traps

Delayed or Missed Diagnosis

- QSS is often a diagnosis of exclusion, and the nonspecific symptoms such as diffuse shoulder pain and paresthesia can mimic other common shoulder pathologies like rotator cuff injuries. A delayed diagnosis leads to prolonged pain, disability, and potentially irreversible damage to the axillary nerve or posterior humeral circumflex artery.
- **Thumb Rule Consideration:** Always consider QSS in athletes and individuals with repetitive overhead activities, particularly when there is unexplained shoulder pain and deltoid or teres minor muscle atrophy. Early MRI and EMG studies can aid in faster diagnosis.

Overlooking Coexisting Conditions

- Patients with QSS may also present with concurrent rotator cuff injuries, degenerative shoulder changes, or acromioclavicular joint pathologies. Focusing solely on these more common conditions while overlooking QSS can result in incomplete treatment and poor outcomes.

- **Thumb Rule Consideration:** Even if other shoulder conditions are diagnosed, keep QSS in mind if there is unexplained deltoid or teres minor atrophy. Careful evaluation of the entire clinical picture and comprehensive imaging studies are essential.

Inappropriate Use of Diagnostic Imaging

- Failure to order advanced imaging like MRI when QSS is suspected can result in misdiagnosis. X-rays or standard shoulder imaging may miss critical findings such as neural or vascular compression in the quadrilateral space.
- **Thumb Rule Consideration:** Always include MRI when QSS is suspected, as it provides better visualization of soft tissues, muscular atrophy, and neurovascular structures. Early and precise imaging can prevent complications from delayed diagnosis.

Inadequate Early Intervention

- Given the progressive nature of QSS, a delay in surgical intervention for patients with confirmed neurovascular compression can lead to permanent muscle atrophy and functional deficits. Mismanaging the condition conservatively without proper follow-up can increase legal risk.
- **Thumb Rule Consideration:** Once QSS is confirmed, prompt referral to a specialist for surgical decompression should be considered, especially in cases of muscle atrophy or vascular compromise. Conservative measures should only be pursued in carefully selected cases with regular monitoring.

Failure to Recognize Non-Surgical Candidates

- Not every case of QSS requires surgery. Misjudging a patient's condition and proceeding with unnecessary surgical intervention can lead to avoidable complications, patient dissatisfaction, and potential legal repercussions.
- **Thumb Rule Consideration:** Surgery is indicated when there is confirmed neurovascular compression and conservative treatment has failed. Always balance the decision for surgery with a thorough evaluation of the patient's overall condition, including the severity of symptoms and functional impairment.

REFERENCES

- Chautems R.C., Glauser T., Waeber-Fey M.C., Rostan O., Barraud G.E. Quadrilateral space syndrome: Case report and review of the literature. Ann. Vasc. Surg. 2000;14:673–676.
- Hoskins W.T., Pollard H.P., McDonald A.J. Quadrilateral space syndrome: A case study and review of the literature. Br. J. Sports Med. 2005;39:e9.

- Brown S.A., Doolittle D.A., Bohanon C.J., Jayaraj A., Naidu S.G., Huettl E.A., Renfree K.J., Oderich G.S., Bjarnason H., Gloviczki P., et al. Quadrilateral space syndrome: The mayo clinic experience with a new classification system and case series. Mayo Clin. Proc. 2015;90:382–394.
- Cahill B.R., Palmer R.E. Quadrilateral space syndrome. J. Hand Surg. Am. 1983;8:65–69.
- Flynn L.S., Wright T.W., King J.J. Quadrilateral space syndrome: A review. J. Shoulder Elbow Surg. 2018;27:650–956.
- Cothran R.L., Helms C. Quadrilateral space syndrome: Incidence of imaging findings in a population referred for MRI of the shoulder. Am. J. Roentgenol. 2005;184:989–992.
- Feng S.-H., Hsiao M.-Y., Wu C.-H., Özçakar L. Ultrasound-guided diagnosis and management for quadrilateral space syndrome. Pain Med. 2017;18:184–186.
- Wilson L., Sundaram M., Piraino D.W., Ilaslan H., Recht M.P. Isolated teres minor atrophy: Manifestation of quadrilateral space syndrome or traction injury to the axillary nerve? Orthopedics. 2006;29:447–450.
- Lopez Ovenza J.M., Ranalletta M., Alonso Hidalgo I., Tanoira I., Bongiovanni S., Maignon G. Quadrilateral space syndrome with compromise of the teres minor muscle. Medicina. 2011;71:49.

RADIAL TUNNEL SYNDROME

Radial tunnel syndrome is a disease which we should consider it in elbow and forearm pains. It is diagnosed with lateral elbow and dorsal forearm pain may radiate to the wrist and dorsum of the fingers. The disease is more prevalent in women with the age of 30 to 50 years old. It occurs by intermittent compression on the radial nerve from the radial head to the inferior border of the supinator muscle, without obvious extensor muscle weakness. Compression could happen in five different sites but the arcade of Frose is the most common area that radial nerve is compressed. To diagnosis radial tunnel syndrome, clinical examination is more important than paraclinic tests such as electrodiagnsic test and imaging studies.

Arch Bone Jt Surg. 2015 Jul; 3(3): 156–162.

Clinical Description

Intermittent compression of the radial nerve through the radial tunnel is thought to be the pathological basis for radial tunnel syndrome (RTS). The condition is not associated with extensor muscle weakness and due to the fact that the diagnosis is mostly clinical so, the existence of RTS remains controversial (1). However, those authors who support the diagnosis have identified a number of potential etiologies including compression of the nerve due to the bands of fascia, radial recurrent vessels, edge of supinator and rarely a haemangioma, lipoma, dislocated head of radius, inflamed synovium or accessory muscles.

Those clinicians who do not support the diagnosis note that the only constant symptom is pain. Yet if thought to be a compressive neuropathy of the posterior interosseouus nerve, why would the EMG universally be negative. To refute this, the fact that motor nerves can provide pain stimuli and unmyelinated and small myelinated fibers are not generally assessed with the EMG. Moreover, the existence of define anatomic space, definitive tenderness in anterior and distal of elbow and the fact motor nerve can provide pain stimuli support the PIN as the responsible factor in RTS.

Pearls & Oysters

Radial tunnel syndrome is a disease which we should consider as presenting in elbow and forearm pains. It is diagnosed with lateral elbow and dorsal forearm pain which may radiate to the wrist and dorsum of fingers. The disease is more common amongst women aged 30 to 50 years old. A painful point exists one inch distal to the lateral epicondyle and over the radial tunnel which exacerbates with resisted active extension of the wrist and third finger could confirm the diagnosis.

Bottom Line Statement

Determining the exact location of the pain in the forearm, is the primary step in evaluating for RTS. The main clinical feature of RTS is a localized tenderness over the radial nerve 5 cm distal to the lateral epicondyle. Patients typically report aggravated pain at nights that may interfere with sleeping. The pain can also become more severe when increased traction is applied to the nerve by extending the elbow, pronating the forearm, or flexing the wrist.

Injury to the nerve can occur due to a multitude of causes at many potential sites along its course. The most common site of involvement is in the proximal forearm affecting the posterior interosseous branch while the main branch of the radial nerve is injured in fractures of the humeral shaft. Signs and symptoms of radial neuropathy depend upon the site of injury. Injury to the nerve distal to innervation of triceps brachii results in loss of extensor function with sparing of function of the triceps resulting in the characteristic wrist drop. Injury in the mid-arm is associated with loss of sensation in the dorsolateral aspect of the hand, the dorsal aspect of the radial three-and-a-half digits and in the first web space. Involvement of only the posterior interosseous nerve (PIN) results in weakness of the wrist and digit extensors.

Medico-Legal Traps

Failure to Differentiate from Lateral Epicondylitis

- One of the most common medico-legal traps is misdiagnosing RTS as lateral epicondylitis (tennis elbow). Both conditions present with lateral elbow pain, but mismanagement due to this confusion can result in prolonged suffering and ineffective treatment.
- **Thumb Rule Consideration:** Distinguish RTS by focusing on tenderness approximately 4-5 cm distal to the lateral epicondyle, not directly on the lateral epicondyle, and confirm with exacerbation of pain during resisted extension of the middle finger.

Neglecting a Thorough Clinical Examination

- RTS diagnosis relies heavily on clinical examination, but it is often overlooked in favor of imaging and EMG tests, which are frequently negative for RTS. Relying solely on these paraclinical tests can lead to misdiagnosis and subsequent legal challenges.
- **Thumb Rule Consideration:** Always prioritize a thorough physical exam to identify tender points and pain patterns, and use imaging or EMG tests only as supplementary tools.

Delaying Surgical Intervention

- Failure to recognize cases of RTS that require early surgical decompression can lead to worsening pain and dysfunction, potentially resulting in legal action from patients who suffer prolonged, unnecessary pain.
- **Thumb Rule Consideration:** If conservative management fails after a reasonable period (typically 3-6 months), refer the patient to a specialist for possible surgical decompression to prevent progression of symptoms and nerve damage.

Misinterpretation of EMG Findings

- RTS often presents without EMG abnormalities, as the posterior interosseous nerve is difficult to assess with standard EMG studies. Misinterpretation of a normal EMG as ruling out RTS can delay diagnosis and appropriate care.
- **Thumb Rule Consideration:** Remember that a negative EMG does not exclude RTS; rely on clinical findings rather than EMG results alone when assessing patients with suspected RTS.

Improper Physical Therapy or Overuse of Affected Arm

- Overaggressive physical therapy or continued overuse of the affected arm without recognizing the diagnosis of RTS can exacerbate the condition, leading to worsened outcomes and potential medico-legal consequences.
- **Thumb Rule Consideration:** Advise patients to limit repetitive pronation, supination, and wrist extension activities and monitor progress closely to adjust therapy as needed.

REFERENCES

- P Bolster MA, Bakker XR. Radial tunnel syndrome: emphasis on the superficial branch of the radial nerve. J Hand Surg Eur. 2009;34(3):343–7.
- Lister GD, Belsole RB, Kleinert HE. The radial tunnel syndrome. J Hand Surg Am. 1979;4(1):52–9.
- Roles NC, Maudsley RH. Radial tunnel syndrome: resistant tennis elbow as a nerve entrapment. J Bone Joint Surg Br. 1972;54(3):499–508.
- Michele AA, Krueger FJ. Lateral epicondylitis of the elbow treated by fasciotomy. Surgery. 1956;39(2):277–84.
- Naam NH, Nemani S. Radial tunnel syndrome. Orthop Clin North Am. 2012;43(4):529–36.
- Eversmann WW. Entrapment and compression neuropathies. In: Green DP, Hotchkiss RN, editors. Operative Hand Surgery. 3rd ed. New York: Churchill Livingstone; 1993. pp. 1341–85.
- Sarhadi NS, Korday SN, Bainbridge LC. Radial tunnel syndrome: diagnosis and management. J Hand Surg Br. 1998;23(5):617–9.
- Lawrence T, Mobbs P, Fortems Y, Stanley JK. Radial tunnel syndrome: A retrospective review of 30 decompressions of the radial nerve. J Hand Surg Br. 1995;20(4):454–9.
- Moradi A, Ebrahimzadeh MH, Ring D. Nonspecific Arm Pain. Arch Bone Jt Surg. 2013;1(2):53–8.
- Ali Moradi, MD; Mohammad H Ebrahimzadeh, MD; Jess B Jupiter, MD. Radial Tunnel Syndrome, Diagnostic and Treatment Dilemma. THE ARCHIVES OF BONE AND JOINT SURGERY. 2015 Jul; 3(3): 156–162.

RADIATION ENTERITIS

Radiation enteritis is damage to the small and/or large intestines secondary to radiation. Different terms like radiation colitis, radiation enteropathy, radiation mucositis, and pelvic radiation disease have been used to describe this phenomenon. Radiation proctitis is a different term that is used to describe the involvement of the rectum and sigmoid colon. Radiotherapy is used as a treatment for many cancers. Radiation enteritis can be acute or chronic. The chronic form usually develops between 3 months to 30 years after treatment.

Stacey R, Green JT. Radiation-induced small bowel disease: latest developments and clinical guidance. Ther Adv Chronic Dis. 2014 Jan;5(1):15-29.

Clinical Description

Radiation enteritis is an unavoidable side effect of radiotherapy, although its development is highly variable, depending on the duration, dosage, and gut sensitivity to radiation. Radiation enteritis is very common; studies have reported a permanent change in bowel habits in 90% of patients that undergo pelvic radiotherapy. Some evidence shows that it may be more common in patients getting radiation therapy for gastrointestinal (GI) and gynecological tumors than urological tumors. Chronic radiation enteritis occurs in approximately 5% to 55% of patients post-radiotherapy.

The repetitive injuries caused to the intestinal mucosa by ionizing radiation, as well as its complex mechanism of healing, are proposed to cause radiation enteritis. Exposure of normal tissues to radiation leads to the production of reactive ions that combine with intracellular water molecules to form radicals like hydroxyl and other free radicals. These radicals are deemed responsible for causing breaks in DNA and causing cell death. Secondary to radiation exposure, activation of genes that are responsible for the translation of transforming growth factor (TGF-beta) takes place. This activation stimulates collagen and fibronectin genes promoting fibrosis. Tissues with rapid proliferation are sensitive to radiation, and thus, cell membrane disruption is also responsible for the cell death observed. The epithelial cells of the small intestine are more radiosensitive as compared to the colon and rectum. Studies show that the presence of Bcl2 in the rectum is the reason for this discrimination. The most characteristic pathologic changes observed are fibrosis and obliterative endarteritis in the intestinal epithelium.

Pearls & Oysters

Radiation enteritis is an unavoidable side effect of radiotherapy; however, its development is highly variable.

It is becoming more common with the advent of new treatment regimens for different cancers including radiotherapy.

Diarrhea, abdominal pain, intestinal hemorrhage, intestinal obstruction, intestinal perforation, fistulas, malabsorption, rectal pain, and rectal bleeding secondary to ulceration are some of the common symptoms.

It can be treated with supportive measures or surgically.

Prognosis varies in different patients, and they should be followed regularly to observe for recurrence of malignancy.

Bottom Line Statement

The care of patients with radiation enteritis is interprofessional. Besides the surgeon, radiation oncologist, gastroenterologist, and radiologist, the nurse and dietitian is a vital member of the team. While not all complications of radiation enteritis can be prevented, the patient's nutritional state should be improved prior to any surgery. The patient should be educated about the potential complications and the need for repeat surgery. The patient should be seen by a stoma nurse in case a colostomy or ileostomy is performed during surgery. More important the patient should be told about the short bowel syndrome and the need for long-term parenteral nutrition. After surgery, routine surgical complications like deep vein thrombosis and atelectasis should be prevented with prophylactic treatment with LWMH and the use of the incentive spirometer, respectively. Finally, the family and the patient should be educated on end-of-life preparation and designation of a power of attorney.

Medico-Legal Traps

Delayed Diagnosis and Mismanagement

- Chronic radiation enteritis can manifest up to 30 years after radiation treatment, and its symptoms often overlap with other gastrointestinal conditions. A failure to consider previous radiation exposure as a cause of symptoms like diarrhea or abdominal pain can lead to misdiagnosis, delayed treatment, and potential litigation for negligence.
- **Thumb Rule Consideration:** Always ask patients with gastrointestinal complaints about their history of radiation treatment, even if it was years or decades ago.

Inadequate Informed Consent

- Patients undergoing radiotherapy are often not fully informed about the long-term risks, such as chronic radiation enteritis. Failure to thoroughly explain the potential side effects, including delayed gastrointestinal complications, can result in medico-legal repercussions if these complications develop later.
- **Thumb Rule Consideration:** Ensure that informed consent for radiotherapy includes a detailed discussion of potential late-onset complications like chronic radiation enteritis.

Neglecting Multidisciplinary Care

- Radiation enteritis requires a collaborative approach involving surgeons, oncologists, gastroenterologists, and dietitians. Failing to provide comprehensive care or delaying referrals to appropriate specialists can result in worsened outcomes and legal consequences.
- **Thumb Rule Consideration:** Involve a multidisciplinary team early in the diagnosis and management of radiation enteritis, and ensure coordinated care to optimize outcomes.

Failure to Address Nutritional Needs

- Many patients with chronic radiation enteritis suffer from malnutrition due to malabsorption or bowel resection surgery. If nutrition is not adequately managed, this can lead to further health deterioration and claims of substandard care.
- **Thumb Rule Consideration:** Include dietitians in the care plan for all patients with radiation enteritis, and prioritize nutritional support to prevent complications like short bowel syndrome.

Inadequate Patient Education on Long-term Effects

- Radiation enteritis is a chronic condition that may necessitate multiple surgeries, and patients need to be fully aware of potential long-term complications like intestinal obstruction or the need for a stoma. A lack of proper education about these realities can lead to misunderstandings and potential legal disputes over treatment outcomes.
- **Thumb Rule Consideration:** Educate patients thoroughly about the chronic nature of radiation enteritis, including possible long-term treatments like stoma placement and parenteral nutrition.

REFERENCES

- Stacey R, Green JT. Radiation-induced small bowel disease: latest developments and clinical guidance. Ther Adv Chronic Dis. 2014 Jan;5(1):15-29.
- Kountouras J, Zavos C. Recent advances in the management of radiation colitis. World J Gastroenterol. 2008 Dec 28;14(48):7289-301.
- Olopade FA, Norman A, Blake P, Dearnaley DP, Harrington KJ, Khoo V, Tait D, Hackett C, Andreyev HJ. A modified Inflammatory Bowel Disease questionnaire and the Vaizey Incontinence questionnaire are simple ways to identify patients with significant gastrointestinal symptoms after pelvic radiotherapy. Br J Cancer. 2005 May 09;92(9):1663-70.
- Lefevre JH, Amiot A, Joly F, Bretagnol F, Panis Y. Risk of recurrence after surgery for chronic radiation enteritis. Br J Surg. 2011 Dec;98(12):1792-7.
- Anwar M, Ahmad S, Akhtar R, Mahmood A, Mahmood S. Antioxidant Supplementation: A Linchpin in Radiation-Induced Enteritis. Technol Cancer Res Treat. 2017 Dec;16(6):676-691.
- Potten CS, Booth C. The role of radiation-induced and spontaneous apoptosis in the homeostasis of the gastrointestinal epithelium: a brief review. Comp Biochem Physiol B Biochem Mol Biol. 1997 Nov;118(3):473-8.
- MacNaughton WK. Review article: new insights into the pathogenesis of radiation-induced intestinal dysfunction. Aliment Pharmacol Ther. 2000 May;14(5):523-8.
- Sauer R, Becker H, Hohenberger W, Rödel C, Wittekind C, Fietkau R, Martus P, Tschmelitsch J, Hager E, Hess CF, Karstens JH, Liersch T, Schmidberger H, Raab R., German Rectal Cancer Study Group. Preoperative versus postoperative chemoradiotherapy for rectal cancer. N Engl J Med. 2004 Oct 21;351(17):1731-40.
- Huang Y, Guo F, Yao D, Li Y, Li J. Surgery for chronic radiation enteritis: outcome and risk factors. J Surg Res. 2016 Aug;204(2):335-343.
- Pironi L, Arends J, Bozzetti F, Cuerda C, Gillanders L, Jeppesen PB, Joly F, Kelly D, Lal S, Staun M, Szczepanek K, Van Gossum A, Wanten G, Schneider SM., Home Artificial Nutrition & Chronic Intestinal Failure Special Interest Group of ESPEN. ESPEN guidelines on chronic intestinal failure in adults. Clin Nutr. 2016 Apr;35(2):247-307.
- Bowman LC, Williams R, Sanders M, Ringwald-Smith K, Baker D, Gajjar A. Algorithm for nutritional support: experience of the Metabolic and Infusion Support Service of St. Jude Children's Research Hospital. Int J Cancer Suppl. 1998;11:76-80.
- Jayapala Reddy V, Sureshkumar S, Vijayakumar C, Amaranathan A, Sudharsanan S, Shyama P, Palanivel C. Concurrent Chemoradiation Affects the Clinical Outcome of Small Bowel Complications Following Pelvic Irradiation: Prospective Observational Study from a Regional Cancer Center. Cureus. 2018 Mar 13;10(3):e2317.
- Yang X, Wang J, Lin L, Gao D, Yin L. Concomitant chemoradiotherapy versus pure radiotherapy in locally advanced cervical cancer: a retrospective analysis of complications and clinical outcome. Eur J Gynaecol Oncol. 2016 Aug;37(4):499-503.

RAMSAY HUNT SYNDROME

Ramsay Hunt syndrome, also known as herpes zoster oticus, is a late complication of varicella-zoster virus infection that results in inflammation of the geniculate ganglion of cranial nerve VII. Ramsay Hunt is a clinical diagnosis and classically is described as a triad of ipsilateral facial paralysis, otalgia, and vesicles near the ear and auditory canal. Diagnosis is often missed or delayed, which can lead to an increased incidence of long-term complications. The condition is self-limiting, but treatment is targeted at decreasing the total duration of the illness as well as providing analgesia and preventing the complications that can occur.

Sweeney CJ, Gilden DH. Ramsay Hunt syndrome. J Neurol Neurosurg Psychiatry. 2001 Aug;71(2):149-54.

Clinical Description

Ramsay Hunt syndrome is characterized by a classic triad of ipsilateral facial paralysis, otalgia, and vesicles in the auditory canal or on the auricle. Additional symptoms include a change in taste sensation, dry eye, tearing, hyperacusis, nasal obstruction, and dysarthria. Hearing loss, tinnitus, and vertigo can be seen with the involvement of the vestibulocochlear nerve, and hoarseness or aspiration may indicate involvement of the vagus nerve. Vesicles may develop after the onset of neurologic symptoms, but the first presenting symptom is usually pain. The vesicles typically appear on the auricle but can be seen along the affected side of the face, scalp, palate, and tongue. In some cases, no vesicles are present, and the patient's chief complaints are severe pain and facial palsy; this variant is known as zoster sine herpete and can be very difficult to distinguish clinically from Bell palsy.

Pearls & Oysters

Other than the presenting symptoms of pain, rash, facial paralysis, dysgeusia, hearing loss, tinnitus, vertigo, hoarseness, dysarthria, and others mentioned above, short-term complications of Ramsay Hunt syndrome include corneal abrasion and exposure keratopathy, depression and social anxiety, and transmission of chickenpox to unvaccinated or immunocompromised close contacts. While flaccid paralysis in the long-term is unlikely, the development of synkinesis is very common. Other long-term complications include postherpetic neuralgia, scarring from the vesicles, and persistent depression and/or social anxiety due to loss of facial function.

Bottom Line Statement

Ramsay Hunt syndrome affects patients in myriad ways, with pain, paralysis, cochleovestibular symptoms, and behavioral health concerns all occurring commonly in the acute period. In the long term, while most patients do recover the majority of their premorbid function when managed appropriately, pain, facial dysfunction, scarring, and behavioral health concerns may all persist. For this reason, optimal patient outcomes occur when healthcare teams include members with expertise across a broad range of specialties. In the short term, primary care, otolaryngology, neurology, ophthalmology, and psychology/psychiatry are often required. In the long-term, plastic surgery or otolaryngology, pain management, ophthalmology, speech or physical therapy, and psychology/psychiatry may be needed. Other causes of head pain must be ruled out first before invoking this diagnosis. Because of the potential for hearing loss in Ramsay Hunt syndrome, patients should be warned of this possibility to avoid erroneously blaming this complication on a therapeutic intervention, such as stellate ganglion block. Patients who develop synkinesis may require regular visits over the course of years and years with a physician or nurse who can administer botulinum toxin injections; it is critical to surround these patients with an experienced interprofessional team early on in the treatment process in order to provide them the care and support they need to maximize their quality of life outcomes.

Medico-Legal Traps

Delayed or Missed Diagnosis

- Ramsay Hunt syndrome (RHS) is often misdiagnosed as Bell's palsy due to overlapping symptoms, leading to delays in appropriate antiviral treatment. This delay can increase the risk of long-term complications, such as permanent facial paralysis or hearing loss, and expose clinicians to malpractice claims for failing to recognize the condition.
- **Thumb Rule Consideration:** Always consider Ramsay Hunt syndrome in patients presenting with facial paralysis and otalgia, especially if there is a history of vesicles near the ear or auditory canal.

Inadequate Patient Education on Long-Term Risks

- Patients may not be informed about the possibility of permanent complications such as synkinesis, hearing loss, or postherpetic neuralgia. Failure to adequately prepare the patient for these potential outcomes can lead to legal repercussions for negligence or lack of informed consent.

- **Thumb Rule Consideration:** Ensure patients are fully informed about the risks of long-term complications, including facial dysfunction and chronic pain, before starting treatment.

Mismanagement of Pain and Psychological Symptoms

- Postherpetic neuralgia and depression are common long-term complications of RHS, and failure to address these effectively can lead to claims of inadequate pain management and insufficient psychological support. These symptoms require multidisciplinary management.
- **Thumb Rule Consideration:** Incorporate pain management and mental health support early in the treatment plan to avoid neglecting these critical aspects of patient care.

Failure to Refer to Specialists

- Given the potential involvement of multiple cranial nerves, including the vestibulocochlear nerve, failure to refer patients to appropriate specialists such as otolaryngologists, neurologists, or ophthalmologists may worsen patient outcomes and lead to claims of substandard care.
- **Thumb Rule Consideration:** Always refer patients with suspected Ramsay Hunt syndrome to a neurologist or otolaryngologist, and involve an ophthalmologist if there is risk of corneal damage.

Neglecting to Monitor and Prevent Corneal Complications

- Corneal abrasions and exposure keratopathy can occur due to facial nerve paralysis leading to inadequate eye closure. If these complications are not proactively monitored and prevented, legal claims of negligence may arise
- **Thumb Rule Consideration:** In cases of facial paralysis, ensure regular ophthalmology consultations to prevent corneal damage, and educate the patient on eye protection strategies, such as artificial tears and taping the eyelid shut during sleep.

REFERENCES

- Paiva ALC, Araujo JLV, Ferraz VR, Veiga JCE. Facial paralysis due to Ramsay Hunt syndrome - A rare condition. Rev Assoc Med Bras (1992). 2017 Apr;63(4):301-302.
- Rajati M, Zarringhalam MA. Ramsay Hunt Syndrome Associated with True Vocal Cord Palsy- A Case Report. Iran J Otorhinolaryngol. 2019 Mar;31(103):115-118.
- Arya D, Bajaj T, Gonzalez J, Elkin R. Ramsay Hunt Syndrome with Multiple Cranial Neuropathy in an Human Immunodeficiency Virus (HIV) Patient. Am J Case Rep. 2018 Jan 18;19:68-71.
- Bhagra A, Stead LG: Ramsay Hunt syndrome: a rare entity, Ann Emerg Med 47:579, 2006.
- Gantz BJ, Redleaf MI, Perry BP, Gubbels SP: Management of Bell's palsy and Ramsay Hunt syndrome. In Brackmann DE, et al: Otologic surgery, ed 3, Philadelphia, 2010, Saunders, pp 335–346.
- Persson A, Bergström T, Lindh M, Namvar L, Studahl M: Varicella-zoster virus CNS disease: viral load, clinical manifestations and sequels, J Clin Virol 46:249–253, 2009.

RED EAR SYNDROME

The syndrome itself has not been clearly defined. Apart from its unique clinical presentation, characterised by episodes of burning pain and reddening of the external ear, the condition lacks definition in terms of aetiology, pathophysiology and treatments. It is for these reasons that it has yet to be included in the revised International Classification of Headache Disorders.

The International Classification of Headache Disorders. 3nd edition, beta version. Cephalalgia. 2013;14(9):629–808.

Clinical Description

Red Ear Syndrome (RES) is a very rare disorder, with approximately 100 published cases in the medical literature. Red ear (RE) episodes are characterised by unilateral or bilateral attacks of paroxysmal burning sensations and reddening of the external ear. The pain and erythema associated with red ear syndrome have a rapid onset to peak, with attacks lasting 15 seconds to 5 minutes and the frequency of attacks ranging from 20 to 200 attacks per day. In some patients, these attacks can be triggered by sensory stimulation of the affected area, such as when brushing the hair. Although in many ways similar to SUNCT headache (i.e., unilateral, rapid onset to peak, short duration of attacks, pain-free periods between attacks), many dissimilarities also exist, including the location and pronounced autonomic phenomenon manifested by the red ear. The attacks occur with a frequency ranging from several a day to a few per year. Episodes can occur spontaneously or be triggered, most frequently by rubbing or touching the ear, heat or cold, chewing, brushing of the hair, neck movements or exertion. Early-onset idiopathic RES seems to be associated with migraine, whereas late-onset idiopathic forms have been reported in association with trigeminal autonomic cephalalgias (TACs). Secondary forms of RES occur with upper cervical spine disorders or temporo-mandibular joint dysfunction. RES is regarded refractory to medical treatments, although some migraine preventative treatments have shown moderate benefit mainly in patients with migraine-related attacks. The pathophysiology of RES is still unclear but several hypotheses involving peripheral or central nervous system mechanisms have been proposed.

Pearls & Oysters

Due to the association of secondary RES with upper cervical spine pathology, an MRI of the cervical spine should be carried out when RES is suspected. In addition, if TMJ dysfunction is a possibility, an orthodontic assessment is warranted. Lastly, an MRI scan of the brain should be included to rule out thalamic lesions. If skin involvement is more generalized, a complete blood count and thermograph should be completed to rule out other secondary causes.

Failure to diagnose red ear syndrome correctly may put the patient at risk if intracranial pathology or demyelinating disease, which may mimic the clinical presentation of red ear syndrome, is overlooked. MRI is indicated in all patients thought to have red ear syndrome. A careful evaluation of the ear to rule out localized pathological conditions is also indicated, as is laboratory testing for collagen-vascular disease if polychondritis is suspected.

Bottom Line Statement

RES is a rare but probably under-recognised condition characterised by unilateral or bilateral episodes of burning pain and erythema over the external ear. The episodes are usually short-lasting and frequent. On the basis of the clinical features described in literature, the first set of diagnostic criteria for RES has been proposed here.

RES appears generally refractory to medical treatments. Open-label trials have suggested a beneficial effect with in some cases with the use of gabapentin, amitriptyline, imipramine, flunarizine, propranolol, verapamil and pregabalin. Other treatments including NSAIDs, ice-pack use and blockade of the greater auricular nerve can also be considered.

Medico-Legal Traps

Failure to Diagnose Correctly and Early

- Red Ear Syndrome (RES) is frequently misdiagnosed due to its rare nature and overlapping symptoms with other conditions like trigeminal autonomic cephalalgias (TACs) or migraines. Missing the diagnosis can lead to unnecessary treatments and prolonged patient suffering, potentially leading to medico-legal claims of negligence or mismanagement.
- **Thumb Rule Consideration:** Always consider RES in patients presenting with episodes of unilateral or bilateral burning pain and erythema of the external ear, particularly if these symptoms are triggered by sensory stimuli like brushing the hair.

Failure to Investigate Secondary Causes

- RES can be secondary to conditions like cervical spine disorders, temporomandibular joint dysfunction (TMJ), or even demyelinating diseases. Failure to investigate these secondary causes with appropriate imaging and tests (e.g., MRI of the cervical spine or TMJ assessment) may lead to delayed or incorrect diagnosis, resulting in claims of substandard care.

- **Thumb Rule Consideration:** Conduct a thorough evaluation for secondary causes with cervical spine imaging, TMJ assessment, and possibly brain MRI to rule out intracranial pathology in patients with RES.

Lack of Patient Education on Disease Refractoriness

- RES is often refractory to medical treatments, and patients may not be adequately informed about this during treatment discussions. Failing to explain the chronic and treatment-resistant nature of the condition could lead to unrealistic expectations, potential dissatisfaction, and medico-legal risks.
- **Thumb Rule Consideration:** Clearly explain to patients the refractory nature of RES and discuss potential treatment options, including gabapentin, amitriptyline, and NSAIDs, as well as their limited success rates.

Neglecting Neurological or Vascular Workup

- Failure to rule out serious neurological or vascular conditions such as thalamic lesions, multiple sclerosis, or collagen-vascular diseases in patients with RES can lead to significant legal repercussions if these conditions go undiagnosed and untreated.
- **Thumb Rule Consideration:** In cases where RES is suspected, ensure that a neurological workup including MRI of the brain and cervical spine is conducted, alongside blood tests to exclude other systemic causes.

Inappropriate or Risky Treatment Approaches

- Inappropriate or excessive use of invasive treatments, such as nerve blocks or unproven surgical interventions, without exhausting conservative measures like pharmacological treatments or NSAIDs can lead to complications. This may result in medico-legal consequences if the risks of such interventions were not fully disclosed or alternative treatments were not considered first.
- **Thumb Rule Consideration:** Prioritize conservative treatments such as medications, ice packs, and NSAIDs before resorting to more invasive treatments, and ensure patients are well informed about the risks and benefits of each treatment option.

REFERENCES

- Lance JW. The mystery of one red ear. Clin Exp Neurol. 1994;14:13–18.
- Lance JW. The red ear syndrome. Neurology. 1996;14(3):617–620.
- Lambru G, Miller S, Matharu MS. The red ear syndrome. J Headache Pain. 2013;14(1):83. Published 2013 Oct 4.
- Boes CJ, Swanson JW, Dodick DW. Chronic paroxysmal hemicrania presenting as otalgia with a sensation of external acoustic meatus obstruction: two cases and a pathophysiologic hypothesis. Headache. 1998;14(10):787–791.
- Kumar N, Swanson JW: The 'red ear syndrome' revisited: two cases and a review of literature, Cephalalgia 24:305–308, 2004.
- Purdy RA, Dodick DW: Red ear syndrome, Curr Pain Headache Rep 11:313–316, 2007.
- Waldman SD: Cervical facet block. In Waldman SD, editor: Atlas of interventional pain management, ed 3, Philadelphia, 2009, Saunders, pp 165–168.

RUNNER'S KNEE

Pain around the kneecap is often a sign of overuse. In other words, the knee might have been exposed to too much or too frequent strain without being able to adapt to it fast enough. This is particularly common when doing sports such as jogging, mountaineering or intensive cycling. The condition is often referred to as "runner's knee" because of this.

There are currently no treatments that directly target the cause of pain at the front of the knee. But good-quality studies have shown that regularly doing exercises to strengthen the thigh and hip muscles can help.

People who do a lot of sports and develop acute knee pain are also advised to take a break from sports or do less for a while so that their knee can recover.

Collins NJ, Barton CJ, van Middelkoop M, Callaghan MJ, Rathleff MS, Vicenzino BT et al. 2018 Consensus statement on exercise therapy and physical interventions (orthoses, taping and manual therapy) to treat patellofemoral pain: recommendations from the 5th International Patellofemoral Pain Research Retreat, Gold Coast, Australia, 2017. Br J Sports Med 2018; 52(18): 1170-1178.

Clinical Description

Pain at the front of the knee usually occurs just behind or next to the kneecap. Doctors then call it patellofemoral pain or patellofemoral pain syndrome (PFPS). "Patellofemoral" means that it affects the area between the kneecap (patella) and the thigh bone (femur).

The pain is often mild at first and then gets worse over time. It tends to be a dull, aching pain and is particularly noticeable when you put strain on the knee – especially when going up or down stairs or bending the knee a lot. The knee may also hurt and feel stiff after sitting for a long time.

A lot of people who have knee pain can feel or hear crackling, crunching or creaking when they move the affected knee. But this isn't a reason for concern: There's no link between knee sounds and pain or the function of the knee. Many people have "noisy knees" without any pain or other knee problems. One reason why joints sometimes make sounds is because small bubbles of gas form in them and you can hear the bubbles bursting.

People whose knees make sounds can – and should – still move. The knee joint can only stay healthy if it is moved enough. If no pressure is applied to it, the cartilage in the joint isn't supplied with enough nutrients. The bones need to have strain put on them too, to stop them from becoming weaker.

Pearls & Oysters

The doctor first asks about the symptoms and feels the knee. Then she or he asks you to squat down. A different test involves slowly stepping off a step with the healthy leg. If that makes the pain worse, it could be patellofemoral pain. Some medical professionals also use special questionnaires to get a more accurate description of the symptoms.

If necessary, further knee tests are done to rule out other causes. These include things like a torn meniscus, osteoarthritis of the knee, and tendon-related problems. But osteoarthritis is very rare in people under the age of 40. Before the end of puberty, certain growth-related problems can cause knee pain too. These can also be ruled out by examining the knee.

Imaging techniques like x-rays, ultrasound scans or MRIs do not help to diagnose runner's knee. But it can make sense to use them if something else is thought to be causing the pain – such as a tendon overuse injury, osteoarthritis of the knee, or a bone fracture.

Bottom Line Statement

Patellofemoral pain syndrome is usually fully relieved with simple measures or physical therapy. It may recur, however, if you do not make adjustments to your training routine or activity level. It is essential to maintain appropriate conditioning of the muscles around the knee, particularly the quadriceps and the hamstrings.

Runner's knee is dull pain around the front of the knee.

It may be caused by a structural defect, or a certain way of walking or running.

Symptoms include pain, and rubbing, grinding, or clicking sound of the kneecap.

Treatment includes not running until the pain goes away. Also using cold packs, compression, and elevation may help. Medicine such as ibuprofen can lessen pain and reduce inflammation. Stretching and strengthening exercises can help prevent runner's knee.

Medico-Legal Traps

Failure to Diagnose Properly and Early

- Misdiagnosing PFPS or failing to recognize the early signs of "runner's knee" can lead to worsening pain and more significant knee dysfunction over time. Some clinicians might focus on other knee issues like tendonitis or ligament injuries, leading to delayed treatment of PFPS and potential legal claims of negligence.

- **Thumb Rule Consideration:** Always perform a thorough clinical examination, including movement-based tests like squatting or stepping, to accurately diagnose PFPS and differentiate it from other knee pathologies.

Ignoring Non-Surgical Treatment Options

- Many patients may assume that surgery is the best or only option for resolving knee pain, and if a clinician jumps to surgical recommendations without fully exploring conservative therapies such as physical therapy, orthoses, or muscle strengthening exercises, this can result in unnecessary procedures and potential legal repercussions for not adhering to standard treatment protocols.
- **Thumb Rule Consideration:** Prioritize non-surgical treatments, including exercise therapy, strengthening of the quadriceps and hamstrings, and activity modification, before considering invasive procedures for managing runner's knee.

Neglecting to Educate Patients on Long-Term Management

- Failure to inform patients about the chronic nature of PFPS, its tendency to recur, and the importance of long-term muscle conditioning and activity modification can lead to dissatisfaction and claims of inadequate care. Patients need to be educated on how to maintain knee health and prevent future issues.
- **Thumb Rule Consideration:** Clearly explain the importance of continued physical therapy and conditioning exercises even after symptoms resolve to avoid recurrence of pain or dysfunction.

Overlooking the Psychosocial Impact

- Runner's knee can lead to significant disruptions in daily activities, especially for athletes. Ignoring the mental health impact or failing to refer patients for psychological support when needed could result in claims of neglecting comprehensive care. Addressing the emotional and psychological strain of chronic pain is essential.
- **Thumb Rule Consideration:** Consider the psychological aspects of chronic knee pain and provide appropriate referrals for counseling or support when necessary, particularly in athletes or individuals highly impacted by the condition.

Inadequate Documentation and Follow-Up

- Poor documentation of the patient's progress, treatment compliance, and ongoing management plans could expose healthcare providers to legal challenges, especially if the patient's condition worsens or surgical options are later explored. Adequate follow-up is crucial to ensure the patient is responding to treatment.

- **Thumb Rule Consideration:** Maintain detailed records of the diagnosis, treatment plan, patient compliance, and all follow-up care to ensure thorough documentation of the management of runner's knee.

REFERENCES

- Crossley KM, Stefanik JJ, Selfe J, Collins NJ, Davis IS, Powers CM et al. 2016 Patellofemoral pain consensus statement from the 4th International Patellofemoral Pain Research Retreat, Manchester. Part 1: Terminology, definitions, clinical examination, natural history, patellofemoral osteoarthritis and patient-reported outcome measures. Br J Sports Med 2016; 50(14): 839-843.
- Hart HF, Barton CJ, Khan KM, Riel H, Crossley KM. Is body mass index associated with patellofemoral pain and patellofemoral osteoarthritis? A systematic review and meta-regression and analysis. Br J Sports Med 2017; 51(10): 781-790.
- Nascimento LR, Teixeira-Salmela LF, Souza RB, Resende RA. Hip and Knee Strengthening Is More Effective Than Knee Strengthening Alone for Reducing Pain and Improving Activity in Individuals With Patellofemoral Pain: A Systematic Review With Meta-analysis. J Orthop Sports Phys Ther 2018; 48(1): 19-31.
- Neal BS, Lack SD, Lankhorst NE, Raye A, Morrissey D, van Middelkoop M. Risk factors for patellofemoral pain: a systematic review and meta-analysis. Br J Sports Med 2019; 53(5): 270-281.
- Robertson CJ, Hurley M, Jones F. People's beliefs about the meaning of crepitus in patellofemoral pain and the impact of these beliefs on their behaviour: A qualitative study. Musculoskelet Sci Pract 2017; 28: 59-64.
- Rogan S, Haehni M, Luijckx E, Dealer J, Reuteler S, Taeymans J. Effects of Hip Abductor Muscles Exercises on Pain and Function in Patients With Patellofemoral Pain: A Systematic Review and Meta-Analysis. J Strength Cond Res 2018; 33(11): 3174-3187.
- Scali K, Roberts J, McFarland M, Marino K, Murray L. Is multi-joint or single joint strengthening more effective in reducing pain and improving function in women with patellofemoral pain syndrome? A systematic review and meta-analysis. Int J Sports Phys Ther 2018; 13(3): 321-334.
- Smith BE, Moffatt F, Hendrick P, Bateman M, Rathleff MS, Selfe J et al. The experience of living with patellofemoral pain-loss, confusion and fear-avoidance: a UK qualitative study. BMJ Open 2018; 8(1): e018624.
- Smith BE, Selfe J, Thacker D, Hendrick P, Bateman M, Moffatt F et al. Incidence and prevalence of patellofemoral pain: A systematic review and meta-analysis. PLoS One 2018; 13(1): e0190892.

SCAPULOCOSTAL SYNDROME

The scapulocostal syndrome, myofascitis of the shoulder muscles, is caused by altered posture, prolonged immobilization of the shoulder region or fixed scapular/spinal deformities. The author studied 440 patients ranging from 18 to 60 years of age whose altered posture caused deep pain in the shoulder region originating from the medial aspect of the scapular spine.

Va Med Q. 1994 Spring;121(2):105-8.

Clinical Description

Scapulocostal syndrome consists of a constellation of symptoms including unilateral pain and associated paresthesias at the medial border of the scapula, referred pain radiating from the deltoid region to the dorsum of the hand, and decreased range of motion of the scapula. Scapulocostal syndrome is commonly referred to as traveling salesman's shoulder, because it is frequently seen in individuals who repeatedly reach backward to retrieve something from the back seat of a car. Scapulocostal syndrome is an overuse syndrome caused by repeated improper use of the muscles of scapular stabilization-the levator scapulae, pectoralis minor, serratus anterior, rhomboids, and, to a lesser extent, infraspinatus and teres minor.

Scapulocostal syndrome is a chronic myofascial pain syndrome, and the sine qua non of myofascial pain syndrome is the finding of myofascial trigger points on physical examination. Although these trigger points are generally localized to the part of the body affected, the pain is often referred to other areas. This referred pain may be misdiagnosed or attributed to other organ systems, thus leading to extensive evaluation and ineffective treatment. Mechanical stimulation of the trigger point by palpation or stretching produces both intense local pain and referred pain. In addition, involuntary withdrawal of the stimulated muscle, called a jump sign, is often seen and is characteristic of myofascial pain syndrome. Almost all patients with scapulocostal syndrome have a prominent infraspinatus trigger point, which is best demonstrated by having the patient place the hand of the affected side over the deltoid of the opposite shoulder. This maneuver laterally rotates the affected scapula and allows palpation and subsequent injection of the infraspinatus trigger point. Other trigger points along the medial border of the scapula may be present and may be amenable to injection therapy.

Taut bands of muscle fibers are often identified when myofascial trigger points are palpated. Despite this consistent physical finding, the pathophysiology of the myofascial trigger point remains elusive, although trigger points are believed to result from microtrauma to the affected muscle. This trauma may occur from a single injury, repetitive microtrauma, or chronic deconditioning of the agonist and antagonist muscle unit.

Pearls & Oysters

Real-time ultrasound is commonly employed to assess the role of various essentialinternal organs, including the heart, colon, kidneys, spleen, and liver. The advantage of this method is that it is non-invasive and free of ionizing radiation. Additionally, theinformation from real-time ultrasound can be stored for subsequent consideration.

Bottom Line Statement

This syndrome is found in females more than in males. Poor sitting posture while workingor using digital media are risk factors for SCS, as it is an overuse disorder caused by the repeated in adequate use of the muscles around the scapulae. This syndrome can be found at myofascial trigger points (MTrPs) on the muscles around the scapulae, including the levator scapulae, upper trapezius, rhomboid major and minor, teres major and minor, infraspinatus serratus anterior, and serratus posterior superior muscles. Hence, this syndrome affects the biomechanics of the scapulae.

Medico-Legal Traps

Failure to Diagnose Myofascial Pain Syndrome Early

- Scapulocostal syndrome (SCS) is frequently underdiagnosed due to the nonspecific nature of its symptoms and its overlap with other musculoskeletal disorders. Failure to recognize and diagnose the condition early can lead to unnecessary treatments and prolonged patient suffering. This misdiagnosis could result in legal claims of negligence or inadequate care.
- **Thumb Rule Consideration:** Always consider myofascial pain syndromes, particularly in patients presenting with shoulder and upper back pain, and identify myofascial trigger points during physical examination.

Misdiagnosis as Other Conditions

- The pain of SCS can radiate to other areas, including the hand and deltoid region, and may be misattributed to other conditions such as cervical spine disorders, rotator cuff injuries, or even cardiac issues. Misdiagnosis can result in inappropriate interventions and delayed treatment.

- **Thumb Rule Consideration:** Thoroughly evaluate the scapular and shoulder region, and differentiate between SCS and other potential causes of referred pain by ruling out more serious conditions through a complete clinical history and examination.

Overreliance on Imaging and Tests

- While imaging techniques like X-rays and MRIs are commonly used to investigate musculoskeletal complaints, they may not be useful in diagnosing SCS, as it is a clinical diagnosis based on trigger points and myofascial findings. Ordering unnecessary or inconclusive tests may lead to delayed diagnosis and potential claims of excessive diagnostic procedures.
- **Thumb Rule Consideration:** Focus on clinical examination and palpation for trigger points rather than relying solely on imaging for diagnosing SCS.

Failure to Provide Proper Physical Therapy or Rehabilitation

- Scapulocostal syndrome often results from poor posture or repetitive improper use of muscles. If treatment does not include rehabilitation to improve posture and strengthen scapular stabilizers, patients are at risk for chronic pain and recurrence. Failure to provide effective physical therapy could lead to malpractice claims.
- **Thumb Rule Consideration:** Always include physical therapy, postural correction, and exercises that target the affected muscles as part of the treatment plan for SCS.

Neglecting to Inform Patients of Activity Modification

- SCS is often an overuse injury caused by repetitive motions or poor posture, especially in individuals with certain professions or habits. Failing to counsel patients on avoiding aggravating activities can result in persistent symptoms and claims of improper or insufficient care.
- **Thumb Rule Consideration:** Educate patients about modifying activities that exacerbate SCS, such as reaching behind while driving or maintaining poor posture at work, to reduce the risk of recurrence.

REFERENCES

- Abrams, B. Scapulocostal syndrome. In Pain Management; Waldman, S.D., Ed.; Saunders: Philadelphia, PA, USA, 2011; Volume 2,pp. 588–592.2.
- Briggs, A.M.; Smith, A.J.; Straker, L.M.; Bragge, P. Thoracic spine pain in the general population: Prevalence, incidence andassociated factors in children, adolescents and adults. A systematic review. BMC Musculoskelet. Disord. 2009,10, 77. [CrossRef]
- Ozdemir, F.; Karaoglu, L.; Ozfirat, O. The lifetime and point prevalence of neck, upper back and low back

pain of the peopleliving in central Malatya with influencing factors. Agri J. Turk. Soc. Algol. 2013,25, 27–35. [CrossRef]4

- Paine, R.; Voight, M.L. The role of the scapula. Int. J. Sports Phys. Ther. 2013,8, 617–629. [CrossRef]
- Taghizadeh, S.; Pirouzi, S.; Hemmati, L.; Khaledi, F.; Sadat, A. Clinical Evaluation of Scapular Positioning in Patients withNonspecific Chronic Low Back Pain: A Case-Control Study. J. Chiropr. Med. 2017,16, 195–198.

SCAPHOLUNATE LIGAMENT TEAR SYNDROME

Injuries to the scapholunate joint are the most common cause of carpal instability. An isolated injury to the scapholunate ligament may progress to abnormal joint mechanics and degenerative cartilage changes. Treatment for scapholunate instability is aimed at arresting the degenerative process by restoring ligament continuity and normalising carpal kinematics. Early arthroscopic diagnosis of scapholunate injury is mandatory for establishing the prognosis of the injury, as a proper ligament repair is recommended within four to six weeks after trauma.

EFORT Open Rev 2017;2:382–393.

Clinical Description

The scapholunate (SL) ligament (SLL) is the most commonly injured carpal ligament. The SLL is C-shaped and has three structurally distinct parts: volar; membranous; and dorsal. The dorsal part of the SLL is the strongest and the primary stabiliser of the SL joint and can resist forces of up to 260 N. The avascular proximal membranous portion does not provide any significant laxity restraint (63 N), while the volar part of the SLL (118 N) plays an important role in terms of rotational stability. The dorsal part of the SLL measures 2 mm to 3 mm in thickness and is in the range of 2 mm to 5 mm in length. The vascular supply to the scaphoid and SLL is delicate. The main vascular contribution comes from the radial artery. Extra-osseous vessels enter the dorsal ridge of the scaphoid and supply two-thirds of the bone. It also appears that the radio-scapholunate (RSL) ligament provides a vascular supply directed at the SLL complex.

There is a gradient of SL injury severity, when it occurs. It ranges from occult, dynamic SL dissociation (gap), followed by carpal collapse, finally ending up in disabling arthritis (scapholunate advanced collapse (SLAC)) wrist. It often takes three to 12 months after trauma before dynamic instability develops and SL dissociation is noted radiologically (SL angle > 60° and SL gap > 3 mm on clenched-fist or ulnar-deviation radiographs). For this development and progression to occur, an additional tear or gradual, continuous elongation of the secondary ligament stabilisers of the SL ligament is needed.

Approximately 5% of all wrist sprains have an associated SL tear. SLL injuries are often associated with distal radius fracture (40% of the cases on average), particularly fractures of the radial styloid, the so-called Chauffeur's fracture.

Pearls & Oysters

The end result of long-standing SLL injury with dissociation (SLD) is always DISI and a so-called SLAC wrist. SLAC is the most common pattern of degenerative arthritis of the wrist. It develops following SLD with rotary subluxation of the scaphoid. The degenerative changes first affect the radial styloid, then the radio-scaphoid joint, followed by parts of the mid-carpal joints. The head of the capitate, in particular, can erode fairly rapidly when it is subsequently dislocated into the gap between the lunate and the scaphoid. The radiolunate joint is not typically involved in SLAC arthritis, due to the spherical shape of the lunate and the congruity of the joint between the lunate and the lunate fossa of the radius.

Bottom Line Statement

A negative result from MRI is unable to rule out the possibility of a clinically relevant injury to the SLL. Clinical provocation wrist tests are of limited diagnostic value. The current gold standard, wrist arthroscopy, remains the preferred diagnostic technique with sufficient conclusive properties when it comes to wrist ligament injuries.

Four different types of SL injury exist, according to the new classification by Andersson-Garcia-Elias. The type of SL injury can probably be decisive for the choice of surgical approach and for the healing conditions.

According to the literature, the integrity and quality of the dorsal SLL, the posture of the scaphoid (widening and rotatory), carpal alignment and cartilage status contribute to the choice of treatment for SL injury. Early diagnosis is mandatory. Ligament-reconstruction techniques should only be performed when there is easily reducible DISI.

The best treatment of choice in different grades of SL injury is, however, still a matter of discussion and debate. SLL injuries remain a challenging problem, even to experienced hand and upper extremity surgeons. There is still a lack of consensus among hand surgeons as to the appropriate treatment of various stages.

Medico-Legal Traps

Delayed Diagnosis and Missed Early Intervention

- Scapholunate ligament (SLL) tears can be missed or misdiagnosed as simple wrist sprains, leading to delays in proper diagnosis. This can result in progression to scapholunate advanced collapse (SLAC) wrist, which has severe consequences for the patient's hand function. A delay in diagnosis may lead to legal claims of negligence, especially if early arthroscopic intervention could have prevented long-term damage.

- **Thumb Rule Consideration:** Always consider SLL tears in wrist trauma cases and conduct appropriate imaging or arthroscopy early, within 4-6 weeks post-trauma.

Inadequate Imaging and Misinterpretation of Test Results

- A negative MRI result may falsely reassure clinicians and patients that there is no significant injury. However, MRI can miss subtle ligament injuries, and clinical tests for scapholunate ligament injuries are not always reliable. Failure to use wrist arthroscopy, the gold standard, to confirm the diagnosis could result in worsening instability and potential malpractice claims.
- **Thumb Rule Consideration:** Do not rely solely on MRI for SLL injuries; use wrist arthroscopy for definitive diagnosis if clinical suspicion persists despite negative imaging.

Failure to Recognize the Severity of the Injury

- The progression of SLL injury from occult dynamic instability to irreversible SLAC wrist can occur over months. Misjudging the severity of the injury early on or failing to recognize the risk of secondary ligament failure can lead to inadequate or delayed treatment, leaving patients with permanent disability and potential legal consequences.
- **Thumb Rule Consideration:** Monitor patients closely for progression, perform follow-up imaging (radiographs in ulnar deviation/clenched fist positions), and take surgical action before irreversible changes occur.

Improper Surgical Technique and Postoperative Complications

- Scapholunate ligament injuries can be surgically challenging, and improper technique, especially failure to stabilize the dorsal ligament or address carpal misalignment, can lead to persistent instability or early arthritis. Such surgical errors could open practitioners to litigation for improper care.
- **Thumb Rule Consideration:** Only perform surgery if the carpal alignment is correctable, and use evidence-based techniques to stabilize the dorsal ligament and restore proper mechanics.

Lack of Informed Consent and Patient Education

- SLL injuries often lead to long-term complications like degenerative arthritis, even with timely intervention. Failing to properly inform patients about the potential for chronic issues, such as SLAC wrist, and the possible need for future surgeries may lead to allegations of insufficient informed consent.

- **Thumb Rule Consideration:** Fully explain the risks, benefits, and possible outcomes of both conservative and surgical treatments, including the risk of progression to SLAC wrist and the likelihood of future interventions.

REFERENCES

- Kuo CE, Wolfe SW. Scapholunate instability: current concepts in diagnosis and management. J Hand Surg Am 2008;33:998-1013.
- Berger RA. The gross and histologic anatomy of the scapholunate interosseous ligament. J Hand Surg Am 1996;21:170-178.
- Garcia-Elias M. Carpal instability. In: Wolfe SW, Hotchkiss RN, Pederson WC, Kozin SH, eds. Green's operative hand surgery. Vol 1 Sixth ed New York: Elsevier Churchill Livingstone, 2011:465-522.
- Kitay A, Wolfe SW. Scapholunate instability: current concepts in diagnosis and management. J Hand Surg Am 2012;37:2175-2196.
- Corella F, Del Cerro M, Larrainzar-Garijo R, Vázquez T. Arthroscopic ligamentoplasty (bone-tendon-tenodesis). A new surgical technique for scapholunate instability: preliminary cadaver study. J Hand Surg Eur 2011;36:682-689.
- Short WH, Werner FW, Green JK, Sutton LG, Brutus JP. Biomechanical evaluation of the ligamentous stabilizers of the scaphoid and lunate: part III. J Hand Surg Am 2007;32:297-309.
- Chennagiri RJR, Lindau TR. Assessment of scapholunate instability and review of evidence for management in the absence of arthritis. J Hand Surg Eur 2013;38:727-738.
- Geissler WB, Freeland AE, Savoie FH, McIntyre LW, Whipple TL. Intracarpal soft-tissue lesions associated with an intra-articular fracture of the distal end of the radius. J Bone Joint Surg [Am] 1996;78-A:357-365.
- Linscheid RL, Dobyns JH, Beabout JW, Bryan RS. Traumatic instability of the wrist: Diagnosis, classification and pathomechanics. J Bone Joint Surg [Am] 1972;54-A:1612-1632.
- Gilula LA. Carpal injuries: analytic approach and case exercises. AJR Am J Roentgenol 1979;133:503-517.

SECRETAN'S SYNDROME

Secretan's syndrome is a rare clinical condition with recurrent swelling of the forearm and dorsum of the hand, together with flexion contracture of the fingers and a thumb that is spared. The disease is associated with automutilation. The cause is poorly understood but factitious trauma is often suspected.

Acta Chir Belg. 2019 Apr;119(2):123-124.

Clinical Description

Henri Francois Secretan first reported 11 cases of workmen who had a hard swelling of the dorsum of the hand after trauma in 1901. Named after Secrtan, the disease usually occurred after minor trauma of the hand without osseous fracture or repetitive self-inflicted injury, without definitive etiology and pathophysiology. Peritendinous fibrosis on the extensor tendons of the hand is one of the widely recognized histologic feature. The earlier reports indicate the general involvement of adults over the age of 30 and with trauma or repetitive working histories. Secretan's disease, is not only limited to the hands also in the upper and lower extremities including feet was reported.

Since, magnetic resonance imaging (MRI) analyses of Secretan's disease is sparsely studied in the literature. Here, we report a case of Secretan's disease with MRI findings.

Pearls & Oysters

Systemic illnesses such as kidney disease, congestive heart failure and liver diseases are excluded through the clinical assessment. In the musculoskeletal area, most arthropathies and tenosynovial pathologies involving the hands should be differentiated, which include various rheumatologic disorders from common rheumatoid arthritis to remitting seronegative symmetrical synovitis with pitting edema, a widely known rheumatologic pathology. Among the neoplastic conditions occurring around the tendinous structures in the adult population, giant cell tumor of tendon sheath or fibroma of tendon sheath should also be considered as a differential diagnosis. MRI may be helpful to characterize and discriminate this rare disease from others.

Bottom Line Statement

Since its first report of Secretan's disease, the postulated three essential etiologies for this disease are

1) reactive peritendinous fibrosis induced by organizing hematoma after true light trauma,

2) swelling caused by hypersympathetic process related to an injury with neurovascular or neurolymphatic changes, and

3) repeated self-inflicted injury for secondary gain or as the product of an underlying psychiatric problem resulting in factitious edema or hyperplastic fibrosis.

The disease also shows variable clinical manifestations from soft swelling as a benign course to a hyperplastic course with persistent and hard fibrosis that limits the range of motion of fingers.

Secretan's disease was diagnosed based on medical history and physical examination, however, further imaging assessments such as MRI and ultrasonography have not been generally adapted.

Medico-Legal Traps

Misdiagnosis and Failure to Identify Self-Inflicted Injury

- Secretan's syndrome is often associated with factitious trauma, yet the initial swelling may be mistaken for other medical conditions such as rheumatoid arthritis, tenosynovitis, or soft tissue neoplasms. Failure to recognize the possibility of self-inflicted injury can lead to misdiagnosis and inappropriate treatments, causing harm to the patient and potential legal liability for incorrect clinical management.
- **Thumb Rule Consideration:** Always consider factitious or self-inflicted injury in cases of unexplained swelling, especially when there is a lack of objective findings supporting other diagnoses.

Inadequate Differentiation from Other Rheumatologic or Musculoskeletal Disorders

- Secretan's syndrome shares symptoms with other conditions like rheumatoid arthritis, remitting seronegative symmetrical synovitis, or giant cell tumors of the tendon sheath. Misinterpreting clinical findings or MRI results can result in unnecessary invasive treatments or delayed appropriate care, leading to worsening of symptoms and potential litigation for delayed diagnosis.
- **Thumb Rule Consideration:** Use thorough differential diagnosis, including MRI and ultrasonography, to exclude more common rheumatologic or musculoskeletal disorders before diagnosing Secretan's syndrome.

Failure to Recognize Psychiatric Factors and Secondary Gain

- Secretan's syndrome often involves a psychiatric component, including self-inflicted injuries for secondary gain or psychological distress. If this is not recognized, the patient may be subject to inappropriate interventions, which could exacerbate their psychological state. Failure to refer the patient to a mental health professional could lead to legal consequences if the condition worsens.
- **Thumb Rule Consideration:** In cases of recurrent unexplained injuries or edema, consider psychiatric evaluation to address underlying psychological issues contributing to self-harm.

Improper Documentation and Lack of Informed Consent

- Given the potential for factitious causes, it is crucial to document all clinical findings, diagnostic tests, and patient interactions comprehensively. Failure to adequately document the patient's condition, including the suspicion of self-inflicted injury, could expose healthcare providers to legal claims of negligence or failure to provide informed care.
- **Thumb Rule Consideration:** Ensure meticulous documentation of all clinical assessments, including differential diagnoses, psychiatric evaluation considerations, and discussions about treatment risks, especially when factitious behavior is suspected.

Inappropriate or Delayed Use of Diagnostic Imaging

- MRI and ultrasonography are important in diagnosing Secretan's syndrome but are often underutilized. Failure to employ imaging early on can delay proper treatment, leading to unnecessary interventions, worsening fibrosis, or limited mobility of the fingers, which could open the provider to malpractice claims.
- **Thumb Rule Consideration:** Use imaging techniques like MRI early in the diagnostic process to differentiate Secretan's syndrome from other conditions and to confirm peritendinous fibrosis or other structural changes.

REFERENCES

- Reading, George (1980). "Secretan's syndrome: Hard edema of the dorsum of the hand". Plastic and Reconstructive Surgery. 65 (2): 182–7.
- Moretta DN, Cooley RD Jr. Secrétan's disease: a unique case report and literature review. Am J Orthop (Belle Mead NJ). 2002; 31:524–527.
- Whitney TM, Jones NF. Magnetic resonance imaging findings in Secretan's disease. J Hand Surg Am. 1995; 20:464–466.
- Reading G. Secretan's syndrome: hard edema of the dorsum of the hand. Plast Reconstr Surg. 1980; 65:182–187.
- Saferin EH, Posch JL. Secretan's disease: post-traumatic hard edema of the dorsum of the hand. Plast Reconstr Surg. 1976; 58:703–707.
- Ramos JA, Bush D, Harrington TM. Secretan's syndrome. Orthopedics. 2007; 30:239–240.

- Angelini G, Meneghini CL, Vena GA. Secretan's syndrome: an artefact oedema of the hand. Contact Dermatitis. 1982; 8:345–346.
- Abnousi F, Chou LB. Secretan's disease of the foot: a case report and review. Foot Ankle Int. 2008; 29:248–250.

SAPHENOUS NEURALGIA

Saphenous neuralgia describes the symptom complex which includes anaesthesia, hyperaesthesia and pain within the distribution of the saphenous nerve. This sensory nerve is closely related to the great saphenous vein during its subcutaneous course through the medial aspect of the leg, and the continuity of the nerve and its branches are at risk during any surgical procedure in this region.

Adar R., Meyer E., Zweig A.. Saphenous neuralgia: a complication of vascular reconstruction below the inguinal ligament, Ann Surg, 1979, vol. 190 (pg. 609-613).

Clinical Description

Saphenous neuralgia is a rare condition that causes pain in the medial calf, often after vascular surgery on the lower extremity. It can also occur as a result of trauma to the infrapatellar branch of the saphenous nerve during total knee arthroplasty, leading to pain and numbness over the patellar tendon. Patients with saphenous neuralgia may experience a type of pain known as medial pseudoclaudication, which can be mistaken for lumbar spinal stenosis.

Other potential causes of saphenous neuralgia include compression of the nerve by tumors, abscesses, or hemorrhages at the point where the nerve exits from Hunter's canal. Stretch injuries to the saphenous nerve can also occur at this location. The nerve is also prone to compression as it crosses the medial knee, a condition known as surfer's knee due to the similarity to the compression of the saphenous nerve by the edge of a surfboard. While diabetes can affect the saphenous nerve, it is usually in conjunction with neuropathy of other nerves in the lower extremity. It is important for healthcare professionals to consider saphenous neuralgia as a potential diagnosis in patients with medial calf pain, particularly those with a history of vascular surgery or total knee arthroplasty.

Pearls & Oysters

Arterial grafts are the first choice as a conduit for myocardial re-perfusion, however with advances in interventional radiology most coronary artery bypass grafting (CABG) procedures require several grafts. Despite the availability of synthetic conduits autogenous great saphenous vein (GSV) is the most commonly used conduit for myocardial re-perfusion and saphenous neuralgia is therefore seen after harvesting of various lengths of vein from the leg or thigh. It has also been described after varicose vein, arterial and orthopaedic procedures.

Bottom Line Statement

The saphenous nerve is the terminal sensory branch of the femoral nerve (L 2,3,4), supplying the skin of the antero-medial aspect of the leg through its two major divisions: the sartorial and infrapatella nerves. It arises anterior to the femoral artery within the adductor canal, and perforates the anterior wall of the canal, travelling around the medial border of sartorius to become closely associated with the GSV in the subcutaneous tissues of the leg. It gives a medial articular branch to the knee and numerous cutaneous branches as it descends through the leg with the vein, with its terminal branches supplying the skin around the medial malleolus.

Saphenous neuralgia describes the symptom complex of anaesthesia, hyperaesthesia and pain in the area innovated by the saphenous nerve.

It is a recognised complication of CABG, however the actual incidence remains unknown. The mechanism of injury is thought to be from local division of the nerve or its branches, or from compression by post-operative soft tissue swelling. Nair has reported sensory loss after GSV harvesting, documenting 92 and 88% immediately post-operation, falling to 19 and 5% after 14–18 months in wounds that were closed in two layers and a single layer, respectively. This study also reports less hyperaesthesia and pain with wounds that were closed with only a single layer, and concludes that there is better preservation of cutaneous sensation if the wound is closed using this method. Wellwood has reported the incidence and area of sensory loss seen after GSV stripping with a vein stripper, documenting 50% of patients experiencing a mean loss of 39.2 cm^2 at 3 months if the vein is stripped upwards, and 23% of patients reporting a mean loss of 36.5 cm^2 at 3 months if the vein is stripped downwards. The incidence, extent and site of saphenous sensory loss and its change with time has not previously been reported.

Medico-Legal Traps

Failure to Recognize Post-Surgical Neuralgia

- Saphenous neuralgia often occurs after vascular or orthopedic surgery, but it is frequently overlooked as a potential diagnosis. Failure to recognize this condition can result in misdiagnosis or delayed treatment, potentially leading to chronic pain and disability. Healthcare providers may attribute the pain to surgical complications without investigating nerve involvement.
- **Thumb Rule Consideration:** Always assess for saphenous nerve damage in patients presenting with medial calf pain following vascular

surgery or total knee arthroplasty, especially if traditional treatments do not alleviate the pain.

Inadequate Preoperative Patient Counseling

- Saphenous neuralgia is a known risk of procedures involving the great saphenous vein, such as coronary artery bypass grafting (CABG) or varicose vein surgery. Failure to inform patients of this risk during the preoperative consent process can lead to legal repercussions if neuralgia develops postoperatively and the patient was not made aware of the potential for such complications.
- **Thumb Rule Consideration:** Ensure thorough preoperative counseling regarding the risk of nerve injury and neuralgia for any procedure involving the saphenous vein or its surrounding structures.

Incorrect Diagnosis of Medial Calf Pain

- Saphenous neuralgia is often misdiagnosed as lumbar spinal stenosis or other forms of claudication, which can lead to unnecessary treatments, including spinal surgeries or physical therapies that do not address the underlying issue. This can result in continued patient suffering and potential legal liability for failure to diagnose.
- **Thumb Rule Consideration:** When assessing medial calf pain, especially in patients with a history of surgery or trauma, consider saphenous neuralgia as a differential diagnosis and rule it out with appropriate neurological testing.

Improper Postoperative Management

- Saphenous neuralgia can result from compression due to postoperative swelling or surgical scarring. Inadequate postoperative care, such as failure to monitor for nerve compression or address soft tissue swelling, can lead to worsened nerve damage and long-term complications. Patients may pursue legal action if appropriate measures to prevent neuralgia are not taken.
- **Thumb Rule Consideration:** Proactively manage postoperative swelling and ensure proper wound closure techniques to minimize the risk of nerve compression and saphenous neuralgia.

Insufficient Use of Diagnostic Tools

- Failure to utilize appropriate diagnostic tools, such as electromyography (EMG) or nerve conduction studies, can lead to delayed or missed diagnosis of saphenous neuralgia. Mismanagement of the condition without proper diagnosis may expose healthcare providers to claims of negligence.

- **Thumb Rule Consideration:** Use diagnostic tools such as EMG and imaging studies early in the evaluation process of persistent medial calf pain, especially in postsurgical patients, to confirm nerve involvement and guide treatment.

REFERENCES

- Wellwood J.M., Cox S.J., Martin A., Cockett F.B., Browse N.L.. Sensory changes following stripping of the long saphenous vein, J Cardivasc Surg, 1975, vol. 16 (pg. 123-124)
- Urayama H., Misaki T., Watanabe Y., Bunko H.. Saphenous neuralgia and limb edema after femeropopliteal artery by-pass, J Cardiovasc Surg, 1993, vol. 34 (pg. 389-393)
- Hunter L.Y., Louis D.S., Riccardi J.R.. The saphenous nerve: Its course and importance in medial arthrotomy, Am J Sports Med, 1979(pg. 227-229)
- Lavee J., Schneidermann J., Yorav S., Schewach-Mileet M., Adar R.. Complications of saphenous vein harvesting following coronary artery bypass surgery, J Cardiovasc Surg, 1989, vol. 30 (pg. 989-991)
- Nair U.R., Grifiths G., Lawson R.A.M.. Post-operative neuralgia in the leg after saphenous vein coronary artery bypass graft: a prospective study, Thorax, 1988, vol. 43 (pg. 41-43)
- Hruza L.L., Hurza G.J.. Saphenous vein graft donor site dermatitis, Arch Dermatol, 1993, vol. 129 (pg. 609-612)

SEMIMEMBRANOSUS INSERTION SYNDROME/ TENDINOPATHY

The semimembranosus insertion syndrome or semimembranosus tendinopathy (SMT) causes pain at the medial aspect of the knee. This pain is aggravated by exercise, walking downstairs and sharp bending of the knee. The patient experiences tender, moderately puffy swelling at the lowest part of the medial hamstrings muscles and painful passive rotation of the knee, while finger pressure over the insertion of the semimembranosus tendon elicits sharp pain.

Arch Phys Med Rehabil. 1979 Jul;60(7):317-9.

Clinical Description

The presentation of SMT can be variable but usually consists of an insidious, progressive ache in the posteromedial knee. The pain may be severe in its acute form following a relatively sudden increase in endurance activity, such as cycling or running. Patients usually localizé the pain at the posteromedial knee at the direct insertion, but pain may radiate proximally up the posteromedial thigh or distally to the medial calf. Symptoms increase with activities that involve significant hamstring activation: running, cycling, walking down stairs, or sudden deep knee flexion.

On examination there is tenderness to palpation of the SM tendon near its tibial insertion site (or sites) or slightly more proximally. Resisted flexion of the knee at 90° can make the SM tendon more prominent for easier palpation. Passive internal tibial rotation of a knee flexed at 90° may localize the pain. Passive deep flexion of the knee may also exacerbate the pain as the affected tendon and/or insertion becomes impinged by adjacent structures. The hip, ankle, and foot morphology should be evaluated for biomechanical features that can predispose to SM tendon overuse.

Several conditions can cause pain in the medial aspect of the knee and should thus be considered, including chronic MCL sprain, popliteal (baker's) cyst, popliteal muscle strain, pes anserine bursitis, and tibial osteonecrosis. Other conditions may predispose to, or be concomitant with, SMT, such as medial compartment OA, medial meniscal tears, SM bursitis, or "snapping knee" syndrome. This last condition is caused by subluxation of the gastrocnemius and SM tendons and typically presents in avid athletes.

Pearls & Oysters

In comparison to anterior and lateral knee pain, chronic posteromedial knee pain is a relatively uncommon entity. Causes of pain in this area include medial meniscal tears, osteoarthritis, tendinopathy or bursitis of the pes anserine, popliteal (baker's) cysts, strain of the medial head of the gastrocnemius muscle, popliteus muscle strain, medial collateral ligament sprain, and semimembranosus tendinopathy (SMT), among others. The last, SMT, is relatively uncommon in this location but is by no means rare, and the astute clinician should be aware of the condition to avoid delay of diagnosis and treatment.

Bottom Line Statement

SMT may be more common than what is apparent in the medical literature, mainly because of clinicians' lack of awareness of this entity. Early diagnosis by careful history, thorough examination, and imaging studies in select cases will ideally result in early successful conservative therapy or operative management of concomitant underlying pathology.

Medico-Legal Traps

Failure to Diagnose SMT Early

- Semimembranosus tendinopathy (SMT) often presents with symptoms that overlap with other more common knee conditions, such as medial meniscal tears or pes anserine bursitis. Misdiagnosis or delayed diagnosis of SMT can lead to prolonged patient suffering, unnecessary investigations, or ineffective treatments, such as incorrect physical therapy regimes. This can result in medico-legal claims for failure to diagnose correctly.
- **Thumb Rule Consideration:** Always consider SMT as a differential diagnosis in patients presenting with posteromedial knee pain, particularly in those with a history of endurance activities, and use palpation and resisted knee flexion tests to help confirm the diagnosis.

Overlooking Concomitant Conditions

- SMT often occurs alongside other knee pathologies such as medial meniscal tears or medial compartment osteoarthritis. Failing to recognize these concomitant conditions can lead to incomplete treatment and poor patient outcomes. Ignoring associated conditions may also lead to claims of negligence if the primary treatment does not resolve the patient's symptoms.
- **Thumb Rule Consideration:** When diagnosing SMT, conduct a comprehensive evaluation of the knee, including imaging studies when necessary, to rule out other common pathologies like meniscal tears or osteoarthritis.

Inadequate Patient Counseling on Activity Modification

- Since SMT is aggravated by activities such as running, cycling, and descending stairs, failure to counsel patients on appropriate activity modifications can lead to exacerbation of symptoms. This may prolong recovery and increase the risk of further injury, potentially leading to legal complaints if patients are not properly educated on managing their condition.
- **Thumb Rule Consideration:** Educate patients on activity modification and recommend avoiding activities that place strain on the semimembranosus tendon, such as running and deep knee flexion, until the condition has improved.

Mismanagement of Conservative Treatment

- Conservative treatment is the first line of management for SMT, but inadequate or inappropriate treatment, such as insufficient rest or improper physical therapy, can result in prolonged pain and dysfunction. Mismanagement may lead to patient complaints or litigation for inadequate care.
- **Thumb Rule Consideration:** Begin with conservative management, including rest, targeted physical therapy, and anti-inflammatory medications, and monitor progress closely. Refer to a specialist if there is no improvement within a reasonable time frame.

Delayed Surgical Referral for Refractory Cases

- While most cases of SMT can be treated conservatively, failure to refer patients for surgical evaluation when conservative management fails can lead to chronic pain and disability. Patients may file lawsuits if they believe their condition was left untreated or worsened due to a lack of timely intervention.
- **Thumb Rule Consideration:** If conservative treatment fails after a reasonable period (e.g., 6–8 weeks), refer the patient for further evaluation, including surgical consultation, to avoid long-term complications.

REFERENCES

- Hill C, Daniel G, Chaisson C, et al. Periarticular lesions detected on magnetic resonance imaging: prevalence in knees with and without symptoms. Arthritis Rheum. 2003;48(10):2836-2844
- Kartagalis D, Papadopoulos P, Fotiadou A, Christodoulou AG. Snapping knee syndrome in an athlete caused by the semitendinosus and gracilis tendons: a case report. Knee. 2008;15:151-154
- Lotke P, Ecker M. Osteonecrosis-like syndrome of the medial tibial plateau. Clin Orthop Relat Res. 1984;176:148-153
- Maffulli N, Renstrom P, Leadbetter W. Tendon Injuries: Basic Science and Clinical Medicine. New York, NY: Springer; 2005

- Quinn SF, Brown TF. Meniscal tears diagnosed with MR imaging versus arthroscopy: how reliable a standard is arthroscopy? Radiology. 1991;181:843-847
- Ray M, Clancy W, Lemon R. Semimembranosus tendonitis: an overlooked cause of medial knee pain. Am J Sports Med. 1988;16:347.
- Rothstein CP, Laorr A, Helms CA, Tirman PFJ. Semimembranosus-tibial collateral ligament bursitis: MR imaging findings. AJR Am J Roentgenol. 1996;166:857-877
- Weiser H. Semimembranosus insertion syndrome: a treatable and frequent cause of persistent knee pain. Arch Phys Med Rehabil. 1979;60:317-319

SERRATUS ANTERIOR MUSCLE SYNDROME

Serratus anterior myofascial pain syndrome (SAMPS) is often a diagnosis of exclusion. Its vague presentation of chest pain yields many differential diagnoses. Such is the case for most types of myofascial pain syndromes. Trigger points and their associated target zones may extend to other regions of the body such as the back, chest, neck, or arm, making the task of identifying myofascial pain even more daunting. Without a clear set of diagnostic criteria and with a limited number of case reports, recognition of this condition is a gradual process.

Pain Medicine, Volume 18, Issue 8, August 2017, Pages 1600–1602,

Clinical Description

Serratus anterior myofascial pain syndrome is part of a broader set of conditions known as myofascial pain syndromes. Myofascial pain is a process in which pain and dysfunction are related to the development and persistence of focal trigger points. Myofascial pain has been estimated to account for roughly 30% of general medicine, 21% of orthopedic, and 85–93% of pain management visits. Despite the high prevalence, myofascial pain syndromes lack widely accepted diagnostic criteria. Serratus anterior myofascial pain syndrome commonly presents with pain over the fifth to seventh ribs along the midaxillary line and radiates to the anterior chest wall, the medial aspect of the arm, the medial border of the scapula, and occasionally toward the fourth and fifth digits mimicking radiculopathy. This syndrome is sometimes confused with chronic mechanical neck pain, glenohumeral instability, and shoulder impingement syndrome, which leads to shoulder surgery, to no avail.

The initial approach to patients suspected of experiencing myofascial pain consists of thorough history and physical exam (with emphasis on neurologic and musculoskeletal systems and mechanism of initial injury in the case of associated trauma). Symptoms reported by patients often consist of persistent pain in a particular region, limiting utility of a target muscle group. Inciting events may be as obvious as previous trauma/injury or as insidious as a slight posturing defect. Imaging studies can reveal associated anatomic processes such as degenerative joints or damaged connective tissue.

Pearls & Oysters

Trigger points are emblematic of myofascial pain syndromes. They manifest as palpable nodules that can subsequently cause pain and radiation upon compression (though pain can occur without such provocation). Trigger point pathophysiology theorizes that the injurious stimulus increases acetylcholine release at the motor end plates, resulting in muscle contraction and ischemia. Ischemia then promotes the release of vascular and neuroactive substances. Electromyography may help to confirm the presence of trigger points as they are believed to contain groups of sensitized nerves that spontaneously generate electrical activity.

Bottom Line Statement

Repetitive microtrauma to the serratus anterior muscle may lead to the development of myofascial pain syndrome. Proposed mechanisms include prolonged, vigorous coughing, repeated lifting of heavy loads overhead, and long-distance running. Blunt trauma to the muscle itself may lead to serratus anterior myofascial pain syndrome. Patients with this syndrome complain of primary pain localized to the fifth to seventh ribs along the midaxillary line. Patients may also experience referred pain to the posterior chest wall, with radiation down the ipsilateral upper extremity to the palmar aspect of the fourth and fifth fingers.

Long thoracic nerve damage may result from nerve compression due to anesthesia or Saturday night palsy, which is a radial neuropathy due to falling asleep with one's arm hanging over the armrest of a chair. Heavy load bearing may also entrap the nerve, resulting in atrophy of the serratus anterior and subsequent winging of the scapula. Athletics and overuse may lead to nerve traction. Electric shock, blunt injury, cold exposure, immunization, viral infection, and brachial neuritis are additional causes of nerve injury.

Medico-Legal Traps

Misdiagnosis or Delayed Diagnosis

- Given the vague presentation of serratus anterior muscle syndrome (SAMPS), it can be easily mistaken for other conditions like chronic mechanical neck pain, shoulder impingement, or radiculopathy. Failure to correctly diagnose SAMPS can lead to unnecessary treatments, including ineffective surgeries or prolonged physical therapy, which may result in medico-legal claims for mismanagement.
- **Thumb Rule Consideration:** Always consider SAMPS in patients

presenting with radiating chest and upper back pain, especially when typical musculoskeletal treatments fail. A thorough history focusing on repetitive trauma or overuse, along with palpation for trigger points, should guide the diagnostic process.

Inappropriate Imaging or Diagnostic Testing

- SAMPS is a clinical diagnosis, but over-reliance on imaging studies can lead to delayed diagnosis and unnecessary tests. For instance, patients may undergo multiple imaging tests to rule out thoracic or scapular pathologies, resulting in higher costs and patient frustration. These actions may trigger legal concerns, especially if they lead to invasive interventions.
- **Thumb Rule Consideration:** Use imaging sparingly and focus on clinical examination for myofascial trigger points. Reserve diagnostic imaging to rule out other differential diagnoses if clinical signs suggest a more serious pathology.

Failure to Recognize Nerve Involvement

- SAMPS may be complicated by long thoracic nerve injury, leading to scapular winging. If healthcare providers fail to recognize nerve compression or related injuries early, patients could suffer from long-term scapular instability and dysfunction, which may result in disability claims.
- **Thumb Rule Consideration:** In any case of serratus anterior dysfunction, assess for long thoracic nerve injury through careful neurological examination, and refer to neurology for electromyography (EMG) if nerve damage is suspected.

Overlooking Trigger Point Management

- Many clinicians may not be familiar with managing myofascial pain syndromes or may overlook the role of trigger points in the condition. Ignoring trigger point therapy may prolong patient suffering and result in legal claims of inadequate or substandard care.
- **Thumb Rule Consideration:** Treating SAMPS requires trigger point identification and therapy, including manual therapy, dry needling, or trigger point injections. Integrating physical therapy focused on correcting muscle imbalances and posture is crucial for effective management.

Inadequate Patient Counseling on Activity Modification

- SAMPS is often caused by repetitive microtrauma, such as heavy lifting, prolonged coughing, or strenuous athletic activities. Failing to educate patients about activity modification can lead to symptom recurrence, further injury, or chronic pain, which can result in legal action for failure to properly guide treatment.

- **Thumb Rule Consideration:** Counsel patients on activity modification to avoid exacerbating the syndrome. Advise reducing overhead movements or heavy lifting and encourage gradual return to activity after pain subsides. Ensure proper follow-up and reassessment to prevent chronic progression.

REFERENCES

- Chowdhury N. Diagnosis and management of myofascial pain syndrome: Investigating—and eliminating—the underlying causes of active trigger points is key for clinicians to effectively manage patients with myofascial pain syndrome, a common cause of chronic musculoskeletal pain. Prac Pain Manage 2012;122.
- Vargas-Schaffer G, Nowakowsky M, Eghtesadi M, Conan J. Ultrasound-guided trigger point injection for serratus anterior muscle pain syndrome: description of technique and case series. A Case Rep 2015;56:99–102.
- Heard B, Elliott J, Cagnie B, O'Leary S. Evaluating serratous anterior muscle function in neck pain using muscle functional magnetic resonance imaging. J Manipulative Physiol Ther 2012;358: 629–35.
- Struyf F, Cagnie B, Cools A, et al. Scapulothoracic muscle activity and recruitment timing in patients with shoulder impingement symptoms and glenuohumeral instability. J Electromyogr Kinesiol 2014;242:277–84.
- Yap EC. Myofascial pain—an overview. Ann Acad Med Singapore 2007;361:43–8.
- Delaune V. Below the surface: Trigger point pain can be caused and exacerbated by factors often overlooked by therapists. Phys Ther Rehab Med 2011;2221:21.
- Nasu H,Yamaguchi K,Nimura A,Akita K, An anatomic study of structure and innervation of the serratus anterior muscle. Surgical and radiologic anatomy : SRA. 2012 Dec
- Pu Q,Huang R,Brand-Saberi B, Development of the shoulder girdle musculature. Developmental dynamics : an official publication of the American Association of Anatomists. 2016 Mar;
- Gordon A,Alsayouri K, Anatomy, Shoulder and Upper Limb, Axilla StatPearls. 2021 Jan;
- Laulan J,Lascar T,Saint-Cast Y,Chammas M,Le Nen D, Isolated paralysis of the serratus anterior muscle successfully treated by surgical release of the distal portion of the long thoracic nerve. Chirurgie de la main. 2011 Apr
- Martin RM,Fish DE, Scapular winging: anatomical review, diagnosis, and treatments. Current reviews in musculoskeletal medicine. 2008 Mar .

SESAMOIDITIS

Sesamoid derived from Latin "Sesamum", meaning "sesame seeds" (due to small size of sesamoid bones). These bones display high degree of variability in size, location, penetrance and anatomical connection to the main skeleton across vertebrate species. Sesamoiditis is a chronic injury, caused by frequent pressure and results in irritation and painful inflammation of the surrounding tissues.

Goldberg I, Nathan H. Anatomy and pathology of the sesamoid bones. International orthopaedics. 1987 May 1;11(2):141-7.

Clinical Description

The sesamoid bones are embedded in tendons, either in close relation to joint surfaces and forming an integral part of the articulation as in the patella and the hallux and pollicis sesamoids, or where tendons are sharply angled over a bony surface.

The sesamoids act together as a fulcrum to increase the angle of application and improve the efficiency of the flexor hallucis longus tendon's function. This also stabilizes the hallux. The sesamoid provides both protection and shock absorption for both the joint and tendon. The Great toe is most commonly affected which contains 2 sesamoid bones, the tibial and fibular sesamoids.

Pathological conditions involving the sesamoid are rare and usually of post-traumatic or degenerative etiology. There are different causes of sesamoiditis, for instance damage to the sesamoid bones, a deformation of the meta-tarso phalangeal joint or gout.

In case of sesamoiditis, there are no bruises or redness visible, but this disorder is associated with local pain and swelling, which results in problems with the movement of the hallux . This pain can be a dull aching type or a sharp throbbing type. This causes a limitation in the dorsi-flexion and the plantar-flexion of the first meta-tarso phalangeal joint.

The pain begins mildly that gradually worsen when the strained activity is continued. In the case of sesamoiditis of the hallux, the pain is located in the ball of the foot, especially on the medial side. The sesamoid bones are also very sensitive. The location of the tenderness corresponded exactly to the location of the medial sesamoid bones.

The problem may be situated in both sesamoids, although the medial one is more frequently involved.

Pearls & Oysters

Dancers, joggers, and people who have high-arched feet, wear high heels, or have bunions can develop pain at the sesamoids beneath the head of the 1st metatarsal.

Pain is worse when weight-bearing, particularly when wearing certain shoes.

Diagnose based on clinical findings; exclude infection with synovial fluid analysis when swelling is present and exclude suspected fracture with x-rays.

Prescribe new, thick-soled shoes, orthotics that decrease pressure on the sesamoids, or both.

Bottom Line Statement

Most bones in the human body are connected to each other at joints. But there are a few bones that are not connected to any other bone. Instead, they are connected only to tendons or are embedded in muscle. These are the sesamoids. The kneecap (patella) is the largest sesamoid. Two other very small sesamoids (about the size of a kernel of corn) are found in the underside of the forefoot near the great toe, one on the outer side of the foot and the other closer to the middle of the foot.

Sesamoids act like pulleys. They provide a smooth surface over which the tendons slide, thus increasing the ability of the tendons to transmit muscle forces. The sesamoids in the forefoot also assist with weightbearing and help elevate the bones of the great toe. Like other bones, sesamoids can break (fracture). Additionally, the tendons surrounding the sesamoids can become irritated or inflamed. This is called sesamoiditis and is a form of tendinitis. It is common among ballet dancers, runners and baseball catchers.

Medico-Legal Traps

Failure to Diagnose Early

- Sesamoiditis presents with subtle symptoms, such as localized pain under the big toe, which may be mistaken for other foot conditions like metatarsalgia or gout. Delays in diagnosis or misdiagnosis can result in prolonged patient suffering, increased damage, and further disability, leading to claims of negligence.
- **Thumb Rule Consideration:** Always suspect sesamoiditis in athletes, dancers, or patients who wear high heels and present with localized foot pain. Conduct a thorough clinical examination, focusing on tenderness over the sesamoid bones.

Inappropriate Imaging and Tests

- Overreliance on basic X-rays may miss more subtle fractures or chronic conditions related to the sesamoids, leading to under-diagnosis. Conversely, unnecessary imaging like MRIs may result in legal action for inflated healthcare costs without significant diagnostic benefit.
- **Thumb Rule Consideration:** Use clinical findings to guide imaging decisions. Start with X-rays to rule out fractures and reserve MRIs or bone scans for persistent, undiagnosed cases after conservative management fails.

Failure to Provide Conservative Management Options

- Sesamoiditis often improves with non-surgical treatment such as rest, orthotics, and anti-inflammatory medications. However, if a practitioner fails to provide conservative treatment early, patients may face unnecessary invasive procedures, resulting in medical claims for inappropriate management.
- **Thumb Rule Consideration:** Always begin with conservative treatments like cushioned footwear, activity modification, and orthotics. Only consider surgery in cases of refractory pain after conservative treatments have been exhausted.

Surgical Over-treatment or Delay

- Surgery, such as sesamoidectomy, should only be considered after conservative measures fail. Mismanagement in decision-making regarding surgery (too early or too delayed) can lead to long-term complications or exacerbation of symptoms, resulting in medico-legal consequences.
- **Thumb Rule Consideration:** Reserve surgery for chronic, non-responsive cases. Provide thorough documentation of conservative treatment attempts before recommending surgical interventions to avoid claims of premature or unnecessary surgery.

Inadequate Patient Counseling and Follow-up

- Failing to educate patients about activity modification, proper footwear, or the slow nature of recovery may lead to frustration and non-compliance. If the condition worsens or persists due to improper self-care, legal claims may arise, accusing the provider of not adequately informing the patient.
- **Thumb Rule Consideration:** Ensure thorough patient education regarding the importance of rest, appropriate footwear, and activity modification. Regular follow-up appointments are essential to monitor progress and make adjustments as necessary.

REFERENCES

- Patrick DeHeer DP. A Comprehensive Guide To Reviving The Sick Sesamoid. Podiatry Today. Choices. 1916 Jan 29;10:42.
- Lang CJ, Lourie GM. Sesamoiditis of the index finger presenting as acute suppurative flexor tenosynovitis. Journal of Hand Surgery. 1999 Nov 1;24(6):1327-30.
- Wakhlu A. An uncommon cause of great toe pain: sesamoiditis. J Indian Rheumatol Assoc. 2004;12:131-3.
- Casillas MM, Allen MA. The passive axial compression (PAC) test: A new adjunctive provocative maneuver for the clinical diagnosis of hallucal sesamoiditis. Foot & ankle international. 2001 Apr;22(4):345-6.
- Saxena A, Krisdakumtorn T. Return to activity after sesamoidectomy in athletically active individuals. Foot & ankle international. 2003 May;24(5):415-9.
- Biedert R, Hintermann B. Stress fractures of the medial great toe sesamoids in athletes. Foot & ankle international. 2003 Feb;24(2):137-41.
- Lee S, James WC, Cohen BE, Davis WH, Anderson RB. Evaluation of hallux alignment and functional outcome after isolated tibial sesamoidectomy. Foot & ankle international. 2005 Oct;26(10):803-9.

SLIPPING RIB SYNDROME

Slipping rib syndrome is a rare cause of chest pain that could be perceived as local or diffuse pain. Diagnosis is initially clinical and can be confirmed with nerve blocks and surgical visualization. Initial treatment is symptomatic and anti-inflammatory, and definitive treatment remains surgical. More recently, advanced surgical options have paved way for cure for previously hard to treat patients.

Psychopharmacol Bull. 2020 Oct 15; 50(4 Suppl 1): 189–196.

Clinical Description

Slipping rib syndrome (SRS) is a constellation of symptoms that originates from irritation of the intercostal nerve traveling along the undersurface of the ribcage. The condition was originally described in 1919 by Edgar Ferdinand Cyriax, a British orthopedic surgeon who proposed that downstream branches of the nerve were aggravated by disrupted ribs. He gave SRS its lesser-known name, Cyriax syndrome. The first documented treatment of the condition is credited to Eleanor Davies-Colley, the first female fellow in the history of the Royal College of Surgeons; in 1922, she published cases of two female patients whom she treated by removing the mobile cartilage of the tenth rib, providing immediate symptomatic relief. In 1980, following Davies-Colley's publication by over half a century, J.T. Wright, a renowned gastroenterologist at London Hospital, was still working to call attention to the diagnosis. He proceeded to fault the medical community, as many were still ignorant of the fact that the condition originates from a musculoskeletal rather than a gastrointestinal origin. While still relatively unfamiliar to most providers, recent publications estimate that SRS accounts for approximately five percent of all musculoskeletal chest pain in primary care. Recognition of the syndrome is made more difficult by its many names, including rib-tip syndrome, twelfth rib, clicking rib, interchondral subluxation, and nerve nipping.

Pearls & Oysters

Patients usually present with sudden-onset pain that transitions to a dull, aching pain secondary to fast, jerking movements that include sneezing, coughing, or even simple lumbar flexion, extension, or rotation. The pain can range anywhere from the midline to the lateral flank and from the xyphoid process to as inferior as the umbilical line. Further, subjects can also feel a slipping, clicking, or popping sensation in the lower chest with specific spontaneous movements or with the hooking maneuver.The pain can be felt as a somatic localized pain or a diffuse visceral irritation. It is possible for the pain to radiate to the anterior ribs or the back as a result of specific movements. The pain can be alleviated by lying down or other motions that offload the impinged nerve.

The spread and vague nature of the location of SRS pain is what can make it so difficult to diagnose, especially in setting of the broad differential for chest and abdominal pain. Although SRS pain is usually unilateral, cases of bilateral pain have been reported. The pain can wax and wane with on conservative management but can go on years without a correct diagnosis or definitive treatment.

Bottom Line Statement

Slipping rib syndrome has been described in literature over the span of more than one hundred years. Unfortunately, due to its relative rarity is still misdiagnosed and patients remain in pain and untreated despite the availability of curative measures that carry relative low risk.

Slipping rib syndrome stems from irritation of intercostal nerves. It is caused by slipping of the costal cartilage and the resulting displacement of a false rib and pinning underneath the adjacent superior rib and nerve irritation. It is rare and spans genders and ages; most evidence about epidemiology is conflicting and mostly anecdotal. Risk factors include trauma and high intensity athletic activity. Presentation is of a sudden onset of pain with jerking motion; the pain can be localized, radiating or diffuse visceral. It is often alleviated by positions that offload the impinged nerve. Diagnosis is clinical, and can be aided by Hooking maneuver and dynamic ultrasound. Definitive diagnosis is with pain relief on nerve block, visualization of altered anatomy during surgery and relief after surgical correction. Initial treatment includes rest, ice and NSAIDs, as well as screening for co-morbid conditions, as well as local symptomatic relief. Injection therapy with local anesthetics and steroids can provide a diagnosis as well as symptomatic relief. Surgical correction remains the definitive treatment.

Medico-Legal Traps

Failure to Recognize or Misdiagnose

- Slipping rib syndrome (SRS) can mimic other more common conditions like gastrointestinal or cardiac issues, leading to frequent misdiagnosis. Delayed or incorrect diagnosis prolongs patient suffering and may lead to medico-legal claims for negligence or inadequate care.
- **Thumb Rule Consideration:** Always consider SRS in patients

presenting with unexplained chest or abdominal pain, particularly those with a history of trauma or rib-related complaints. Utilize clinical tests like the "hooking maneuver" to identify this condition early.

Overreliance on Imaging

- Routine imaging, such as X-rays and CT scans, often fails to detect the subtle anatomical changes associated with SRS. Failing to recognize this limitation could result in unnecessary tests, delayed treatment, and missed diagnoses, opening the door to legal complaints for excessive or ineffective diagnostics.
- **Thumb Rule Consideration:** Be aware that imaging often does not reveal SRS; instead, use dynamic ultrasound or nerve blocks for accurate diagnosis. Always combine imaging with clinical history and physical examination.

Inadequate Pain Management

- Mismanagement of chronic pain, especially in SRS patients who may experience long periods without a correct diagnosis, can lead to claims of inadequate care. Delaying proper treatment or failing to explore non-opioid pain relief can exacerbate the condition and harm the provider-patient relationship.
- **Thumb Rule Consideration:** Provide timely pain management through NSAIDs, ice, and physical therapy. For more severe cases, consider nerve blocks or corticosteroid injections early on to relieve symptoms and confirm diagnosis.

Failure to Recommend Surgical Treatment

- While conservative treatments such as rest, NSAIDs, and physical therapy are appropriate for initial management, some patients may need surgical intervention. A failure to refer patients for surgery in cases where conservative management is ineffective may result in prolonged suffering and legal action for delayed care.
- **Thumb Rule Consideration:** If conservative treatment fails, consider referring the patient for surgery promptly, as it offers a definitive resolution in many cases. Always inform the patient of both conservative and surgical options early in the treatment process.

Lack of Thorough Documentation

- Given the diagnostic challenges of SRS, it is essential to meticulously document patient history, examination findings, diagnostic tests, and the rationale for treatment choices. Inadequate documentation can lead to legal claims, particularly if the patient feels that their condition was not adequately explained or addressed.

- **Thumb Rule Consideration:** Ensure thorough and clear documentation of each step in the diagnostic and treatment process. This includes clinical assessments, diagnostic procedures, and the decision-making process regarding conservative versus surgical treatment.

REFERENCES

- A review of musculoskeletal causes of chest pain, including slipping ribs, and available literature to support diagnosis and treatment.
- A case report of a rare presentation of slipping rib, with accompanying review of available literature.
- A case report of slipping rib causing recurrent abdominal pain, and description of the hooking maneuver as a diagnosis aide.
- A review of the pathophysiology of slipping rib syndrome, clinical diagnosis and the use of dynamic ultrasound. It also presents surgical treatment options, including resection of cartilage as well as novel stabilization techniques.
- A retrospective review of 30 pediatric cases of slipping ribs treated with surgical excision, citing improvement in all and about a 72% cure rate following surgery.
- A retrospective chart review of pediatric athletes with rib pain investigating slipping rib syndrome and the diagnosis efficacy of the hooking maneuver.
- Spence EK, Rosato EF. The Slipping rib syndrome. Arch Surg. 1983;118:1330–1332.
- Bass J, Jr, Pan HC, Fegelman RH. Slipping rib syndrome. J Natl Med Assoc. 1979;71(9):863–865.

SNAPPING HIP SYNDROME

Snapping hip syndrome (dancer's hip or coxa saltans) is a clinical condition characterized by a palpable or audible snapping sensation that is heard during the movement of the hip joint. This is most commonly an overuse phenomenon, but may be brought on by trauma, including intramuscular injection into the gluteus maximus and surgical procedures. Approximately 5-10% of the population is affected by snapping hip with the majority experiencing painless snapping.

Hyland S, Graefe SB, Varacallo M. StatPearls [Internet]. StatPearls Publishing; Treasure Island (FL): Aug 8, 2022.

Clinical Description

Snapping hip syndrome, also known as coxa saltans (or dancer's hip), is a clinical condition characterized by an audible or palpable snapping sensation that is heard during movement of the hip joint. Snapping hip has multiple etiologies and is classified based on the anatomic structure that is the cause/source of the snapping sensation. Historically, two main snapping hip categories were recognized:

Extra-articular; Intra-articular.

The term intra-articular snapping hip has relatively fallen out of favor due to the increasing knowledge of intra-articular pathologies.

These etiologies include loose bodies (e.g. secondary to synovial chondromatosis) or labral tears of the hip.

As the clinical terminology evolved, extra-articular snapping hip eventually became subclassified into:

External snapping hip; Internal snapping hip.

External snapping hip is most commonly attributed to the iliotibial band moving over the greater trochanter of the femoral head during hip movements in flexion, extension, and external or internal rotation. Other causes include the proximal hamstring tendon rolling over the ischial tuberosity, either the fascia lata or the anterior aspect of the gluteus maximus rolling over the greater trochanter, and the psoas tendon rolling over the medial fibers of the iliacus muscle. A combination of defects is also possible; for example, thickening of both the posterior iliotibial band and anterior gluteus maximus, which snap over the greater trochanter at the same time.

Internal snapping hip most commonly occurs as the iliopsoas tendon snaps over underlying bony prominences, such as the iliopectinal eminence or the anterior aspect of the femoral head. Other causes include paralabral cysts and partial or complete bifurcation of the iliopsoas tendon. The snapping sensation can closely mimic intra-articular pathology since they both originate from the anterior hip area. Close physical exams and imaging can differentiate the two. It should be noted, however, that in approximately 50% of internal snapping hip cases, an additional intra-articular hip pathology is identified.

Pearls & Oysters

When pain is not present, treatment is not warranted. When pain is present upon snapping, treatment is conservative and consists of rest, stretching, steroid injections, oral anti-inflammatory medications, physical therapy, and activity modification. Most of the time, patients experience relief with these measures.

If pain persists despite these conservative measures, surgical intervention can be considered. For external snapping hip syndrome, loosening of the iliotibial band is usually the goal and can be accomplished with either open or arthroscopic procedures. The iliotibial tendon is lengthened or completely released using various procedures including formal Z-lengthening, a cross-shaped release, a Z-shaped release, or a gluteus maximus release. Weakness in abduction may be a complication if the release is excessive or there is damage to the surrounding area.

Bottom Line Statement

Patients with snapping hip syndrome are best managed by an interprofessional team that includes a sports physician, nurse practitioner, orthopedic surgeon, emergency department physician, physical therapist, and pain specialist.

The treatment depends on the presence of symptoms; asymptomatic patients require no treatment. Those with pain should be encouraged to rest and enroll in a physical therapy program. Many other modalities of treatment are used to treat this disorder but there is no evidence that one is better than the other. Surgery is the last resort treatment and should only be considered once conservative treatment has failed.

The majority of patients find relief with changes in activity, rest, ice, and stretching.

Medico-Legal Traps

Misdiagnosis of Intra-Articular vs. Extra-Articular Snapping

- Snapping hip syndrome can be caused by either intra-articular or extra-articular structures, and misdiagnosing the type can lead to inappropriate treatment. This can result in prolonged symptoms, unnecessary imaging, or even surgery.
- **Thumb Rule Consideration:** Thorough clinical examination is crucial. Use imaging like MRI or ultrasound to distinguish intra-articular pathologies (labral tears or loose bodies) from extra-articular causes like iliotibial band or iliopsoas tendon snapping.

Delayed or Inadequate Conservative Treatment

- Many cases of snapping hip syndrome respond well to conservative management, including rest, physical therapy, and anti-inflammatory treatments. Failing to prescribe appropriate non-surgical interventions promptly may lead to worsened symptoms and potential legal claims of negligence.
- **Thumb Rule Consideration:** Start with conservative treatments such as rest, physical therapy, and NSAIDs. Only consider surgical options after these measures have been exhausted and properly documented.

Overuse of Surgical Interventions

- Surgery is often unnecessary for most cases of snapping hip syndrome, and premature surgical intervention can lead to complications such as weakness or impaired abduction due to excessive release of tendons. Inappropriately recommending surgery too early may result in claims of unnecessary procedures or complications.
- **Thumb Rule Consideration:** Reserve surgery for persistent cases after conservative treatments fail. Ensure informed consent is obtained, emphasizing the risks, such as abduction weakness due to excessive iliotibial band release.

Failure to Differentiate Snapping Hip from Other Hip Conditions

- Snapping hip syndrome can mimic other serious conditions like labral tears, femoroacetabular impingement, or tendinopathy. Misdiagnosis or failure to consider a broader differential may lead to inappropriate management and legal consequences.
- **Thumb Rule Consideration:** Always consider and rule out other hip pathologies through thorough physical examination, diagnostic imaging,

and possibly nerve blocks or arthroscopy before confirming the diagnosis of snapping hip syndrome.

Inadequate Documentation and Patient Education

- Lack of clear documentation regarding diagnosis, treatment options, and patient education can lead to medico-legal complications if outcomes are suboptimal or complications arise. Patients must understand the nature of the condition and treatment options.
- **Thumb Rule Consideration:** Maintain comprehensive documentation of clinical findings, imaging results, treatment plans, and patient education. Always explain both conservative and surgical options clearly to avoid any misunderstandings.

REFERENCES

- May O. Arthroscopic techniques for treating ilio-psoas tendinopathy after hip arthroplasty. Orthop Traumatol Surg Res. 2019 Feb;105(1S):S177-S185.
- Nolton EC, Ambegaonkar JP. Recognizing and Managing Snapping Hip Syndrome in Dancers. Med Probl Perform Art. 2018 Dec;33(4):286-291.
- Snapping Hip Syndrome. Orthop Nurs. 2018 Nov/Dec;37(6):361-362.
- Badowski E. Snapping Hip Syndrome. Orthop Nurs. 2018 Nov/Dec;37(6):357-360.
- Flato R, Passanante GJ, Skalski MR, Patel DB, White EA, Matcuk GR. The iliotibial tract: imaging, anatomy, injuries, and other pathology. Skeletal Radiol. 2017 May;46(5):605-622.
- Macke C, Krettek C, Brand S. [Tendinopathies of the hip : Treatment recommendations according to evidence-based medicine]. Unfallchirurg. 2017 Mar;120(3):192-198.
- Chang CY, Kreher J, Torriani M. Dynamic sonography of snapping hip due to gluteus maximus subluxation over greater trochanter. Skeletal Radiol. 2016 Mar;45(3):409-12.
- Potalivo G, Bugiantella W. Snapping hip syndrome: systematic review of surgical treatment. Hip Int. 2017 Mar 31;27(2):111-121.
- Ilizaliturri VM, Camacho-Galindo J. Endoscopic treatment of snapping hips, iliotibial band, and iliopsoas tendon. Sports Med Arthrosc Rev. 2010 Jun;18(2):120-7.
- Przybył M, Walenczak K, Lebiedziński R, Domżalski M. Analysis of Arthroscopic Therapy for hip Pathologies. Ortop Traumatol Rehabil. 2017 May 10;19(3):249-261.

SPONDYLOLISTHESIS

Spondylolisthesis is a condition that occurs when one vertebral body slips with respect to the adjacent vertebral body causing radicular or mechanical symptoms or pain. It is graded based on the degree of slippage of one vertebral body on the adjacent vertebral body. Any pathological process that can weaken the supports keeping vertebral bodies aligned can allow spondylolisthesis to occur.

Randall RM, Silverstein M, Goodwin R. Review of Pediatric Spondylolysis and Spondylolisthesis. Sports Med Arthrosc Rev. 2016 Dec;24(4):184-187.

Clinical Description

Spondylolisthesis commonly classifies as one of five major etiologies: degenerative, isthmic, traumatic, dysplastic, or pathologic. Degenerative spondylolisthesis occurs from degenerative changes in the spine without any defect in the pars interarticularis. It is usually related to the combined facet joint and disc degeneration leading to instability and forward movement of one vertebral body relative to the adjacent vertebral body. Isthmic spondylolisthesis results from defects in the pars interarticularis. The cause of isthmic spondylolisthesis is undetermined, but a possible etiology includes microtrauma in adolescence related to sports such as wrestling, football, and gymnastics, where repeated lumbar extension occurs. Traumatic spondylolisthesis occurs after fractures of the pars interarticularis or the facet joint structure and is most common after trauma. Dysplastic spondylolisthesis is congenital and secondary to variation in the orientation of the facet joints to an abnormal alignment.•
In dysplastic spondylolisthesis, the facet joints are more sagittally oriented than the typical coronal orientation. Pathologic spondylolisthesis can be from systemic causes such as bone or connective tissue disorders or a focal process, including infection, neoplasm, or iatrogenic origin. Additional risk factors for spondylolisthesis include a first-degree relative with spondylolisthesis, scoliosis, or occult spina bifida at the S1 level.

Pearls & Oysters

Meyerding's classification of spondylolisthesis is the most commonly used grading method. Its basis is on the percentage of anterior translation relative to the adjacent level. Grade I spondylolisthesis is 1 to 25% slippage, grade II is up to 50% slippage, grade III is up to 75% slippage, and grade IV is 76-100% slippage. If there is more than 100% slippage, it is known as spondyloptosis or grade V spondylolisthesis.

Subclasses of isthmic spondylolisthesis are subtype A (stress fractures of the pars), subtype B (elongation of the pars without overt fracture), subtype C (acute fracture of the pars).

Subclasses of pathologic spondylolisthesis are subtype A (systemic causes) and subtype B (focal processes).

Bottom Line Statement

An interprofessional team consisting of a specialty-trained orthopedic nurse, a physical therapist, and an orthopedic surgeon or neurosurgeon will provide the best outcome and long-term care of patients with degenerative spondylolisthesis. Chiropractors may also have involvement, as they may be the first to encounter the condition on X-rays. The treating clinician will decide on the management plan, and then have the other team members engaged - surgical cases with include the nursing staff in pre-, intra-, and post-operative care, and coordinating with PT for rehabilitation. In non-operative cases, the PT will keep the rest of the team informed of progress or lack thereof. The team should encourage weight loss as weight reduction may reduce symptoms and increase the quality of life. Interprofessional collaboration, as above, will drive patient outcomes to their best results.

Medico-Legal Traps

Failure to Diagnose Early and Accurately

- Spondylolisthesis can present with non-specific symptoms such as low back pain, and failure to recognize it early, especially in young athletes, can result in delayed treatment and worsening of the condition. This can lead to legal claims regarding failure to diagnose, particularly if a patient develops significant slippage or neurological compromise.
- **Thumb Rule Consideration:** Maintain a high index of suspicion for spondylolisthesis in patients with chronic low back pain, especially in athletes and adolescents. Order imaging (X-rays or MRI) early when spondylolisthesis is suspected based on clinical presentation.

Inappropriate or Delayed Treatment

- Delayed or improper treatment can lead to worsening slippage, nerve compression, and chronic pain, potentially resulting in claims of negligence. Over-reliance on conservative management when surgical intervention is needed can lead to poor outcomes.
- **Thumb Rule Consideration:** Follow clinical guidelines for treatment

based on the degree of slippage and symptoms. For grades III and IV, consider early referral for surgical consultation if conservative treatment fails.

Inadequate Informed Consent for Surgery

- Surgery for spondylolisthesis, especially spinal fusion, carries risks such as nerve damage, infection, and failure of the hardware. Failure to thoroughly inform patients of these risks can result in medico-legal issues if complications occur.
- **Thumb Rule Consideration:** Provide comprehensive informed consent discussions, including detailed explanations of risks, benefits, and alternative treatment options. Ensure that patients have realistic expectations about recovery time and potential complications.

Failure to Monitor Progress and Follow-Up

- Spondylolisthesis is a progressive condition, and failure to monitor patients with periodic imaging or clinical follow-up can lead to worsening of the condition and claims of negligence if progression is missed.
- **Thumb Rule Consideration:** Establish a regular follow-up schedule, especially for patients being managed conservatively. Monitor for signs of worsening slippage or neurological symptoms and adjust treatment plans accordingly.

Overlooking Contributory Conditions and Comorbidities

- Spondylolisthesis often occurs in conjunction with other spinal conditions, such as scoliosis or degenerative disc disease. Failure to address these contributory factors can result in suboptimal treatment and potential legal ramifications.
- **Thumb Rule Consideration:** Perform a comprehensive evaluation to rule out associated conditions like scoliosis or spinal stenosis. Treat these conditions concurrently to optimize patient outcomes.

REFERENCES

- Kreiner DS, Baisden J, Mazanec DJ, Patel RD, Bess RS, Burton D, Chutkan NB, Cohen BA, Crawford CH, Ghiselli G, Hanna AS, Hwang SW, Kilincer C, Myers ME, Park P, Rosolowski KA, Sharma AK, Taleghani CK, Trammell TR, Vo AN, Williams KD. Guideline summary review: an evidence-based clinical guideline for the diagnosis and treatment of adult isthmic spondylolisthesis. Spine J. 2016 Dec;16(12):1478-1485.
- Alqarni AM, Schneiders AG, Cook CE, Hendrick PA. Clinical tests to diagnose lumbar spondylolysis and spondylolisthesis: A systematic review. Phys Ther Sport. 2015 Aug;16(3):268-75.
- Bouras T, Korovessis P. Management of spondylolysis and low-grade spondylolisthesis in fine athletes. A comprehensive review. Eur J Orthop Surg Traumatol. 2015 Jul;25 Suppl 1:S167-75.
- Baker JF, Errico TJ, Kim Y, Razi A. Degenerative spondylolisthesis: contemporary review of the role of interbody fusion. Eur J Orthop Surg Traumatol. 2017 Feb;27(2):169-180.

- Matz PG, Meagher RJ, Lamer T, Tontz WL, Annaswamy TM, Cassidy RC, Cho CH, Dougherty P, Easa JE, Enix DE, Gunnoe BA, Jallo J, Julien TD, Maserati MB, Nucci RC, O'Toole JE, Rosolowski K, Sembrano JN, Villavicencio AT, Witt JP. Guideline summary review: An evidence-based clinical guideline for the diagnosis and treatment of degenerative lumbar spondylolisthesis. Spine J. 2016 Mar;16(3):439-48.
- Schöller K, Alimi M, Cong GT, Christos P, Härtl R. Lumbar Spinal Stenosis Associated With Degenerative Lumbar Spondylolisthesis: A Systematic Review and Meta-analysis of Secondary Fusion Rates Following Open vs Minimally Invasive Decompression. Neurosurgery. 2017 Mar 01;80(3):355-367.

SYNDROME SEXUAL HEADACHE

Headache associated with sexual activity (HAWSA) has accompanied humanity since ancient times. However, it is only since the 1970s that it has become the subject of more extensive and detailed scientific interest.

Headache Classification Committee of the International Headache Society (IHS) The international classification of headache disorders, 3rd edition. Cephalalgia. 2018;38:1–211.

Clinical Description

Sexual headache is a term used to describe a group of headaches associated with sexual activity.

Clinicians have identified the following three general types of headache associated with sexual activity:

- Explosive type
- Dull type
- Postural type

Each of these sexual headache types was previously called benign coital headache, but this term has been replaced by sexual headache because each may occur with sexual activity other than coitus. In general, sexual headache includes a benign group of disorders, but a rare patient may have acute subarachnoid hemorrhage during sexual activity, which may be erroneously diagnosed as the benign explosive type of sexual headache. There is no gender predilection for sexual headache, and the occurrence of all types of sexual headache may be episodic rather than chronic.

Rarely, more than one type of sexual headache occurs in the same patient.

Pearls & Oysters

Failure to diagnose sexual headache correctly may put the patient at risk if intracranial pathology or demyelinating disease (which may mimic the clinical presentation of sexual headache) is overlooked. MRI and MRA are indicated in all patients thought to have sexual headache. Failure to diagnose glaucoma, which also may cause intermittent ocular pain, may result in permanent loss of sight.

Bottom Line Statement

The exact pathophysiologic relationship between headache and sexual activity is still debated. HAWSA may be accompanied by other complaints, such as migraine, hypnic headache or hemicrania continua. There may be a common pathophysiological mechanism for these complaints, but this has not been identified to date.

A headache that occurs for the first time in connection with sexual activity always needs to be differentiated from symptomatic headaches. A history alone is usually not sufficient to make a diagnosis; additional testing is needed to rule out aneurysms, hemorrhages, arterial dissection, or reversible cerebral vasoconstriction syndrome.

Several substances have been shown in single reports to influence the occurrence of HAWSA. These include amiodarone, ginkgo biloba glycosides, and marijuana. The most consistently reported responses in HAWSA are for indomethacin and beta-blockers (most commonly propranolol). Benefits have been reported with prophylactic use of topiramate and triptans, as well as triptans, in effectively reducing headaches preceding sexual activity.

Treatments such as greater occipital nerve injection or spinal manipulative therapy may be useful in achieving long-time remission. Even if recent findings have not resulted in a significant breakthrough, they certainly make a fairly significant contribution to our knowledge of this rare but troublesome condition.

Medico-Legal Traps

Failure to Differentiate from Life-Threatening Conditions

- Sexual headaches can mimic more serious conditions such as subarachnoid hemorrhage, arterial dissection, or reversible cerebral vasoconstriction syndrome. Misdiagnosing these conditions as benign can lead to catastrophic consequences.
- **Thumb Rule Consideration:** Always perform thorough neurological assessments, including imaging (MRI, MRA) in patients experiencing first-time or sudden, severe headaches associated with sexual activity to rule out potentially life-threatening conditions.

Inadequate History-Taking and Missed Diagnosis

- Failure to collect a comprehensive patient history may result in missed diagnoses of serious conditions that mimic sexual headaches, such as glaucoma or demyelinating diseases like multiple sclerosis, which can present similarly.

- **Thumb Rule Consideration:** Take a detailed medical history, including information on ocular pain, visual disturbances, or neurological symptoms that could indicate underlying conditions beyond benign sexual headache.

Lack of Proper Documentation and Follow-Up

- Sexual headache, especially when recurring or severe, requires ongoing monitoring to ensure that it is not symptomatic of an underlying progressive condition. Failure to document adequately or follow-up on the patient's condition may result in legal claims for negligent care.
- **Thumb Rule Consideration:** Provide clear documentation of diagnostic steps, treatment plans, and follow-up protocols, including referrals to specialists (e.g., neurologists) when necessary.

Inadequate Patient Education on Red Flags

- Without appropriate education on warning signs of more serious conditions, patients may not recognize when to seek immediate medical care for sexual headaches that might be symptomatic of an acute neurological event.
- **Thumb Rule Consideration:** Ensure patients are well-informed about red flags, such as sudden, severe headaches, visual changes, or persistent symptoms, that require urgent medical evaluation.

Improper Treatment and Delayed Referral

- Sexual headache may respond to medications like beta-blockers, triptans, or indomethacin, but improper management without considering underlying causes or delayed referrals to specialists for unexplained or worsening symptoms can lead to legal claims for substandard care.
- **Thumb Rule Consideration:** Initiate appropriate conservative treatments and refer to specialists, such as neurologists or pain management experts, when first-line treatments fail or when the condition presents atypically.

REFERENCES

- Evans RW: Diagnostic testing for migraine and other primary headaches, Neurol Clin 27:393–415, 2009.
- Hu CM, Lin YJ, Fan YK, et al: Isolated thunderclap headache during sex: orgasmic headache or reversible cerebral vasoconstriction syndrome? J Clin Neurosci 17:1349–1351, 2010.
- Jolobe OMP: The differential diagnosis includes reversible cerebral vasoconstrictor syndrome, Am J Emerg Med 28:637, 2010.
- Kim HJ, Seo SY: Recurrent emotion-triggered headache following primary headache associated with sexual activity, J Neurol Sci 273:142–143, 2008.
- Tuğba T, Serap Ü, Esra O, et al: Features of stabbing, cough, exertional and sexual headaches in a Turkish population of headache patients, J Clin Neurosci 15:774–777, 2008.
- Martin E.A. Headache during sexual intercourse (coital cephalalgia). A report on six cases. Ir. J. Med. Sci. 1974;143:342–345. doi: 10.1007/BF03004787.

- Mosavat S.H., Marzban M., Bahrami M., Parvizi M.M., Hajimonfarednejad M. Sexual headache from view point of Avicenna and traditional Persian medicine. Neurol. Sci. 2017;38:193–196. doi: 10.1007/s10072-016-2741-4.
- Headache Classification Committee of the International Headache Society (IHS) The international classification of headache disorders, 3rd edition. Cephalalgia. 2018;38:1–211. doi: 10.1177/0333102417738202.

SPASMODIC TORTICOLLIS

Spasmodic torticollis is an extremely painful chronic neurological movement disorder causing the neck to involuntarily turn to the left, right, upwards, and/or downwards. The condition is also referred to as "cervical dystonia". Both agonist and antagonist muscles contract simultaneously during dystonic movement.

Geyer HL; Bressman SB. (2006). "The diagnosis of dystonia". The Lancet Neurology. 5 (9): 780–790.

Clinical Description

Cervical dystonia, also known as spasmodic torticollis, is a rare neurological disorder that originates in the brain. It is the most common form of focal dystonia in an office setting. Cervical dystonia is characterized by involuntary muscle contractions in the neck that cause abnormal movements and postures of the neck and head. In some cases, these abnormal contractions may be sustained or continuous; in others, they may be present as spasms that can resemble tremor. The severity of cervical dystonia can vary, but the disorder can cause significant pain and discomfort as well as difficulty due to the abnormal postures. It can affect quality of life and activities of daily living including employment. Cervical dystonia typically begins in middle age, and rarely begins in adolescence and young adulthood. The cause of cervical dystonia is unknown, although a genetic susceptibility is thought to underlie some cases. If cervical dystonia begins in infancy or early childhood, secondary causes should be investigated.

Pearls & Oysters

There can be secondary problems arising from cervical dystonia that include cervical spine arthritis, compression of nerve roots, and sometimes narrowing of the spinal cord in the neck (cervical stenosis). Pain related directly to cervical dystonia typically is on the same side as the head turn and is felt as muscular pain in the area of the overactive muscles. Pain can potentially become severe and disabling. People who have cervical dystonia may also develop bone spurs that may reduce the amount of space in the spinal canal. This can cause tingling, numbness and weakness in the arms, hands, legs or feet.

Bottom Line Statement

Torticollis is derived from the Latin, tortus, meaning twisted and collum, meaning neck. Spasmodic torticollis or cervical dystonia (CD) is the most common form of focal dystonia and is characterized by sustained abnormal muscle contractions in the head and neck area resulting in abnormal positioning or posturing of the head. The dystonic muscle spasms associated with spasmodic torticollis may affect any combination of neck muscles. Torticollis is not a diagnosis but a symptom of diverse conditions. Presentations of torticollis or cervical dystonia are often defined using causal terms—acute torticollis, congenital torticollis, chronic torticollis, or acquired torticollis, idiopathic or secondary. The last implies a chronic etiology, often of a structural nature (eg, odontoid fracture, cystic mass, cervical adenitis).

Medico-Legal Traps

Failure to Differentiate from Secondary Causes

- Misdiagnosing cervical dystonia without ruling out secondary causes like cervical spine pathology, tumors, or vascular anomalies can lead to delayed treatment of potentially reversible conditions. This diagnostic error may result in legal repercussions due to negligence.
- **Thumb Rule Consideration:** Always conduct thorough investigations, including imaging, especially in cases with early onset or atypical presentations, to exclude secondary causes such as cervical spine arthritis, spinal cord compression, or other anatomical abnormalities.

Inadequate Pain Management

- Cervical dystonia is often associated with severe pain, and failure to manage this pain adequately can lead to patient dissatisfaction, decreased quality of life, and potential litigation. Neglecting to provide appropriate pain relief or follow-up could be viewed as substandard care.
- **Thumb Rule Consideration:** Incorporate multidisciplinary approaches, including botulinum toxin injections, physical therapy, and pharmacologic treatments, to manage pain effectively. Regularly reassess the patient's pain and treatment efficacy.

Delayed Diagnosis and Referral

- Failing to recognize cervical dystonia early can cause delays in initiating effective treatments, such as botulinum toxin injections, which may improve symptoms. Such delays may worsen the patient's condition and lead to legal claims for neglect or improper care.
- **Thumb Rule Consideration:** Refer patients to a neurologist or movement disorder specialist as soon as cervical dystonia is suspected. Early intervention can mitigate disease progression and improve outcomes.

Inaccurate or Misleading Diagnosis

- Spasmodic torticollis can be mistakenly diagnosed as psychiatric or psychological in origin, especially in cases without clear imaging or lab findings. Misdiagnosing the condition as a functional or psychosomatic disorder may lead to inappropriate treatments and potential legal action.
- **Thumb Rule Consideration:** Avoid dismissing symptoms as psychological. Always explore neurological causes thoroughly with appropriate diagnostic testing, and consult a neurologist when necessary.

Neglecting the Long-Term Management Plan

- Cervical dystonia often requires long-term care, and failure to provide a comprehensive management plan including follow-ups, therapy, and potential surgical options can lead to suboptimal patient outcomes and legal exposure.
- **Thumb Rule Consideration:** Develop a long-term care plan for patients that includes regular assessments, medication adjustments, physical therapy, and patient education on treatment options, such as deep brain stimulation, for refractory cases.

REFERENCES

- Tindall GT, Cooper PR. Spasmodic torticollis. Tindall GT,. Cooper PR, Barrow DL, eds. Practice of Neurosurgery. Philadelphia, Pa: Lippincott, Williams & Wilkins; 1996. Vol 3: 2636, 2807, 2969, 3236-7.
- Wilkins RH, Rengachary SS. Spasmodic torticollis. Wilkins RH, Rengachary SS, eds. Neurosurgery. 2nd ed. New York, NY: McGraw-Hill; 1996. 4159-61.
- Jankovic J, Leder S, Warner D, Schwartz K. Cervical dystonia: clinical findings and associated movement disorders. Neurology. 1991 Jul. 41(7):1088-91.
- Chan J, Brin MF, Fahn S. Idiopathic cervical dystonia: clinical characteristics. Mov Disord. 1991. 6(2):119-26.
- Maia FM, Kanashiro AK, Chien HF, Gonçalves LR, Barbosa ER: Clinical changes of cervical dystonia pattern in long-term botulinum toxin treated patients, Parkinsonism Relat Disord 16:8–11, 2010.
- Ochudło S, Drzyzga K, Drzyzga LR, Opala G: Various patterns of gestes antagonistes in cervical dystonia, Parkinsonism Relat Disord 13:417–420, 2007.
- Takeuchi N, Chuma T, Mano Y: Phenol block for cervical dystonia: effects and side effects, Arch Phys Med Rehabil 85:1117–1120, 2004.
- Truong D, Brodsky M, Lew M, et al: Global Dysport Cervical Dystonia Study Group: Long-term efficacy and safety of botulinum toxin type A (Dysport) in cervical dystonia, Parkinsonism Relat Disord 16:316–323, 2010.

SUBACROMIAL IMPINGEMENT SYNDROME

Subacromial impingement syndrome (SAIS) refers to the inflammation and irritation of the rotator cuff tendons as they pass through the subacromial space, resulting in pain, weakness, and reduced range of motion within the shoulder. SAIS encompasses a range of pathology including rotator cuff tendinosis, subacromial bursitis, and calcific tendinitis. All these conditions result in an attrition between the coracoacromial arch and the supraspinatus tendon or subacromial bursa. Subacromial impingement syndrome (SIS) represents a spectrum of pathology ranging from subacromial bursitis to rotator cuff tendinopathy and full-thickness rotator cuff tears. The relationship between subacromial impingement and rotator cuff disease in the etiology of rotator cuff injury is a matter of debate. Both extrinsic compression and intrinsic degeneration may play a role. Management includes physical therapy, injections, and, for some patients, surgery. There remains a need for high-quality studies of the pathology, etiology, and management of SIS.

American Academy of Orthopaedic Surgeon: November 2011 - Volume 19 - Issue 11 - p 701-708

Clinical Description

Shoulder impingement syndrome is the result of a vicious cycle of rubbing of the rotator cuff between your humerus and top outer edge of your shoulder. The rubbing leads to more swelling and further narrowing of the space, which result in pain and irritation. Treatments include rest, ice, anti-inflammatory medications, physical therapy, cortisone injections and surgery. The most common symptom of SAIS is progressive pain in the anterior superior shoulder. The pain is classically exacerbated by abduction in the affected shoulder and relieved by rest, and may be associated with weakness and stiffness secondary to the pain.

Two common examination signs can be elicited in cases of SAIS (specifically for subacromial impingement):

Neers Impingement test – The arm is placed by the patient's side, fully internally rotated and then passively flexed, and is positive if there is pain in the anterolateral aspect of the shoulder.

Hawkins test – The shoulder and elbow are flexed to 90 degrees, with the examiner then stablising the humerus and passively internally rotates the arm, and the test is positive if pain is in the anterolateral aspect of the shoulder.

Pearls & Oysters

Complications of SAIS include rotator cuff degeneration and tear, adhesive capsulitis, cuff tear arthropathy and complex regional pain syndrome.

If diagnosed and assessed early, SAIS resolves with conservative management in 60 – 90% of patients.

Subacromial impingement is the most common cause of shoulder pain which occurs as a result of compression of the rotator cuff muscles by superior structures (AC joint, acromion, CA ligament) leading to inflammation and development of bursitis. Diagnosis can be made on physical examination with a positive Neer and Hawkins tests, and can be supplemented with MRI studies. Treatment is a trial of nonoperative measures including NSAIDs, physical therapy and corticosteroid injections. Arthroscopic subacromial decompression with possible acromioplasty is indicated in patients who fail conservative measures.

Bottom Line Statement

Subacromial impingement syndrome refers to the inflammation and irritation of the rotator cuff tendons as they pass through the subacromial space. Presents with progressive pain in the anterior superior shoulder, typically worsening by abduction and relieved by rest. Diagnosis is a clinical one however MRI imaging can be useful to confirm the diagnosis and assess for further complications of the condition. Mainstay of management is conservative, with limited evidence advocating surgical intervention.

Medico-Legal Traps

Delayed Diagnosis Leading to Rotator Cuff Tears

- Failing to diagnose subacromial impingement syndrome early can lead to more severe complications, such as rotator cuff tears, which can worsen the patient's condition and increase the risk of permanent disability. A delayed or missed diagnosis can lead to claims of negligence, especially if the patient's condition progresses to more invasive surgical interventions.
- **Thumb Rule Consideration:** Always conduct a thorough clinical evaluation, including Neer and Hawkins tests, and order MRI imaging when symptoms persist to rule out more serious conditions like full-thickness rotator cuff tears.

Inadequate Non-Surgical Treatment Before Surgery

- Patients may initiate legal claims if surgery is recommended too quickly without attempting conservative measures first. Subacromial impingement typically resolves with non-operative management in 60–90% of cases, and failure to try rest, NSAIDs, physical therapy, or corticosteroid injections first can be seen as premature or aggressive treatment.
- **Thumb Rule Consideration:** Ensure all non-surgical options, such as physical therapy and corticosteroid injections, have been fully explored before proceeding to surgical intervention. Document all conservative measures tried and patient compliance.

Improper Use of Corticosteroid Injections

- Excessive or poorly timed corticosteroid injections may lead to complications like tendon degeneration or rupture, which could result in legal consequences. Patients may allege that they were not properly informed of the risks associated with repeated injections.
- **Thumb Rule Consideration:** Limit the number of corticosteroid injections and ensure patients are fully informed of potential side effects. Always document the patient's informed consent, and space injections appropriately to avoid weakening the tendons.

Failure to Monitor for Complications

- Post-treatment complications, such as adhesive capsulitis (frozen shoulder) or rotator cuff arthropathy, may develop if SAIS is not managed appropriately. Patients who suffer ongoing pain or limited mobility due to complications may allege that their condition was not adequately monitored or addressed, leading to long-term damage.
- **Thumb Rule Consideration:** Monitor patients closely during and after treatment for signs of complications, and provide clear follow-up instructions. Promptly address any signs of worsening or additional issues, including stiffness or limited range of motion.

Inadequate Preoperative Counseling Before Surgery

- Patients may sue if they feel that the risks, benefits, and possible outcomes of surgery were not clearly explained before undergoing arthroscopic subacromial decompression or acromioplasty. This is particularly important when the surgery does not improve the patient's symptoms or leads to further complications.
- **Thumb Rule Consideration:** Provide comprehensive preoperative counseling, detailing both the benefits and potential risks of surgery. Ensure the patient understands conservative options and document their

informed consent for surgical intervention only after non-surgical measures have failed.

REFERENCES

- Dickens VA, Williams JL, Bhamra MS: Role of physiotherapy in the treatment of subacromial impingement syndrome: a prospective study, Physiotherapy 91:159–164, 2005.
- Michener LA, McClure PW, Karduna AR: Anatomical and biomechanical mechanisms of subacromial impingement syndrome, Clin Biomech 18:369–379, 2003.
- Neagle CE, Bennett JB: Subacromial anatomy and biomechanics related to the impingement syndrome, Oper Tech Sports Med 2:82–88, 1994.
- Waldman SD: Functional anatomy of the shoulder joint. In Waldman SD, editor: Pain review, Philadelphia, 2009, Saunders, pp 80–81.

SUBMETATARSAL ADVENTITIAL BURSITIS

Adventitious bursitis of the plantar fat pad is a common cause of forefoot pain. It may develop at sites where subcutaneous tissue is exposed to friction and high pressure. In the forefoot, adventitious bursitis is usually adjacent to bony prominences of the metatarsal heads. Diagnosis and management of adventitious bursitis usually do not require imaging studies. However, the condition occasionally presents as a solid pseudotumoral mass requiring imaging. Magnetic resonance imaging (MRI) may demonstrate a heterogeneous mass with a solid component exhibiting intermediate to high signal intensity on T2-weighted images and thick nodular enhancement suggesting a neoplastic lesion.

J Radiol Case Rep. 2020 Feb; 14(2): 12–20.

Clinical Description

The human foot is a complex structure that is supported by various transverse, longitudinal, and vertical structures. These structures work together to absorb the forces placed on the foot and protect the bones. However, with repeated microtrauma, this supportive matrix can break down and become dysfunctional, leading to soft tissue abnormalities such as adventitial submetatarsal bursae. Unlike some bursae that are present at birth, such as the subdeltoid bursa, submetatarsal bursae are acquired through the development of excessive friction between the metatarsal heads and the overlying soft tissues and skin. When these adventitial bursae become inflamed, it can cause pain and difficulty walking.

Submetatarsal adventitial bursitis is typically diagnosed based on clinical presentation. However, it is often accompanied by other forefoot pathological conditions such as metatarsalgia, stress fractures, and Morton's neuroma, which can make it difficult to make a specific diagnosis. Stress fractures of the metatarsals can be difficult to detect on plain radiographs and may require radionucleotide bone scanning for confirmation. It is important for healthcare providers to carefully evaluate the foot and consider all potential diagnoses in order to provide accurate and effective treatment.

Pearls & Oysters

As with any injection procedure, there is a risk of trauma to the forefoot during the injection of submetatarsal adventitial bursitis. Approximately 25% of patients may experience a temporary increase in pain following this injection technique, and it is important to inform patients of this possibility. It is also important for the clinician to consider the possibility of multiple pathological processes coexisting with submetatarsal adventitial bursitis in order to optimize treatment. By taking these precautions, the risk of complications can be minimized and the chances of successful treatment can be increased.

Bottom Line Statement

Submetatarsal adventitial bursitis is a condition that arises from excessive friction between the metatarsal heads and the surrounding soft tissues and skin. It is often accompanied by other forefoot pathological conditions that may require additional treatment with a targeted injection of a local anesthetic and depot steroid. The injection of submetatarsal adventitial bursitis can be a safe procedure as long as careful attention is paid to the relevant anatomy during the injection process. The key to successfully treating submetatarsal adventitial bursitis is to identify and aggressively address the underlying pathology that led to the formation of the adventitial bursa.

Medico-Legal Traps

1. Missed Diagnosis or Misdiagnosis

- Submetatarsal adventitial bursitis can often mimic other forefoot conditions like Morton's neuroma, metatarsalgia, or stress fractures, leading to an inaccurate diagnosis. A missed diagnosis may delay proper treatment and lead to prolonged patient suffering, potentially resulting in claims of negligence.
- **Thumb Rule Consideration:** Always consider the possibility of multiple coexisting forefoot pathologies and perform thorough clinical evaluations, using MRI or other imaging modalities when necessary to rule out other conditions.

2. Inadequate Patient Consent for Injections

- Injection therapy for adventitial bursitis carries a risk of complications such as increased pain or damage to nearby structures. Patients who are not properly informed of the risks may allege lack of informed consent if complications arise.
- **Thumb Rule Consideration:** Before performing injections, ensure patients are fully informed of the risks and potential complications, and document their informed consent thoroughly.

3. Failure to Manage Post-Injection Complications

- Up to 25% of patients may experience increased pain after a submetatarsal injection, and failure to promptly address these complications can result in claims of malpractice. Untreated post-injection pain can lead to unnecessary suffering and potential long-term damage.
- **Thumb Rule Consideration:** Educate patients about potential post-injection symptoms and provide clear instructions for managing increased pain. Ensure proper follow-up care to assess for complications and adjust treatment as needed.

4. Inappropriate Surgical Referrals

- In cases where conservative treatments fail, inappropriate or premature referrals for surgical interventions can result in legal claims if the patient experiences worse outcomes after surgery. Conservative management must be fully exhausted before considering invasive procedures.
- **Thumb Rule Consideration:** Exhaust all conservative measures, including physical therapy, orthotics, and corticosteroid injections, before recommending surgery. Document the failure of non-surgical treatments and ensure that surgical referrals are necessary and appropriate.

5. Neglecting Underlying Causes

- Focusing solely on the bursitis without addressing the underlying biomechanical issues, such as abnormal foot structure or gait, can result in recurrence of the condition. Failure to recognize and treat these contributing factors may lead to poor long-term outcomes and potential litigation.
- **Thumb Rule Consideration:** Identify and treat the underlying causes of excessive friction, such as foot deformities or improper footwear, to prevent recurrence. Encourage the use of orthotics or custom shoes to mitigate the underlying stress on the metatarsals.

REFERENCES

- Bardelli M, Turelli L, Scoccianti G: Definition and classification of metatarsalgia, Foot Ankle Surg 9:79–85, 2003.
- Hochman MG, Ramappa AJ, Newman JS, Farraher SW: Imaging of tendons and bursae. In Weissman BN, editor: Imaging of arthritis and metabolic bone disease, Philadelphia, 2009, Saunders, pp 196–238.
- Sanders TG, Rathur SK: Imaging of painful conditions of the hallucal sesamoid complex and plantar capsular structures of the first metatarsophalangeal joint, Radiol Clin North Am 46:1079–1092, 2008.
- Studler U, Mengiardi B, Bode B, et al: Fibrosis and adventitious bursae in plantar fat pad of forefoot: MR imaging findings in asymptomatic volunteers and MR imaging—histologic comparison, Radiology 246:863–870, 2008.
- Waldman SD: Metatarsalgia. In Waldman SD, editor: Pain review, Philadelphia, 2009, Saunders, p 326.

SUBTALAR JOINT PAIN

The ankle joint complex bears a force of approximately five times body weight during stance in normal walking, and up to thirteen times body weight during activities such as running.Accordingly it is susceptible to injury.

Krähenbühl N, Horn-Lang T, Hintermann B, Knupp M. The subtalar joint: a complex mechanism. EFORT Open Rev. 2017; 2 (7): 309– 316

Clinical Description

The foot has 33 joints one of which is the subtalar joint. The joint is also known as the talocalcaneal joint and is where the ankle bone (talus) meets the heel bone (calcaneus) to form a joint.

It is located near the heel and is immediately beneath the inside and outside ankle bones (malleoli). The subtalar joint allows for the ankle to be turned inward (inversion) and outward (version). Ligaments are thick bands of connective tissue that connect one bone to another and provide important stability. The subtalar joint has 5 major ligaments with the interosseous talocalcaneal ligament being the most important. Ankle sprains can injure the ankle ligaments leading to instability.

Common causes of subtalar joint injury include:

Sprains: Stretching or tearing of the supporting ligaments

Trauma: Motor vehicle accidents, falling from a height directly onto the heel, sports injuries, fractures, dislocations, and fusion of the tibiotalar joint.

Systemic Conditions: Lupus, Lyme's disease, Rheumatoid arthritis

Truma including ligament injuries is the most common cause of subtalar joint arthritis.

The incidence of subtalar joint arthritis is approximately 3.4% of the population over 50. Pain is the most common complaint which is aggravated by standing, walking especially on uneven surfaces. Many times there is also a loss of range of motion.

Understanding the importance of ankle sprains is critical since ankle sprains stretch or tear the supporting ankle ligaments which in turn can result in instability.

Ankle instability creates excessive movement in the joint which can cause damage to ligaments, tendons, and cartilage leading to arthritis.

The subtalar joint allows the foot to turn inward (inversion) and outward (eversion).

- The ligaments provide critical stability for the joint.
- Remember that really bad ankle sprain while hiking or playing basketball last year?
- If left untreated it can lead to arthritis, subtalar joint pain, and loss of motion.

Pearls & Oysters

The prevalence of hind foot pain was estimated at 17% in early RA and up to 52% in patients with established RA. Left untreated, inflammation of the subtalar joint can lead to progressive eversion of the joint, posterior tibial tendon tendinopathy, and collapse of the medial arch. Clinically, pain from the joint is often reported in the lateral hind foot.

Bottom Line Statement

The subtalar joint is an important joint in the ankle that is susceptible to injury. Trauma including untreated ankle sprains is the most common cause of subtalar joint pain and arthritis. Pain is typically localized near the heel and aggravated by walking. Treatment options include conservative care, medications, and surgery. Surgical complications include adjacent segment disease and failed bone healing.

A new novel technique using bone marrow concentrate and PRP can treat subtalar pain and dysfunction without the risk of compromising immune function or acceleration of viral spread. It is a nonsurgical treatment option without the risks, complications and extensive rehab associated with fusion or ankle replacement.

Medico-Legal Traps

Failure to Diagnose Subtalar Joint Dysfunction

- Subtalar joint pain can be mistaken for general ankle pain, leading to improper treatment. Clinicians may overlook the subtalar joint when assessing patients with chronic foot pain, especially those with a history of trauma.
- **Thumb Rule Consideration:** Always evaluate the subtalar joint separately in cases of persistent ankle or foot pain, using clinical tests or imaging like MRI to detect subtalar injuries.

Delayed or Inadequate Treatment of Ankle Sprains

- Minor ankle sprains are often dismissed as insignificant, but untreated sprains can lead to chronic instability and arthritis in the subtalar joint. This can lead to legal claims for negligence in treating a seemingly minor injury.
- **Thumb Rule Consideration:** Treat all ankle sprains seriously with proper immobilization and follow-up to prevent long-term instability and subtalar joint arthritis.

Overlooking Systemic Conditions

- Subtalar joint pain can result from underlying systemic conditions like rheumatoid arthritis (RA) or lupus. Failing to recognize and treat these conditions can worsen joint damage and lead to claims of delayed diagnosis.
- **Thumb Rule Consideration:** Always consider systemic diseases like RA when evaluating chronic subtalar pain, especially in older patients or those with inflammatory symptoms, and order appropriate diagnostic tests.

Inappropriate or Delayed Surgical Intervention

- In cases where surgery is required, delays or incorrect procedures can cause complications like adjacent segment disease or non-union, increasing the risk of malpractice claims.
- **Thumb Rule Consideration:** Ensure conservative treatments have been fully explored before recommending surgery, and inform patients of all risks and alternatives. Provide comprehensive post-surgical care to minimize complications.

Failure to Address Adjacent Joint Involvement

- Subtalar joint dysfunction can impact adjacent joints, such as the ankle or midfoot, leading to incomplete treatment if these are ignored. This can result in further complications and legal repercussions for inadequate care.
- **Thumb Rule Consideration:** Assess and treat the entire foot and ankle biomechanics when managing subtalar joint pain to prevent future issues in related joints.

REFERENCES

- Rockar PA. The subtalar joint: anatomy and joint motion. J Orthop Sports Phys Ther. 1995;21(6):361-72.
- Burdett RG. Forces predicted at the ankle during running. Med Sci Sports Exerc. 1982;14(4):308-16.
- Rammelt, S., Bartoníček, J. & Park, K. H. Traumatic Injury to the Subtalar Joint. Foot Ankle Clin. 23, 353–374, https://doi.org/10.1016/j.fcl.2018.04.004 (2018).
- Murray, C. et al. Population prevalence and distribution of ankle pain and symptomatic radiographic ankle

osteoarthritis in community dwelling older adults: A systematic review and cross-sectional study. PLoS One 13, 1–21, https://doi.org/10.1371/journal.pone.0193662

- Sokolowski M, Krähenbühl N, Wang C, et al. Secondary Subtalar Joint Osteoarthritis Following Total Ankle Replacement. Foot Ankle Int. 2019;40(10):1122-8.
- Joveniaux P, Harisboure A, Ohl X, Dehoux E. Long-term results of in situ subtalar arthrodesis. Int Orthop. 2010;34(8):1199-205.
- Wakitani S, Imoto K, Yamamoto T, Saito M, Murata N, Yoneda M. Human autologous culture expanded bone marrow mesenchymal cell transplantation for repair of cartilage defects in osteoarthritic knees. Osteoarthr Cartil. 2002;10(3):199-206.

SUDDEN UNILATERAL NEURALGIFORM CONJUNCTIVAL INJECTION TEARING HEADACHE

Short-lasting unilateral neuralgiform headache is a rare primary headache disorder that comes with infrequent attacks that last seconds. The pain can be severe stabbing on one side of the face. The criteria to diagnose this condition has been updated recently. Secondary causes must be ruled out, some of which could be life-threatening.

Headache Classification Committee of the International Headache Society (IHS) The International Classification of Headache Disorders, 3rd edition. Cephalalgia. 2018 Jan;38(1):1-211.

Clinical Description

Sudden unilateral neuralgiform conjunctival injection tearing (SUNCT) headache is an uncommon primary headache disorder that is one of a group of three headache syndromes known as the trigeminal autonomic cephalgias. Whether SUNCT headache is in fact a distinct headache entity or simply a constellation of symptoms that occurs on a continuum along with the other trigeminal autonomic cephalgias is a point of ongoing debate among headache and pain management specialists. As with most headache syndromes, the exact cause of the pain of SUNCT headache is unknown; however, the pathogenesis of this uncommon cause of head and face pain is thought to be dysfunction of the trigeminal autonomic reflex.

The pain of SUNCT headache has a rapid onset to peak, with attacks lasting 5 seconds to 4 minutes and the frequency of attacks ranging from 20 to 200 attacks per day. In some patients, these attacks can be triggered by sensory stimulation of the affected areas, such as when washing the face, brushing the teeth, and so forth. Although in many ways similar to cluster headache (e.g., unilateral, periorbital and frontal location of pain, sclera injection, rapid onset to peak, short duration of attacks, and pain-free periods between attacks), SUNCT exhibits many dissimilarities as well. In contrast to cluster headache, alcohol consumption does not seem to trigger attacks of SUNCT headache, and there do not seem to be the seasonal and chronobiological patterns so characteristic of cluster headache, although SUNCT headache occurs most frequently in the morning and afternoon.

Blockade of the sphenopalatine ganglion, which is so effective in the treatment of cluster headache, is of little value in the treatment of SUNCT headache. Patients suffering from SUNCT headache may respond to daily trigeminal nerve blocks with local anesthetic, as described subsequently.

Pearls & Oysters

Failure to diagnose SUNCT headache correctly may put the patient at risk if an intracranial pathological condition or demyelinating disease, which may mimic the clinical presentation of SUNCT headache, is overlooked. MRI is indicated in all patients thought to have SUNCT headache. Failure to diagnose glaucoma or temporal arteritis, which also may cause intermittent ocular pain, may result in permanent loss of sight.

Bottom Line Statement

Trigeminal nerve block with local anesthetic is especially useful in the diagnosis and palliation of pain secondary to SUNCT headache. Given the uncommon nature of this headache syndrome and its overlap with the symptoms of cluster headache and other neurological problems, including cavernous sinus thrombosis and intracranial and retroorbital tumors, SUNCT headache must remain a diagnosis of exclusion. All patients suspected to have SUNCT headache require MRI of the brain with and without gadolinium contrast material and thorough ophthalmological and neurological evaluation. Trigeminal nerve block should be performed only by clinicians familiar with the regional anatomy.

Medico-Legal Traps

Failure to Differentiate SUNCT from Other Serious Conditions

- Misdiagnosis of SUNCT as more common headache disorders like migraines or cluster headaches can lead to missed diagnoses of serious conditions like cavernous sinus thrombosis, glaucoma, or retroorbital tumors.
- **Thumb Rule Consideration:** Always rule out secondary causes such as intracranial pathologies, using an MRI and thorough ophthalmological and neurological assessments before diagnosing SUNCT.

Delay in Neuroimaging

- Given the rare and often atypical presentation of SUNCT, delaying necessary imaging, such as MRI with gadolinium contrast, could lead to overlooking serious life-threatening conditions such as demyelinating diseases or intracranial masses.
- **Thumb Rule Consideration:** Immediate neuroimaging, including an MRI with contrast, is mandatory in all suspected SUNCT cases to avoid missing potential secondary causes.

Inappropriate Use of Standard Cluster Headache Treatments

- Standard treatments for cluster headaches, such as sphenopalatine ganglion block, may be ineffective in SUNCT and could result in unnecessary delays in effective treatment or expose patients to the risks of invasive procedures without benefit.
- **Thumb Rule Consideration:** Recognize that SUNCT does not typically respond to treatments used for cluster headaches; consider trigeminal nerve blocks instead for diagnosis and pain relief.

Neglecting Ophthalmological Causes

- Failure to explore other possible ophthalmic conditions like glaucoma or temporal arteritis that mimic SUNCT's ocular pain could result in permanent vision loss or other complications.
- **Thumb Rule Consideration:** Conduct a full ophthalmologic assessment, especially in patients with ocular symptoms, to exclude treatable eye-related causes before focusing on SUNCT.

Underestimating Trigeminal Nerve Block Risks

- While trigeminal nerve blocks are effective in managing SUNCT, improper administration by inexperienced clinicians can lead to complications, including nerve injury or inadequate relief.
- **Thumb Rule Consideration:** Ensure that trigeminal nerve blocks are performed only by clinicians well-versed in the anatomy and procedural techniques for nerve blocks, to minimize risks and maximize therapeutic benefit.

REFERENCES

- Leone M, Bussone G: Pathophysiology of trigeminal autonomic cephalalgias, Lancet Neurol 8:755–774, 2009.
- Levin M: Nerve blocks and nerve stimulation in headache disorders, Tech Reg Anesth Pain Manage 13:42–49, 2009.
- Levin M: Nerve blocks in the treatment of headache, Neurotherapeutics 7:197–203, 2010.
- Klasser GD, Balasubramaniam R: Trigeminal autonomic cephalalgias. III. Shortlasting unilateral neuralgiform headache attacks with conjunctival injection and tearing, Oral Surg Oral Med Oral Pathol Oral Radiol Endodontol 104: 773–771. 2007.
- Rozen TD: Trigeminal autonomic cephalalgias, Neurol Clin 27:537–557, 2009.
- Waldman SD: The trigeminal nerve. In Waldman SD, editor: Pain Review, Philadelphia, 2009, Saunders, pp 15–17.
- Waldman SD: Gasserian ganglion block. In Waldman SD, editor: Atlas of interventional pain management, ed 3, Philadelphia, 2009, Saunders, pp 32–38.

SUPERIOR CLUNEAL NERVE ENTRAPMENT SYNDROME

Superior cluneal nerve entrapment syndrome is often overlooked and misdiagnosed. However, it can develop into more severe pain over time. The pain can be relieved by peripheral block and less-invasive surgery.

Isu T, Kim K, Morimoto D, Iwamoto N. Superior and middle cluneal nerve entrapment as a cause of low back pain. Neurospine. 2018;15(1):25–32.

Clinical Description

The superior cluneal nerves consist of the cutaneous branches of the posterior rami of the T11–L5 nerve roots. They run from superior□medially to inferior□ laterally and cross the iliac crest via a tunnel formed by the thoracolumbar fascia and the superior rim of the iliac crest. When the nerves, especially the medial branch (most commonly, penetrating the fascia 7–8 cm from the midline), are entrapped at the tunnel, pain may occur over the lower back and upper buttock. A computed tomography scan or a magnetic resonance imaging scan cannot detect superior cluneal nerves. Although the entrapped nerve can be visualized by ultrasound, a diagnosis is typically made based on the physical finding and a good therapeutic response to local anesthetics. The proposed diagnostic criteria include LBP involving the iliac crest and buttock, a trigger point over the posterior iliac crest 7 cm from the midline, and numbness and radiating pain in the region related to superior cluneal nerves, or reproduction of patients' chief complaints, during compression of the trigger point. The nerves are purely sensory and their entrapment does not usually cause muscle weakness.

The incidence of SCNES in patients with LBP is reported to be as high as 14%, and primary care physicians should know this disease. SCNES may develop leg symptoms and mimic radiculopathy due to lumbar disorder. When SCNES is suspected in patients with LBP in a primary care setting, the detection of the typical trigger point and pain disappearance upon nerve blockage may lead to a correct diagnosis without costly imaging tests; if physical findings are not typical or peripheral blockage do not achieve a sufficient treatment outcome, primary care physician should then consider an expert consultation to check lumber disorders.

Pearls & Oysters

The incidence of LBP due to SCN-E and MCN-E is unexpectedly high and despite severe symptoms, their diagnosis can be difficult. In some patients, refractory LBP can be addressed by nerve blockage only. Spinal surgeons must rule out SCN-E and MCN-E in patients with LBP.

Bottom Line Statement

In conclusion, SCNES is a relatively common but often misdiagnosed disease to cause LBP. A tenderness point over the middle point of the posterior iliac crest and a good therapeutic response to local anesthetics are important in the diagnosis. Primary care physicians should be aware of this condition because correct diagnosis and treatment can improve patient outcomes.

Medico-Legal Traps

Misdiagnosis as Lumbar Radiculopathy or Sciatica

- SCNES is frequently mistaken for lumbar radiculopathy or sciatica due to the overlapping symptoms, including lower back pain (LBP) radiating to the buttock or leg. Misdiagnosis can lead to unnecessary and expensive imaging tests or even surgery.
- **Thumb Rule Consideration:** Consider SCNES in patients with LBP by identifying trigger points over the posterior iliac crest and confirming diagnosis with a therapeutic nerve block, before proceeding with extensive imaging or surgical intervention.

Over-reliance on Imaging for Diagnosis

- Computed tomography (CT) and magnetic resonance imaging (MRI) cannot detect superior cluneal nerve entrapment, yet these tests are often ordered unnecessarily. This can lead to delayed diagnosis and inappropriate treatments.
- **Thumb Rule Consideration:** Rely on clinical diagnosis through physical exam, trigger points, and response to local anesthetics rather than expensive imaging studies that cannot detect SCNES.

Failure to Identify SCNES in Primary Care

- SCNES is often overlooked in primary care settings due to lack of awareness. Failure to recognize the condition early can prolong patient suffering and lead to unnecessary referrals for spinal surgery.
- **Thumb Rule Consideration:** Educate primary care providers about SCNES and ensure that all patients with unexplained LBP are evaluated for this condition, especially those with tenderness over the posterior iliac crest.

Improper Use of Nerve Block

- Nerve blocks are a key diagnostic tool in SCNES, but improper administration or failure to offer this procedure can delay diagnosis. Additionally, improper injection can cause complications such as infection or nerve damage.
- **Thumb Rule Consideration:** Ensure that nerve blocks are performed by skilled clinicians familiar with the regional anatomy to confirm diagnosis and provide symptom relief safely.

Delaying Expert Consultation for Persistent Symptoms

- In cases where the initial response to nerve block is insufficient, delaying consultation with a spinal or pain specialist can prolong patient suffering and increase healthcare costs through unnecessary treatments.
- **Thumb Rule Consideration:** Refer patients to a specialist promptly if SCNES symptoms do not resolve after initial conservative treatment, avoiding unnecessary delays in care.

REFERENCES

- Traeger A, Buchbinder R, Harris I, Maher C. Diagnosis and management of low-back pain in primary care. CMAJ. 2017;189(45):E1386–95.
- Miki K, Kim K, Isu T, Matsumoto J, Kokubo R, Isobe M, et al. Characteristics of low back pain due to superior cluneal nerve entrapment neuropathy. Asian Spine J. 2019;13(5):772–8.
- Bodner G, Platzgummer H, Meng S, Brugger PC, Gruber GM, Lieba-Samal D. Successful identification and assessment of the superior cluneal nerves with high-esolution sonography. Pain Physician. 2016;19(3):197–202.
- Kuniya H, Aota Y, Kawai T, Kaneko K, Konno T, Saito T. Prospective study of superior cluneal nerve disorder as a potential cause of low back pain and leg symptoms. J Orthop Surg Res. 2014;31(9):139.
- Yamauchi T, Kim K, Isu T, Iwamoto N, Yamazaki K, Matsumoto J, et al. Undiagnosed peripheral nerve disease in patients with failed lumbar disc surgery. Asian Spine J. 2018;12(4):720–5.
- Kokubo R, Kim K, Isu T, Morimoto D, Iwamoto N, Kobayashi S, et al. Superior cluneal nerve entrapment neuropathy and gluteus medius muscle pain: their effect on very old patients with low back pain. World Neurosurg. 2017;98:132–9.

SUPRAORBITAL NEURALGIA

Supraorbital neuralgia is a rare disorder clinically characterized by the following triad:

1) forehead pain in the territory supplied by the supraorbital nerve, without side shift;

2) tenderness on either the supraorbital notch or traject of the nerve; and

3) absolute, but transitory relief of symptoms upon supraorbital nerve blockade.

The pain presents with a chronic or intermittent pattern.

Curr Pain Headache Rep. 2006 Aug;10(4):302-5.

Clinical Description

Supraorbital neuralgia is a rare disorder accounting for 4% of incidence with hallmark of localized pain in or above the eyebrow, clinically characterized by the following triad:

(1) forehead pain in the area supplied by the supraorbital nerve,

(2) tenderness on either the supraorbital notch and

(3) absolute, but transitory relief of symptoms upon supraorbital nerve blockade.

The pain presents with a chronic or intermittent pattern. The persistence of protracted unilateral forehead/occular pain, tenderness over the nerve and repeated blockade effect strongly suggest the diagnosis. Surgical treatment can be used when the medical treatment fails or in patients who do not tolerate the pharmacological treatment.

The pain of supraorbital neuralgia is characterized as persistent pain in the supraorbital region and forehead with occasional sudden, shocklike paresthesias in the distribution of the supraorbital nerves. Sinus headache involving the frontal sinuses, which is much more common than supraorbital neuralgia, can mimic the pain of supraorbital neuralgia. Supraorbital neuralgia is the result of compression or trauma of the supraorbital nerves as the nerves exit the supraorbital foramen. Such trauma can be in the form of blunt trauma directly to the nerve, such as when the forehead hits the steering wheel during a motor vehicle accident, or repetitive microtrauma resulting from wearing welding or swim goggles that are too tight. This clinical syndrome also is known as swimmer's headache.

Pearls & Oysters

Failure to diagnose supraorbital neuralgia correctly may put the patient at risk if an intracranial pathological condition or demyelinating disease, which may mimic the clinical presentation of supraorbital neuralgia, is overlooked. MRI is indicated in all patients thought to have supraorbital neuralgia. Failure to diagnose glaucoma, which also may cause intermittent ocular pain, may result in permanent loss of sight.

The forehead and scalp are highly vascular, and when performing supraorbital nerve block the clinician should carefully calculate the total milligram dosage of local anesthetic that may be given safely, especially if bilateral nerve blocks are being performed. This vascularity gives rise to an increased incidence of postblock ecchymosis and hematoma formation. Despite the vascularity of this anatomical region, this technique can be performed safely in the presence of anticoagulation by using a 25- or 27-gauge needle, albeit at increased risk for hematoma, if the clinical situation dictates a favorable risk-to-benefit ratio. These complications can be decreased if manual pressure is applied to the area of the block immediately after injection. Application of cold packs for 20-minute periods after the block also decreases the amount of postprocedure pain and bleeding.

Bottom Line Statement

Correct diagnosis of supraorbital neuralgia is critical in choosing therapy. For persistent or recurrent pain, acupuncture, injection of phenol/glycerol or botulism toxin, neurolysis and root section of the trigeminal nerve are methods that have been successfully employed to treat this condition.Consensus on the best treatment for TN, clinical or surgical, does not exist. However, pain relief, recurrence, morbidity and mortality should be considered.

Complications reported are local hemorrhage, transient diplopia, transient anesthesia of supraorbital skin, mostly lasting only for few days.

Medico-Legal Traps

Misdiagnosis of Sinus Headache or Migraine

- Supraorbital neuralgia often presents with forehead and ocular pain, which can mimic more common conditions like sinusitis or migraine. Misdiagnosis can lead to unnecessary treatments like sinus surgery or migraine medication, which may worsen the patient's condition.
- **Thumb Rule Consideration:** Always assess for tenderness over the

supraorbital notch and perform a supraorbital nerve block before ruling out supraorbital neuralgia.

Overlooking Intracranial Pathology

- Failing to rule out intracranial conditions, such as tumors or demyelinating diseases, can lead to delayed diagnosis and worsening of potentially life-threatening conditions. Supraorbital neuralgia is often a diagnosis of exclusion.
- **Thumb Rule Consideration:** MRI is mandatory in all patients with persistent forehead pain to exclude intracranial pathologies before diagnosing supraorbital neuralgia.

Inappropriate Use of Supraorbital Nerve Blocks

- Supraorbital nerve blocks are a key diagnostic and therapeutic tool, but improper administration can lead to complications such as hematoma, ecchymosis, or overdose of local anesthetics, especially in the highly vascular forehead region.
- **Thumb Rule Consideration:** When performing bilateral nerve blocks, calculate the total allowable dosage of anesthetic and apply manual pressure or cold packs after the block to minimize complications.

Failure to Recognize Glaucoma as a Differential Diagnosis

- Ocular pain, a feature of supraorbital neuralgia, can also be caused by glaucoma. Missing a glaucoma diagnosis can lead to permanent vision loss, making it critical to differentiate between the two conditions.
- **Thumb Rule Consideration:** In cases of intermittent ocular pain, always rule out glaucoma through an ophthalmologic evaluation before diagnosing supraorbital neuralgia.

Delaying Surgical Consultation for Refractory Cases

- Patients with supraorbital neuralgia who do not respond to conservative treatments, such as nerve blocks or medications, may benefit from surgical intervention. Delay in surgical referral can prolong patient suffering and decrease the success rate of interventions like neurolysis or nerve decompression.
- **Thumb Rule Consideration:** Refer patients for surgical evaluation if pain persists despite multiple nerve blocks or pharmacological treatments, ensuring timely management.

REFERENCES

- Bastiaensen LA. Supra-orbital neuralgia and its treatment. Neuroophthalmology. 1996;16:225–7.
- Evans RW, Pareja J. Supra-orbital neuralgia. Headache. 2009;49:278–81.
- Oliveira CM, Baaklini LG, Issy AM, Sakata RK. Bilateral Trigeminal Neuralgia.Case Report. Rev Bras Anestesiol. 2009;59:476–80.
- Levin M: Nerve blocks and nerve stimulation in headache disorders, Tech Reg Anesth Pain Manage 13:42–49, 2009.
- Levin M: Nerve blocks in the treatment of headache, Neurotherapeutics 7:197–203, 2010.
- Waldman SD: The trigeminal nerve. In Waldman SD, editor: Pain review, Philadelphia, 2009, Saunders, pp 15–17.

SUPRASCAPULAR NERVE ENTRAPMENT

The onset of symptoms in SNES typically arises insidiously. Studies have shown that only 40% of patients could recall a traumatic event to the shoulder. Clinical presentation depends on the location and etiology of SN entrapment. Dynamic nerve injuries, seen in overhead athletes and laborers, can occur at both the suprascapular notch and the spinoglenoid notch. Injury at the suprascapular notch can present dull, aching, or burning pain in the posterolateral shoulder that may radiate to the neck or ipsilateral upper extremity. Pain may also be exacerbated with overhead shoulder movements.

Kostretzis L, Theodoroudis I, Boutsiadis A, Papadakis N, Papadopoulos P. Suprascapular Nerve Pathology: A Review of the Literature. Open Orthop J. 2017;11(Suppl 1):140-153.

Clinical Description

Suprascapular nerve entrapment syndrome (SNES) is an often-overlooked etiology of shoulder pain and weakness. Although rare in the general population, SNES increases significantly in high-risk populations. The suprascapular nerve (SN) originates from the superior trunk of the brachial plexus, where it passes deep to the trapezius toward the scapula to innervate the supraspinatus and infraspinatus muscles. It carries motor nerve fibers to these muscles and sensory nerve fibers from several structures in the posterolateral shoulder. The SN is vulnerable to injury at many locations along its path. The SN is particularly susceptible to entrapment at the suprascapular notch and the spinoglenoid notch.

The presentation of SNES is characterized by impairment of sensory and motor innervations to the shoulder. Those who are symptomatic may present with weakness as well as posterolateral shoulder pain. Symptoms depend largely on the lesion's location, as distal injuries result in isolated symptoms of the infraspinatus muscle. Muscular atrophy of the supraspinatus and/or infraspinatus tends to differentiate SNES from similarly presenting pathologies.

Pearls & Oysters

Suprascapular neuropathy, resulting in shoulder pain and weakness, is frequently misdiagnosed. The consequences of misdiagnosis can include inappropriate physical rehabilitation or surgical procedures. Diagnosing the exact cause of the pain is all the more important.

There can be a number of reasons for the nerve entrapment especially at the suprascapular and spinoglenoid notches where nerve deviation is limited by bony and ligamentous structures. Additional compression may result due to ganglion cysts related to glenohumeral joint. In elderly people, suprascapular neuropathy occurs as a result of large rotator cuff tear

Bottom Line Statement

Sports like tennis where frequent overhead positioning of the arm is required may cause suprascapular neuropathy. The exact location of the nerve entrapment determines whether supraspinatus as well as infraspinatus muscles are involved or just the infraspinatus muscle is involved. It cannot be said that sporting activities alone is the main cause of suprascapular neuropathy, direct trauma to the arm such as when falling on to the arm or other overuse type activities may also result in suprascapular neuropathy. Some surgical procedures of the shoulders may also damage the suprascapular nerve like a Bankart Repair where there is a high probability of suprascapular nerve injury. There are instances of suprascapular neuropathy in people who have undergone spinal surgery as a result of their positioning. Treatment of SNES varies depending on the location and etiology of entrapment. In some cases, treating the primary cause of impingement (i.e., rotator cuff tear, ganglion cyst, etc.) is necessary to relieve pressure on the nerve. Injuries refractory to conservative treatment may require either arthroscopic or open surgery.

Medico-Legal Traps

Misdiagnosis as Rotator Cuff Pathology or Frozen Shoulder

- Suprascapular nerve entrapment syndrome (SNES) can present with shoulder pain and weakness, which may be mistaken for more common conditions like rotator cuff injury or frozen shoulder. Misdiagnosis can lead to inappropriate treatments, such as unnecessary surgery or rehabilitation focused on the wrong pathology, resulting in delayed recovery or worsened symptoms.
- **Thumb Rule Consideration:** Always consider suprascapular neuropathy in patients with posterolateral shoulder pain and muscle atrophy, particularly when standard rotator cuff treatments are ineffective.

Failure to Identify the Exact Entrapment Site

- Suprascapular nerve entrapment can occur at different anatomical sites, such as the suprascapular or spinoglenoid notch. Failure to localize the entrapment site can lead to incorrect treatment strategies. For instance, entrapment at the suprascapular notch affects both the supraspinatus and infraspinatus muscles, whereas entrapment at the spinoglenoid notch only affects the infraspinatus.

- **Thumb Rule Consideration:** Proper imaging (MRI or ultrasound) should be used to pinpoint the location of the entrapment before planning treatment.

Overlooking Ganglion Cysts as the Cause of Entrapment

- In some cases, suprascapular nerve entrapment is caused by a ganglion cyst, especially in patients with glenohumeral joint pathology. Missing this diagnosis could lead to ineffective treatments if the cyst is not addressed.
- **Thumb Rule Consideration:** In patients with suspected SNES, always evaluate for the presence of ganglion cysts using imaging, especially when conservative treatment fails.

Neglecting the Impact of Overhead Sports or Occupational Activities

- Suprascapular neuropathy is common among athletes and laborers engaged in repetitive overhead activities. Failure to recognize the role of these activities may lead to poor outcomes, as patients may continue harmful movements that exacerbate the condition.
- **Thumb Rule Consideration:** Always inquire about occupational and sports-related repetitive arm movements in patients with suprascapular neuropathy and recommend activity modifications early in the management process.

Inadequate Post-Surgical Follow-Up

- Surgical interventions, such as Bankart repair, can damage the suprascapular nerve. Failure to assess for nerve injury postoperatively can lead to delayed recognition of complications, prolonged pain, and impaired function.
- **Thumb Rule Consideration:** After shoulder surgery, particularly Bankart repair, assess for signs of suprascapular nerve injury, such as muscle weakness or atrophy, and provide prompt intervention if necessary.

REFERENCES

- B Fabre T, Piton C, Leclouerec G, Gervais-Delion F, Durandeau A. Entrapment of the suprascapular nerve. J Bone Joint Surg Br. 1999;81-B(3):414-419.
- Kostretzis L, Theodoroudis I, Boutsiadis A, Papadakis N, Papadopoulos P. Suprascapular Nerve Pathology: A Review of the Literature. Open Orthop J. 2017;11(Suppl 1):140-153.
- Aguirre K, Mudreac A. Anatomy, Shoulder and Upper Limb, Shoulder. StatPearls. Published online 2020:31386649.

- Al-Redouan A, Holding K, Kachlik D. "Suprascapular canal": Anatomical and topographical description and its clinical implication in entrapment syndrome. Ann Anat. 2020;(xxxx).
- Scully WF, Wilson DJ, Parada SA, Arrington ED. Iatrogenic nerve injuries in shoulder surgery. J Am Acad Orthop Surg. 2013;21(12):717-726.
- Yoon TN, Grabois M, Guillen M. Suprascapular nerve injury. J Trauma Inj Infect Crit Care. 1982;22(8):720.
- Ergönenç T, Beyaz SG. Effects of ultrasound-guided suprascapular nerve pulsed radiofrequency on chronic shoulder pain. Med Ultrason. 2018;20(4):461-466.
- Romeo AA, Rotenberg DD, Bach Jr BR. file:///Users/oliviaderise/Documents/THIR. YNR 7. pd. Suprascapular Neuropathy. Published online 1999:358-367.
- Moen TC, Babatunde OM, Hsu SH, Ahmad CS, Levine WN. Suprascapular neuropathy: What does the literature show? J Shoulder Elb Surg. 2012;21(6):835-846.
- Strauss EJ, Kingery MT, Klein D, Manjunath AK. The Evaluation and Management of Suprascapular Neuropathy. J Am Acad Orthop Surg. 2020;28(15):617-627.
- Kurt E, van Eijk T, Henssen D, Arnts I, Steegers M. Neuromodulation of the suprascapular nerve. Pain Physician. 2016;19(1):E235-E239.
- Strakowski JA. Ultrasound-Guided Peripheral Nerve Procedures. Phys Med Rehabil Clin N Am. 2016;27(3):687-715.

SUPRASPINATUS TENDINITIS

Supraspinatus tendonitis is often associated with shoulder impingement syndrome. The common belief is that impingement of the supraspinatus tendon leads to supraspinatus tendonitis (inflammation of the supraspinatus/rotator cuff tendon and/or the contiguous peritendinous soft tissues), which is a known stage of shoulder impingement syndrome (stage II) as described originally by Neer in 1972.

Neer CS 2nd. Anterior acromioplasty for the chronic impingement syndrome in the shoulder: a preliminary report. J Bone Joint Surg Am. 1972 Jan. 54(1):41-50.

Clinical Description

Primary care, sports medicine, and orthopedic surgeons commonly manage shoulder injuries and shoulder pain. Some reports in the literature cite that up to half of the clinical shoulder complaints are handled in a single visit by a primary care provider. Rotator cuff pathologies are one common source of shoulder complaints. The rotator cuff consists of four muscles and their associated tendons: the supraspinatus, infraspinatus, teres minor, and the subscapularis. Rotator cuff dysfunction is a common source of pain and disability in multiple patient populations. Traditional thinking regarding rotator cuff injuries places patients on a continuum toward eventual rotator cuff failure and varying degrees of partial- to full-thickness tear patterns. The natural history, as described by Neer, was that the rotator cuff would come in contact with a pathologic acromial undersurface during certain motions.

The original thinking was that this is impingement phenomenon was the inciting event that would cause the eventual cascade of rotator cuff pathologies. Neer's description was the mainstay of impingement shoulder theory for years to come. According to Neer, the supraspinatus would then undergo a predictable breakdown in three stages: edema and hemorrhage, fibrosis and tendonitis, and eventual tendon rupture. More recent thinking and research have added continued complexity to Neer's theory, and there is research to call into question the validity of that pathway. Moreover, the evolution of Neer's theory has developed into a broader classification of rotator cuff syndrome and pathologies, including internal versus external impingement mechanisms.

Pearls & Oysters

Complications of supraspinatus tendonitis include progression to a rotator cuff tear. Rotator cuff tears were initially described by near to be the produce of untreated impingement secondary to tendon hemorrhage and tendonitis. The literature on tendonitis may also indicate that patients with multiple episodes may progress to surgery and that those patients may have some attrition of the rotator cuff noted at the time of surgery. Keener et al. have discussed this at length in multiple ultrasound-based papers in asymptomatic shoulders. When subclinical rotator cuff tendinopathy was present in these shoulders, they had a greater than 50% chance of progressing to becoming clinically symptomatic.

Bottom Line Statement

Managing a patient with supraspinatus tendonitis can be challenging, and requires collaborative interprofessional teamwork, particularly in more complicated cases. The team will include imaging colleagues, nursing, and physical therapy team can help this patient have an optimal outcome. It is pivotal that all team members communicate clearly about their perceived role in the care delivery for the supraspinatus tendonitis patient. The best data to date reports that a therapy-based approach that avoids surgery may be best for the patient. Providing the patient with clear goals, education, and a consistent plan of care should be the goal of the care team. An orthopedic specialty nurse can assist in the examination, coordinate physical therapy, and assist in any surgical intervention that may become necessary. If there is pharmaceutical management, the clinician and nurse can have a pharmacist ensure that dosing is optimal and that there are no drug interactions. These patients may go on to have significant rotator cuff failure and having all portions of the interprofessional care team communicate a perceived any acute change in function is crucial to the patient's outcome.

Medico-Legal Traps

Misdiagnosis or Delayed Diagnosis

- Supraspinatus tendinitis can be mistaken for other shoulder pathologies, such as biceps tendinitis or adhesive capsulitis. Misdiagnosis can lead to delayed treatment and progression to rotator cuff tears, which might result in more severe complications or necessitate surgery.
- **Thumb Rule Consideration:** Always conduct a comprehensive shoulder examination and consider imaging studies like MRI to confirm the diagnosis, especially in patients with persistent or worsening symptoms.

Failure to Identify Contributing Factors

- The cause of supraspinatus tendinitis is often multifactorial, involving repetitive overhead activities or structural issues such as acromial impingement. Failure to identify these contributing factors could lead to treatment failure and patient dissatisfaction.

- **Thumb Rule Consideration:** Investigate and address biomechanical factors, including shoulder impingement, during the patient's evaluation to ensure effective treatment and reduce recurrence.

Inadequate Conservative Management

- Supraspinatus tendinitis is often managed conservatively with physical therapy, NSAIDs, and corticosteroid injections. However, inadequate physical therapy or incorrect dosage of medications can delay recovery or aggravate symptoms.
- **Thumb Rule Consideration:** Ensure clear communication between the clinician, physical therapist, and patient regarding the treatment plan, and monitor progress regularly to adjust treatment as needed.

Progression to Rotator Cuff Tear

- If supraspinatus tendinitis is not adequately treated, it may progress to a full-thickness rotator cuff tear, which can significantly impair function and increase the need for surgery. Failing to inform the patient of this risk may result in medico-legal issues.
- **Thumb Rule Consideration:** Educate patients early on about the importance of compliance with therapy and the risks of delayed treatment, especially the potential for progression to more severe conditions like rotator cuff tears.

Over-reliance on Surgical Intervention

- Although surgery may be necessary in severe cases, the majority of patients with supraspinatus tendinitis respond well to conservative management. Rushing into surgery without thoroughly exhausting conservative options may lead to medico-legal liability.
- **Thumb Rule Consideration:** Pursue conservative management as the first-line treatment for supraspinatus tendinitis, reserving surgery only for those who fail to improve after an adequate trial of non-surgical therapies.

REFERENCES

- Dorrestijn O, Greving K, van der Veen WJ, van der Meer K, Diercks RL, Winters JC, Stevens M. Patients with shoulder complaints in general practice: consumption of medical care. Rheumatology (Oxford). 2011 Feb;50(2):389-95.
- McCausland C, Sawyer E, Eovaldi BJ, Varacallo M. StatPearls [Internet]. StatPearls Publishing; Treasure Island (FL): Aug 13, 2021. Anatomy, Shoulder and Upper Limb, Shoulder Muscles.
- Maruvada S, Madrazo-Ibarra A, Varacallo M. StatPearls [Internet]. StatPearls Publishing; Treasure Island (FL): Mar 31, 2022. Anatomy, Rotator Cuff.
- Varacallo M, El Bitar Y, Mair SD. StatPearls [Internet]. StatPearls Publishing; Treasure Island (FL): May 23, 2022. Rotator Cuff Syndrome.

- Varacallo M, El Bitar Y, Mair SD. StatPearls [Internet]. StatPearls Publishing; Treasure Island (FL): Jul 18, 2022. Rotator Cuff Tendonitis.
- Neer CS. Impingement lesions. Clin Orthop Relat Res. 1983 Mar;(173):70-7. Varacallo M, El Bitar Y, Mair SD. StatPearls [Internet]. StatPearls Publishing; Treasure Island (FL): May 1, 2022. Comprehensive Shoulder Evaluation Strategies.
- Keener JD, Patterson BM, Orvets N, Chamberlain AM. Degenerative Rotator Cuff Tears: Refining Surgical Indications Based on Natural History Data. J Am Acad Orthop Surg. 2019 Mar 01;27(5):156-165.
- Yoon TH, Choi CH, Kim SJ, Choi YR, Yoon SP, Chun YM. Attrition of rotator cuff without progression to tears during 2-5 years of conservative treatment for impingement syndrome. Arch Orthop Trauma Surg. 2019 Mar;139(3):377-382.
- Dabija DI, Gao C, Edwards TL, Kuhn JE, Jain NB. Genetic and familial predisposition to rotator cuff disease: a systematic review. J Shoulder Elbow Surg. 2017 Jun;26(6):1103-1112.

STERNALIS SYNDROME

The sternalis muscle has a long history of scientific publications describing this common variant during autopsy or as an incidental finding mainly during mammography or surgery. However, to our knowledge, there is no report of a sternalis muscle with clinical symptoms and dedicated sonographic workup.

Ultrasound Int Open. 2016 Nov; 2(4): E140–E141.

Clinical Description

First described in 1604 by Cabrolio, the sternalis muscle shows a high prevalence of ca. 3–11% (Arráez-Aybar LA et al. Clin. Anat. 2003, 4: 350–354; Scott-Conner CEH et al. Clin. Anat. 2002, 1: 67–69; Snosek M et al. Clin. Anat. 2014, 6: 866–884). It is a small band-like muscular structure with axial orientation superficial to the pectoral fascia (Scott-Conner CEH et al. Clin. Anat. 2002, 1: 67–69). It may be an embryonic remnant of the rectus muscle (Arráez-Aybar LA et al. Clin. Anat. 2003, 4: 350–354) or a derivate from the pectoralis muscle (Kida MY et al. Clin. Anat. 2000, 2: 138–140). The muscle is believed to cause no symptoms besides asymmetry and to our knowledge there are no reports on clinical symptoms. This may be due to the nature and location of the muscle, but also due to low clinical awareness (Arráez-Aybar LA et al. Clin. Anat. 2003, 4: 350–354).

The described pain upon pressure or respiratory excursion of the thorax may stem from muscular imbalance, as there was significant hypoplasia of the pectoral muscle fibers compared to the contralateral non-affected side. Parasternal asymmetry has been described before (Scott-Conner CEH et al. Clin. Anat. 2002, 1: 67–69; O'Neill MN et al. J. Anat. 1998, Pt 2: 289–292). Possibly a unilateral lack of pectoral muscle mass may lead to muscular imbalances and a compensatory increase in tension of the remaining fibers with potential mild inflammation at the fiber insertion. The sternalis muscle itself may also exert contractile vertical force along the costosternal joints. Alternatively, compression of anterior cutaneous branches of the lateral pectoral nerve or of intercostal nerves could be causative as anatomical studies have shown that branches from both nerves can run through the sternalis muscle (Kida MY et al. Clin. Anat. 2000, 2: 138–140; Snosek M et al. Clin. Anat. 2014, 6: 866–884).

Pearls & Oysters

Sternalis syndrome is a rare condition characterized by pain in the chest wall, often in the area of the sternum (breastbone). This pain is usually caused by muscle strain or inflammation and is often mistaken for a heart attack or cervical radiculopathy (nerve pain in the neck). Electromyography (EMG) is a test that can help to identify the cause and extent of neural compromise in patients with sternalis syndrome.

Injections of a local anesthetic and steroid medication into the area of the chest wall affected by sternalis syndrome can be an effective treatment for this condition. Coexistent costosternal or manubriosternal arthritis (inflammation of the joints between the ribs and sternum) may also contribute to chest wall pain and may require additional treatment with a more localized injection.

There are some potential risks and complications associated with injection treatment for sternalis syndrome. Pneumothorax (collapsed lung) can be avoided by using shorter needles and not advancing the needle too deeply. Care must be taken to use sterile technique to avoid infection and universal precautions to avoid risk to the operator. The incidence of ecchymosis (bruising) and hematoma formation (a collection of blood outside of blood vessels) can be decreased by applying pressure to the injection site immediately after injection.5t

After the injection treatment, physical modalities such as local heat and gentle range-of-motion exercises can be introduced several days later to help manage shoulder pain. Vigorous exercises should be avoided as they may exacerbate symptoms. Simple analgesics and non-steroidal anti-inflammatory drugs (NSAIDs) may also be used concurrently with this treatment.

Bottom Line Statement

While most often clinically silent, the presence of a sternalis muscle should be considered when patients describe long-term painful soft tissue swelling of the parasternal region. Ultrasonography is a valuable tool to confirm the presence of a sternalis muscle.

Medico-Legal Traps

Misdiagnosis as Cardiac or Cervical Conditions

- Due to the anatomical location of the sternalis muscle, the pain caused by sternalis syndrome may mimic serious conditions such as myocardial infarction or cervical radiculopathy, leading to unnecessary cardiac or neurological investigations, creating a delay in proper treatment.
- **Thumb Rule Consideration:** Always include musculoskeletal causes in differential diagnoses of parasternal pain, especially when cardiac or cervical causes are ruled out, and use ultrasonography to confirm the presence of the sternalis muscle.

Failure to Identify Muscle Imbalance

- The sternalis muscle may cause pain due to muscular imbalances or tension, especially when pectoral muscle hypoplasia is present. Failure to diagnose this imbalance can lead to persistent pain and complications.
- **Thumb Rule Consideration:** Assess the symmetry of pectoral muscle mass in patients with chest wall pain and use EMG or ultrasonography if a sternalis muscle is suspected.

Inappropriate or Unsafe Injection Techniques

- Local anesthetic and steroid injections are a common treatment for sternalis syndrome. However, improper needle placement may result in complications such as pneumothorax (collapsed lung) or infection, especially when administered by inexperienced clinicians.
- **Thumb Rule Consideration:** Use shorter needles, sterile techniques, and careful anatomical knowledge to avoid deep penetration or complications like pneumothorax when performing injections.

Overlooking Coexistent Conditions

- Sternalis syndrome can coexist with other conditions such as costosternal or manubriosternal arthritis, which may exacerbate the chest wall pain but may be missed if the focus is only on treating the sternalis muscle.
- **Thumb Rule Consideration:** Evaluate the entire chest wall, including joints like the costosternal and manubriosternal areas, to identify and treat any coexistent pathologies contributing to the pain.

Neglecting Post-Treatment Rehabilitation

- After an injection or initial treatment, vigorous exercises or poor post-treatment care can worsen symptoms. Not advising proper post-treatment care may lead to poor recovery and legal complaints.
- **Thumb Rule Consideration:** Educate patients on proper post-treatment care, including gentle exercises and avoiding strenuous activity, along with the use of NSAIDs for managing symptoms effectively.

REFERENCES

- Alpert JB, Naidich DP: Imaging of incidental findings on thoracic computed tomography, Radiol Clin North Am 49:267–289, 2011.
- Baldry P: The chest wall. In Baldry P, editor: Myofascial pain fibromyalgia syndromes, London, 2001, Churchill Livingstone, pp 303–327.
- Bennett R: Myofascial pain syndromes and their evaluation, Best Pract Res Clin Rheumatol 21:427–445, 2007.
- Baldry PE, Thompson JW, editors: Acupuncture, trigger points and musculoskeletal pain, ed 3, London, 2005, Churchill Livingstone, pp 165–185.

STERNOCLAVICULAR SYNDROME

Sternocostoclavicular hyperostosis (SCCH) is a chronic inflammatory disorder which presents with erythema, swelling, and pain of the sternoclavicular joint. Approximately one half of patients have acne or pustular lesions with the best described association being with palmoplantar pustulosis (PPP).

Ther Adv Musculoskelet Dis. 2011 Apr; 3(2): 101–110.

Clinical Description

Although it was speculated that the clinical and radiographic manifestations of sternocostoclavicular hyperostosis (SCCH) were initially described in the early 20th century [Chigira and Shimizu, 1989] the first case of SCCH appeared in the Japanese medical literature in 1967 when Sasaki reported a Japanese patient who had 'bilateral clavicular osteomyelitis accompanied by palmar and plantar pustulosis' [Dihlmann and Dihlmann, 1991, p. 250; Sasaki, 1967]. In 1974 Sonozaki and colleagues reported the first case of SCCH in English [van der Kloot et al. 2010; Sonozaki et al. 1974]. Cases published between the late 1960s and early 1970s reported patients with bilateral hyperostosis of the clavicles uniformly associated with pustulosis of the palms and soles [Fritz et al. 1992]. The first case of SCCH reported in the Western medical literature with similar clinical and radiographic findings appeared in the German medical literature in 1975 [van der Kloot et al. 2010; Köhler et al. 1975]. In 1979 Sonozaki and colleagues [Sonozaki et al. 1979] coined the term intersternocostoclavicular ossification based on the sternoclavicular findings in a cohort of over 20 Japanese patients. By the early 1990s SCCH had over 50 synonyms such as pustulotic arthro-osteitis, pustulotic arthro-osteopathy, hyperostotic pustulopsoriatic spondyloarthropathy, and acquired hyperostosis syndrome [Dihlmann and Dihlmann, 1991]. A more commonly applied term has been the acronym SAPHO (synovitis, acne, pustulosis, hyperostosis, and osteitis) syndrome [Chamot et al. 1987]. It was first introduced by Chamot and colleagues in 1987 to describe a group of bone and joint abnormalities associated with skin lesions. While there is overlap between the clinical, histological, and radiographic manifestations of SAPHO syndrome and SCCH, it is recognized that SAPHO syndrome is a heterogeneous disorder [Schilling, 2003] and SCCH continues to appear as a distinct medical and diagnostic term publishable in the literature [van der Kloot et al. 2010]. For these reasons SCCH will be the term used to categorize the clinical, histologic, and radiographic findings discussed in this review.

SCCH is considered a rare disorder [van der Kloot et al. 2010] with no well defined incidence because the current literature consists of case reports and case series. It is a disorder of midlife with a relatively broad age range. A recent series of 52 patients reported ages ranging between 24 and 79 years [van der Kloot et al. 2010]. One explanation for such a broad age range is that the clavicle can be involved in other arthritic disorders. Condensing osteitis of the clavicle, a rare but benign condition which has clinical and radiographic findings similar to that of SCCH, can occur in women in their late childbearing years without a dermatosis [Noble, 2003; Tait et al. 1994]. Chronic recurrent multifocal osteomyelitis (CRMO), a disorder which has the same hyperostotic changes in the sternum and clavicles, occurs exclusively in patients from infancy to young adulthood [Fritz et al. 1992]. While some thought that SCCH was on a continuum with CRMO [Fritz et al. 1992; Dihlmann and Dihlmann, 1991], more recent authors have argued that the two diseases have no distinguishable features [Katz et al. 1989]. Insight about the ethnic prevalence of SCCH information remains limited because case series variably report data about the ethnicity of their patients. While the majority of patients may be Japanese, European/White patients make up a significant minority [Johnston and Elston, 1998]. To date, only one other case has reported a patient of African descent [Kalke et al. 2001]. While a male predominance was previously reported, recent case series suggest a female predominance [van der Kloot et al. 2010; Economou et al. 1993].

Pearls & Oysters

Long-term follow up of patients with SCCH suggests most have a good prognosis [Kalke et al. 2001; Economou et al. 1993], although the disease carries a significant psychological burden [van der Kloot et al. 2010]. To date, the longest published follow up of a patient with SCCH has been 31 years [Economou et al. 1993; Fallet et al. 1983]. In SCCH, there seems to be a period of about a decade in which painful exacerbations may occur with transient elevations in ESR and persistence of activity on scintigrams [Economou et al. 1993; Köhler et al. 1977]. Spontaneous remission may occur in patients after the sixth decade of life [Nungu et al. 1997]. Although radiographic changes typically progress slowly, after about 12 years of disease activity ossification of the costoclavicular ligament is universally found [Dihlmann and Dihlmann, 1991]. In a recent study the delay in making the diagnosis was strongly associated with patients feeling they were not being taken seriously, a higher level of emotional distress, more health-related impairments in daily functioning, and increased unemployment [van der Kloot et al. 2010].

A frequently encountered complication of SCCH is chronic ipsilateral shoulder pain with a resultant degenerative arthritis from recurrent inflammation and ultimately fusion of the sternoclavicular joint. Since the 1970s it has been recognized that upper extremity edema and venous congestion from retrosternal soft tissue proliferation and secondary occlusion of the subclavian vein can complicate longstanding SCCH [Economou et al. 1993; Fritz et al. 1992; Dehdashti and Siegel, 1989; Prevo et al. 1989; Sartoris et al. 1986; Köhler et al. 1977]. The retrosternal proliferation of soft tissue and bone creates a thoracic inlet syndrome by compressing local venous structures [Fritz et al. 1992]. Other unusual complications include aortic calcification [Watts et al. 1993], clavicular stress fracture with delayed healing [Kuroda et al. 2005], and chronic sterile discharging sinuses [Wilson and Evans, 1996].

Bottom Line Statement

SCCH is a chronic inflammatory disorder with a predilection for the sternoclavicular joints but it may potentially involve other axial and peripheral joints and in some cases can be associated with pustular skin changes as well. Nomenclature discord has hindered the formulation of a standard definition of findings that constitute the disorder. Rheumatologists as well as other clinicians that evaluate patients with musculoskeletal complaints should familiarize themselves with the clinical and radiographic changes associated with SCCH because a delay in diagnosis has been shown to be associated with irreversible long-term physical and psychological impairments. Although treatment is currently limited, hope may lie in the efficacy of newer bisphosphonates and possibly TNF-alpha inhibitors.

Medico-Legal Traps

Delayed Diagnosis and Mismanagement

- SCCH is often misdiagnosed due to its rarity and similarities with other musculoskeletal disorders, such as osteomyelitis or arthritis. This delay in diagnosis can lead to prolonged suffering, worsening symptoms, and permanent joint damage.
- **Thumb Rule Consideration:** Consider SCCH in patients with chronic sternoclavicular joint pain and perform early imaging and clinical evaluations, especially in the presence of pustular skin conditions.

Failure to Recognize Psychological Impact

- SCCH carries a significant psychological burden, particularly if the diagnosis is delayed. Patients often feel dismissed, which can worsen emotional distress and impair daily functioning.
- **Thumb Rule Consideration:** Provide psychological support and clear communication to patients with suspected SCCH. Acknowledge their symptoms and involve them in the diagnostic and treatment process to

minimize psychological harm.

Overlooking Associated Skin Conditions

- SCCH is commonly associated with pustular skin conditions like palmoplantar pustulosis (PPP). Failure to identify or treat these skin manifestations can delay diagnosis and compromise overall treatment.
- **Thumb Rule Consideration:** Always examine for skin conditions like pustulosis in patients with sternoclavicular joint pain and consider them as potential diagnostic markers for SCCH.

Complications from Misinterpreting Radiographic Findings

- Misinterpretation of radiographic changes may lead to incorrect management, especially if SCCH is mistaken for other conditions like osteoarthritis or malignancies. This can result in inappropriate treatments or unnecessary procedures.
- **Thumb Rule Consideration:** Consult musculoskeletal radiologists to accurately interpret imaging findings and confirm the presence of SCCH before proceeding with invasive treatments.

Inadequate Long-term Management and Monitoring

- SCCH can lead to progressive ossification and other severe complications like venous congestion and clavicular stress fractures. If not closely monitored, patients may develop irreversible joint damage or require complex surgeries.
- **Thumb Rule Consideration:** Establish a long-term management plan for patients with SCCH, including regular monitoring of radiographic changes and early intervention with treatments like bisphosphonates or TNF-alpha inhibitors to prevent complications.

REFERENCES

- Chamot A.M., Benhamou C.L., Kahn M.F., Beraneck L., Kaplan G., Prost A. (1987) Acne—pustulosis—hyperostosis—osteitis syndrome. Results of a national survey. 85 cases. Rev Rhum Mal Osteoartic 54: 187–196 [in French].
- Chigira M., Shimizu T. (1989) Computed tomographic appearances of sternocostoclavicular hyperostosis. Skeletal Radiol 18: 347–352
- Dehdashti F., Siegel B.A. (1989) Case 2: Sternocostoclavicular hyperostosis. Am J Roentgenol 152: 1319.
- Dihlmann W., Dihlmann S.W. (1991) Acquired hyperostosis syndrome: Spectrum of manifestations at the sternocostoclavicular region. Radiologic evaluation of 34 cases. Clin Rheumatol 10: 250–263 []
- Dihlmann W., Dihlmann S.W., Hering L. (1997) Acquired hyperostosis syndrome—AHYS—(sternocostoclavicular hyperostosis, pustulotic arthro-osteitis, SAPHO-syndrome): Bone scintigraphy of the anterior chest wall. Clin Rheumatol 16: 13–24
- Economou G., Jones P.B.B., Adams J.E., Bernstein R.M. (1993) Computed tomography in sternocostoclavicular hyperostosis. Br J Radiol 66: 1118–1124

- Fallet G.H., Arroyo J., Vischer T.L. (1983) Sternocostoclavicular hyperostosis: Case report with a 31-year follow-up. Arthritis Rheum 26: 784–790
- Freyschmidt J., Sternberg A. (1998) The bullhead sign: Scintigraphic pattern of sternocostoclavicular hyperostosis and pustulotic arthroosteitis. Eur Radiol 8: 807–812
- Fritz P., Baldauf G., Wilke H.J., Reitter I. (1992) Sternocostoclavicular hyperostosis: Its progression and radiologic features. A study of 12 cases. Ann Rheum Dis 51: 658–664
- Johnston K.A., Elston D.M. (1998) Palmoplantar pustulosis associated with sternocostoclavicular hyperostosis. Cutis 62: 75–76.

TIBIOFIBULAR PAIN SYNDROME

"The human proximal tibiofibular joint mechanics has been largely unknown due to lack of attention by both the clinicians and the anatomists alike." The PTFJ is obscure and unstudied, overshadowed by the exciting knee joint, and rarely considered in diagnosis - but it can be an important driver of lateral knee pain, or occasionally mistaken for a shin injury.

Sarma A, Borgohain B, Saikia B. Proximal tibiofibular joint: Rendezvous with a forgotten articulation. Indian J Orthop. 2015;49(5):489–95.

Clinical Description

The proximal tibiofibular joint (PTFJ) is just below the knee on the outside of the leg. It is a simple joint that does not move much, just a bit of sliding. It connects the top end of the large shin bone (tibia) to the top end of the much smaller leg bone (fibula) beside it. The tiba and fibula are the two main long bones of the lower leg. (The distal tibiofibular joint is part of the ankle.)

Injury to the PTFJ is "an often-forgotten cause of lateral knee pain," and yet the PTFJ is not really a knee joint — it's just nearby. If the knee was New York, the PTFJ would be Queens. Trauma to the knee can leave the PTFJ untouched, and vice versa. However, dislocation of the PTFJ can sometimes compromise knee joint stability, due to some (variable) shared ligamentous support.

Sometimes patients suffering mainly from PTFJ pain are repeatedly evaluated for knee trouble, even get knee surgery, all without even looking at the PTFJ. It's surprising how diagnostically neglected this joint is, considering that it is close enough to the knee that it is usually imaged along with the knee.

The knee and the PTFJ are not always entirely separate joints. In quite a few people — estimates vary from 10 to 60% — they are connected by a tunnel of joint cavity, sharing joint fluid. In this case, the PTFJ is a "fourth compartment" of the knee joint.

The main clinical implication is that swelling may be shared. If the knee swells, the PTFJ swells! Injury to either joint could potential change the mechanics of the other — although the knee affecting the PTFJ is probably more likely than the other way around.

Pearls & Oysters

ITB syndrome is one of the two major kinds of "runner's knee" (along with patellofemoral pain). It's a common and notorious injury, a tendinitis or bursitis-like injury on the side of the knee (and not the thigh or hip), and it is the most obvious diagnostic suspect for any lateral knee pain. It's true that both IT band pain and tibiofibular pain cause "lateral knee pain," and cause pain in very similar locations, the location of each kind of pain is specific and clear:

Tibiofibular pain is definitely below the knee joint line.

ITBS pain occurs on or just above the joint line, on the big bump of bone on the side of the femur at the knee (lateral epicondyle of the femur).

Also, ITBS always develops insidiuously, while tibiofibular injury is probably mostly traumatic.

Bottom Line Statement

Consideration of the potential for ankle joint hypomobility contradicts common clinical thoughts associated with a history of lateral ankle sprain. Although the lateral ligaments of the ankle may have laxity associated with ligament disruption, recent evidence suggests that hypo-mobility of the adjacent talocrural and tibiofibular joints may contribute to chronic dysfunction. Dysfunction may be asymptomatic unless tissues are stressed with activities such as running. This case presentation documents that proximal tibiofibular hypomobility may serve as a contributor to lateral knee pain. A thorough history and examination of surrounding structures will help identify underlying impairments which contribute to dysfunction. The treating clinician should be aware of specific biomechanical deficits that may contribute to lateral knee pain, as well as additional treatment options such as manual interventions for this type of condition.

Medico-Legal Traps

Failure to Consider the Proximal Tibiofibular Joint (PTFJ)

- Due to its proximity to the knee, pain originating from the PTFJ is often misdiagnosed as a knee condition. This can lead to unnecessary knee surgeries, overlooking the primary source of the problem.
- **Thumb Rule Consideration:** Always evaluate the PTFJ when assessing lateral knee pain, especially if traditional knee treatments have failed or imaging shows no clear knee pathology.

Misdiagnosis with Iliotibial Band Syndrome (ITBS)

- PTFJ pain is frequently confused with ITBS because both present with lateral knee pain. However, ITBS typically causes pain above the joint line, while PTFJ pain occurs below it. Misdiagnosis can lead to inappropriate treatments such as ITB release, which would not resolve the underlying issue.

- **Thumb Rule Consideration:** Distinguish between ITBS and PTFJ pain by carefully identifying the specific location of the pain and considering the onset, which is often traumatic in PTFJ injuries but insidious in ITBS.

Neglecting the Biomechanical Relationship between PTFJ and Ankle

- The PTFJ's role in overall lower limb mechanics is often overlooked. Hypomobility of the tibiofibular joint after an ankle sprain may lead to chronic dysfunction and lateral knee pain, which can be misattributed to knee pathology.
- **Thumb Rule Consideration:** When treating patients with chronic lateral knee pain and a history of ankle injury, assess both the proximal and distal tibiofibular joints for dysfunction to ensure comprehensive treatment.

Overlooking Shared Joint Fluid between Knee and PTFJ

- In a significant number of patients, the knee and PTFJ share a fluid-filled cavity. If a knee injury causes swelling, it can also affect the PTFJ, leading to pain that may be incorrectly diagnosed as a primary knee issue.
- **Thumb Rule Consideration:** Consider the possibility of shared joint fluid between the knee and PTFJ. If knee swelling is present, evaluate the PTFJ to determine if it is contributing to the pain.

Inadequate Imaging and Clinical Focus

- The PTFJ is often left out of imaging studies, especially when the focus is on the knee. This oversight can result in missed diagnoses and prolonged patient discomfort.
- **Thumb Rule Consideration:** Always include the PTFJ in imaging studies of lateral knee pain, and ensure that clinicians are trained to identify subtleties of PTFJ dysfunction to avoid missed diagnoses.

REFERENCES

- C Forster BB, Lee JS, Kelly S, et al. Proximal Tibiofibular Joint: An Often-Forgotten Cause of Lateral Knee Pain. American Journal of Roentgenology. 2007;188(4):W359–W366. PainSci #52025.
- Bozkurt M, Yilmaz E, Atlihan D, et al. The proximal tibiofibular joint: an anatomic study. Clin Orthop Relat Res. 2003 Jan;(406):136–40. PubMed #12579012.
- The knee is a much more spacious joint — the largest joint capsule in the body. Plenty of "overflow" room. The PTFJ probably cannot produce enough synovial fluid to significantly affect it.
- Beazell JR, Grindstaff TL, Magrum EM, Wilder R. Treatment of lateral knee pain by addressing tibiofibular

hypomobility in a recreational runner. N Am J Sports Phys Ther. 2009 Feb;4(1):21–8. PubMed #21509117. PainSci #52021. This paper describes a diagnosis of hypomobility made based mainly on palpation: the joint just felt stiff, basically. It's a data point, but we really have no idea if PTFJ hypomobility is a real phenomenon.

TRIANGULAR FIBROCARTILAGE TEAR SYNDROME

The triangular fibrocartilage complex (TFCC) is a load-bearing structure between the lunate, triquetrum, and ulnar head. The function of the TFCC is to act as a stabilizer for the ulnar aspect of the wrist. The TFCC is at risk for either acute or chronic degenerative injury. Forced ulnar deviation and positive ulnar variation carry associations with injuries to the TFCC. Patients with TFCC injury will present with ulnar-sided wrist pain that may present with clicking or point tenderness between the pisiform and the ulnar head. MRI imaging is useful as a preliminary diagnostic tool; arthroscopy is the diagnostic gold standard. Treatment options include conservative therapies such as rest, NSAIDs, corticosteroid injections, and operative management.

Skalski MR, White EA, Patel DB, Schein AJ, RiveraMelo H, Matcuk GR. The Traumatized TFCC: An Illustrated Review of the Anatomy and Injury Patterns of the Triangular Fibrocartilage Complex. Curr Probl Diagn Radiol. 2016 Jan-Feb;45(1):39-50.

Clinical Description

The triangular fibrocartilage complex (TFCC) is a load-bearing structure between the lunate, triquetrum, and ulnar head. The Triangular Fibrocartilage Complex is the ligamentous and cartilaginous structures that separate the radiocarpal from the distal radioulnar joint. The TFCC consists of an articular disc, meniscus homologue, ulnocarpal ligament, dorsal & volar radioulnar ligament and extensor carpi ulnaris sheath. The function of the TFCC is to act as a stabilizer for the ulnar aspect of the wrist. The TFCC is at risk for either acute or chronic degenerative injury. Forced ulnar deviation and positive ulnar variation carry associations with injuries to the TFCC. Patients with TFCC injury will present with ulnar-sided wrist pain that may present with clicking or point tenderness between the pisiform and the ulnar head. TFCC is reported to accompany distal radius fractures in 39 to 84% of cases MRI imaging is useful as a preliminary diagnostic tool; arthroscopy is the diagnostic gold standard. Treatment options include conservative therapies such as rest, NSAIDs, and corticosteroid injections as well as operative management. Prognosis for TFCC injury is generally favorable.

Pearls & Oysters

The pitfalls related to the diagnosis of TFCC injury largely relate to MRI misread. Some examples of common mistakes when reading MRI include:

The prestyloid recess is a normal structure in the wrist near the ulnar styloid filled with fluid and can frequently be mistaken as an indication of injury or mass. Cartilaginous tissue at the ulnar styloid can have a signal intensity that can be misread as a partial tear. The ligamentum subcruentum is a normal structure at the ulnar insertion of the triangular fibrocartilage disc that often has high signal intensity. Similarly, the radial attachment of the triangular fibrocartilage disc is a normal structure that appears with high signal intensity on MRI. Neither of these should be confused as an injury. Another complication regarding reading MRI includes if there is wrist rotation during the timing of the imaging. If this is the case, the central disk can appear thin in the coronal plane. As long as there is no significant signal in addition to the thin-appearing disk, this is non-pathologic. An intermediate signal in the central disk may represent intrinsic degeneration instead of a tear. Chondrocalcinosis can also appear similar to Palmer Class 2 lesions. If this is suspected, CT imaging prior to making the diagnosis of TFCC tear is in order.

Bottom Line Statement

Patients will complain of ulnar-sided wrist pain that often gets worse with activity. There may also be a weakness in the grip, instability, or clicking. There are some elements of the history which can occur in conjunction with individual sports, for example, baseball-specific acute injury can be due to forced wrist extension while doing a head-first slide or when a hitter attempts to hit an inside pitch and gets "jammed."

Chronic injury can occur in baseball players as a result of the heavy load placed on the wrist during the swing. These athletes can sustain TFCC injuries even if they do not have positive ulnar variance In gymnastics the TFCC can be injured through overuse injury (both support skills and hanging elements). With repetitive weight bearing (both compressive and tensile), this area can become inflamed and tendonitis/tendonosis can develop in the anchoring wrist ligaments (often misdiagnosed as a wrist sprain).

Medico-Legal Traps

Misinterpretation of MRI Findings

- A common issue in diagnosing TFCC injuries is misreading MRI scans, particularly mistaking normal anatomical features (e.g., prestyloid recess, ligamentum subcruentum) for pathology. Misinterpretation can lead to unnecessary treatments, including surgery, or failure to address the actual injury.
- **Thumb Rule Consideration:** Ensure that radiologists familiar with

wrist anatomy review imaging, and consider arthroscopy, the gold standard, to confirm the diagnosis before surgical intervention.

Overlooking Degenerative Causes

- Not all TFCC injuries are acute; many arise from chronic degenerative processes. Failing to differentiate between traumatic and degenerative causes may result in improper management strategies, such as overly aggressive surgical interventions for chronic conditions better treated with conservative therapy.
- **Thumb Rule Consideration:** Differentiate between acute and degenerative TFCC injuries by combining clinical history with imaging to guide appropriate management.

Failure to Assess for Associated Injuries

- TFCC tears often accompany distal radius fractures or ulnar impaction syndrome. Overlooking associated conditions may result in incomplete treatment, leading to persistent pain or long-term disability.
- **Thumb Rule Consideration:** Always assess for concurrent injuries such as distal radius fractures and ulnar variance, as these can affect both diagnosis and treatment decisions.

Underestimating the Importance of Early Diagnosis

- Delayed or missed diagnosis of TFCC tears, especially in athletes or laborers, can lead to worsening instability and chronic pain, necessitating more invasive surgical interventions later. This delay may lead to claims of negligence or malpractice.
- **Thumb Rule Consideration:** Prioritize early and accurate diagnosis of TFCC injuries, particularly in high-risk patients such as athletes, and initiate appropriate conservative treatment to prevent progression.

Neglecting Proper Postoperative Care and Rehabilitation

- Inadequate postoperative care or improper rehabilitation protocols following TFCC repair can result in suboptimal outcomes, including chronic pain, loss of function, or reinjury. This could lead to patient dissatisfaction and legal disputes over postoperative management.
- **Thumb Rule Consideration:** Collaborate with a multidisciplinary team to ensure patients receive a comprehensive postoperative rehabilitation plan, including physical therapy and regular follow-up assessments.

REFERENCES

- Im J, Kang SJ, Lee SJ. A comparative study between conservative and surgical treatments of triangular fibrocartilage complex injury of the wrist with distal radius fractures. Clin Orthop Surg. 2021 Mar;13(1):105-9.
- Casadei K, Kiel J. Triangular fibrocartilage complex (TFCC) injuries. InStatPearls [Internet] 2020 Jan 20. StatPearls Publishing. Available from:https://www.ncbi.nlm.nih.gov/books/NBK537055/ (last accessed 5.4.2020).
- Marpole Physio What is a Triangular Fibrocartilage Complex Injury of the Wrist Available from: https://www.youtube.com/watch?v=pnk9cB9kMy8 (last accessed 5.4.2020).
- Verheyden JR, Palmer AK. EMedicine. Triangular Fibrocartilage Complex. http://emedicine.medscape.com/article/1240789-overview. (accessed 25 June 2009).
- Wheeless CR. Wheeless' Textbook of Orthopaedics. Triangular Fibrocartilage Complex. http://www.wheelessonline.com/ortho/triangular_fibrocartilage_complex (accessed 25 June 2009).
- UK Orthopaedic Surgery & Sports Medicine. Health in Sports Report-Issue 6: Triangular Fibrocartilage Complex (TFCC) Injury. http://ukhealthcare.uky.edu/sportsmedicine/health_in_sports/issue6.asp (accessed 25 June 2009).
- Gymnastics Injuries TFCC Available from:https://gymnasticsinjuries.wordpress.com/tag/tfcc/ (last accessed 6.4.2020)
- Reiter A, Wolf MB, Schmid U, Frigge A, Dreyhaupt J, Hahn P, et al. Arthroscopic repair of palmer 1B triangular fibrocartilage complex tears. Arthroscopy. 2008;24(11):1244-1250.
- Estrella EP, Hung LK, Ho PC, Tse WL. Arthroscopic repair of triangular fibrocartilage complex tears. Arthroscopy. 2007;23(7):729-737.
- Parmelee-Peters, K., & Eathorne, S. (2005). The Wrist: Common Injuries and Management. Primary Care, Clinics in Office Practice, 35-70.

TRICEPS TENDINITIS

Elbow extension is very critical for the throwing athlete. The extensor mechanism of the elbow is a relativelyuncommon source of clinical dysfunction. However, two primary processes may affect the triceps tendon, triceps tendonitis, and triceps avulsion injuries. Triceps tendonitis, the more common of the two, is manifested by chronic posterior elbow pain with extension activities. It occurs almost exclusively in males, usually in the fourth decade of life, and especially in individuals who perform forceful repetitive extension activities, eg, throwing athletes. Two distinct subsets of patients exist: those with and those without an olecranon traction spur.

Operative Techniques in Sports Medicine Volume 9, Issue 4, October 2001, Pages 217-221

Clinical Description

Triceps tendonitis is a condition characterized by tissue damage to the triceps tendon causing pain in the back of the elbow. The muscle at the back of the upper arm is known as the triceps. The triceps originates from the shoulder blade and humerus (upper arm bone) and inserts into the ulna (forearm bone) via the triceps tendon. The triceps muscle is primarily responsible for straightening the elbow and assisting certain shoulder movements. During contraction of the triceps, tension is placed through the triceps tendon. When this tension is excessive due to too much repetition or high force, damage to the triceps tendon may occur. Triceps tendonitis is a condition whereby there is damage to the triceps tendon with subsequent degeneration and inflammation. This may occur traumatically due to a high force going through the triceps tendon beyond what it can withstand, or more commonly, due to gradual wear and tear associated with overuse.

Patients with this condition typically experience pain in the back of the elbow. In less severe cases, patients may only experience an ache or stiffness in the elbow that increases with rest following activities requiring strong or repetitive contraction of the triceps muscle. These activities may include performing push ups, bench presses or dips, using a hammer repetitively or punching excessively (e.g. boxing).

In more severe cases, patients may experience an ache that increases to a sharper pain with activity. Occasionally patients may notice swelling at the back of the elbow and experience weakness when attempting to straighten the elbow against resistance and pain or tightness when performing a triceps stretch. Pain may also increase when firmly touching the affected triceps tendon. Most patients with this condition heal well with appropriate physiotherapy and return to normal function in a number of weeks. Occasionally, rehabilitation can take significantly longer and may take many months in those who have had the condition for a long period of time. Early physiotherapy treatment is vital to hasten recovery.

Pearls & Oysters

Management of triceps tendinopathies depends on the mechanism of injury and the patient's motor examination. Triceps tendinopathies and partial tendon tears with intact strength can be managed conservatively with rest, ice, immobilization, nonsteroidal anti-inflammatory drugs, and physical therapy. If conservative management fails for 6 months or there are strength deficits on examination, surgery should be considered. Based on the current evidence, there are no clear guidelines for "best" surgical approach. Although rare, the most significant surgical complication to be concerned about is rerupture.

Bottom Line Statement

The term tendonitis refers to acute inflammation of the tendon (triceps tendon inflammation). Inflammation occurs in the first few days following injury as part of the natural healing process. However, more long-term injuries are more likely to have passed the 'inflammation' stage and the term tendinopathy is probably more accurate.

This is because degeneration of the tendon is more likely rather than the presence of acute inflammation. The term 'tendinopathy' more accurately describes this. Triceps tendinopathy is the least common tendon injury of the elbow, and most commonly presents as rupture.

Medico-Legal Traps

Misdiagnosis Due to Overlapping Symptoms

- Triceps tendinitis can often be confused with other elbow pathologies, such as olecranon bursitis or lateral epicondylitis, especially since they can cause similar pain patterns. Misdiagnosing the condition can lead to ineffective treatments and prolonged recovery, potentially escalating to litigation if chronic pain or disability ensues.
- **Thumb Rule Consideration:** Conduct a thorough differential diagnosis using imaging modalities like ultrasound or MRI to distinguish between triceps tendinitis and other elbow conditions.

Delayed Diagnosis of Triceps Rupture

- In severe cases, triceps tendinitis can progress to a partial or complete rupture. Failure to identify and address a triceps tendon rupture promptly may result in poor functional outcomes, increased recovery time, and potential legal action due to perceived negligence.
- **Thumb Rule Consideration:** When symptoms worsen or fail to improve after conservative treatment, suspect tendon rupture and confirm with imaging. Early intervention is critical to avoid complications.

Inadequate Documentation of Treatment Plan

- Inconsistent or poorly documented management of the patient's condition, especially in long-term cases, can expose healthcare providers to medico-legal risks. Lack of clear records can make it difficult to defend the rationale for treatment choices if the patient claims inadequate care.
- **Thumb Rule Consideration:** Maintain detailed documentation of the patient's symptoms, progress, and response to treatments, especially when conservative measures are prolonged.

Failure to Inform Patients About Activity Modification

- Patients with triceps tendinitis, especially athletes or laborers, may fail to adhere to recommendations regarding rest and activity modification. This can delay recovery or worsen the injury. If patients are not clearly advised on the importance of modifying activities, this can lead to a claim of negligence.
- **Thumb Rule Consideration:** Provide clear, written instructions on activity modification and the potential risks of non-compliance to ensure patients understand the impact of continued strain on the tendon.

Inappropriate Surgical Indications

- Surgery is generally a last resort for triceps tendinitis but may be considered if conservative treatments fail. However, rushing into surgery without exhausting non-invasive options, or performing surgery without clear indications, could lead to negative outcomes and potential legal repercussions.
- **Thumb Rule Consideration:** Ensure surgery is only recommended after a minimum of 6 months of conservative treatment, unless there is clear evidence of tendon rupture or significant functional deficits.

REFERENCES

- Curr Sports Med Rep. 2020 Sep;19(9):367-372.
- Badia A, Stennett C: Sports-related injuries of the elbow, J Hand Ther 19:206–227, 2006.
- Jafarnia K, Gabel GT, Morrey BF: Triceps tendinitis, Oper Tech Sports Med 9:217–221, 2001.
- Potter HG, Schachar J, Jawetz S: Imaging of the elbow, Oper Tech Orthop 19:199–208, 2009.
- Waldman SD: Functional anatomy of the elbow. In Waldman SD, editor: Pain review, Philadelphia, 2009, Saunders, pp 76–77.

TRIGGER WRIST

Trigger wrist is a relatively rare condition compared with trigger finger, which is the most common disorder of the hand. To avoid inadequate and ineffective treatment of patients with trigger wrist, careful examination and proper diagnosis are vital.

Indian J Orthop. 2021 Apr; 55(2): 492–497.

Clinical Description

One of the common causes of a painful clicking finger is trigger finger. This is a common condition often seen at the clinic. While it may seem to be a simple problem, one has to be careful before any surgical intervention not to miss triggering occurring due to pathology at the wrist.

Trigger wrist or snapping wrist are two commonly used names that describe a pathology at the wrist that can cause painful clicking or snapping wrist on either wrist or even fingers movement. This will mimic the presentation of trigger finger. The definition of trigger wrist is still controversial. Historically trigger wrist had been first reported by Marti et al. and Eibel et al. and these include cases in which movement of the wrist or fingers leads to triggering of the wrist. However, in 1986, Desai et al. suggested the term trigger wrist should only be applied when the triggering occurred in relation to the wrist movement and not the fingers. This is considered as "true trigger wrist". In most of the trigger wrist cases, it was associated with finger movement, not wrist movement. This group of presentation is more accurately described as "trigger finger at the wrist". Both groups, the true trigger wrist and the trigger fingers at the wrist will be combined as trigger wrist in this discussion. The differences are the causative pathology and its location. Some of these patients also may present with carpal tunnel syndrome. This is due to the mass effect within the carpal tunnel that compresses the median nerve. This need to be addressed during carpal tunnel release.

As trigger wrist is an uncommon presentation compared to trigger finger, trigger wrist might be missed and to some extent, patients may be advised to undergo unnecessary medical procedures such as steroid injection and even unnecessary surgical procedures such as A1 pulley release. A detailed history and complete physical examination are mandatory to decide on a further plan of action especially in the atypical presentation of trigger finger or trigger finger in association with carpal tunnel syndrome. Inappropriate management will lead to worsening of symptoms such as severe tenosynovitis, flexor tendon adhesion, or advanced carpal tunnel syndrome with thenar muscle atrophy which requires more extensive exploration or reconstructive surgery.

Pearls & Oysters

Patients presenting with trigger wrist occurring during movement of the fingers are more common compared to patients with trigger wrist occurring with wrist movements. We need to differentiate whether it is a trigger finger, true trigger wrist, or trigger finger at the wrist. Triggering of the fingers may occur several weeks before the trigger wrist phenomenon. It is difficult to differentiate between trigger wrist or finger in the absence of typical triggering or snapping around the wrist, the patient may present with discomfort or pain caused by finger movement and not occurring with wrist movement. Persistent pain and decreased range of motion of the wrist may suggest entrapment of the tendon. Patients may also present with symptoms of carpal tunnel syndrome. Paraesthesia may be brought about by flexion of the fingers

Bottom Line Statement

Due to it is an uncommon presentation of trigger wrist and various possible pathologies, detailed history taking, and examination is mandatory. In patients presenting with an unusual presentation of trigger finger, assessment of lesions proximal to A1 pulley is indicated. Cardinal symptoms of trigger wrist are more than two fingers triggering at the wrist with mild to moderate carpal tunnel syndrome and palpable mass or crepitus felt over the wrist. Subsequent investigations such as plain radiograph or ultrasound will guide for further detailed radiological investigation such as MRI or CT Scan to delineate the extension and origin of the lesion before definitive surgery.

Medico-Legal Traps

Misdiagnosis as Trigger Finger

- Trigger wrist is often mistaken for the more common condition of trigger finger. Failing to differentiate between the two conditions can lead to ineffective treatments, such as unnecessary A1 pulley release, which would not address the underlying issue. This can result in prolonged patient discomfort and potential legal claims for misdiagnosis.
- **Thumb Rule Consideration:** Always consider trigger wrist in patients with atypical trigger finger symptoms and evaluate the wrist as a potential source of the problem.

Inadequate Examination for Proximal Pathology

- Trigger wrist is a rare condition that can be associated with other pathologies, such as carpal tunnel syndrome or flexor tendon entrapment. Failing to perform a comprehensive assessment of the wrist, in addition to the fingers, could lead to overlooking these associated conditions. This can cause further complications and may result in litigation if more extensive surgical interventions are required later.
- **Thumb Rule Consideration:** Perform a detailed clinical examination of both the wrist and fingers, especially in cases of suspected trigger wrist, to rule out proximal pathology.

Overlooking the Possibility of Carpal Tunnel Syndrome

- Some cases of trigger wrist are associated with carpal tunnel syndrome due to mass effect within the carpal tunnel. Ignoring this association could lead to worsening symptoms, such as thenar muscle atrophy and advanced nerve damage, which could result in a claim of negligence.
- **Thumb Rule Consideration:** In cases of trigger wrist, always evaluate for carpal tunnel syndrome and consider combined surgical interventions if needed.

Failure to Use Appropriate Imaging Modalities

- Relying solely on clinical findings without confirming the diagnosis through imaging can result in missing critical details, such as tendon entrapment or the presence of a mass. Failing to use MRI or ultrasound when indicated could lead to an incomplete diagnosis and legal claims for inadequate evaluation.
- **Thumb Rule Consideration:** When the diagnosis is unclear or when surgical intervention is being considered, use imaging modalities like ultrasound or MRI to confirm the diagnosis and assess the extent of pathology.

Performing Unnecessary Surgical Procedures

- Without a clear understanding of the pathology, patients with trigger wrist may undergo unnecessary surgeries, such as A1 pulley release or steroid injections, which may fail to resolve the condition and worsen symptoms. This exposes healthcare providers to the risk of malpractice claims.
- **Thumb Rule Consideration:** Ensure a correct diagnosis before proceeding with any invasive treatments, and prioritize conservative therapies unless absolutely necessary.

REFERENCES

- Ryzewicz M, Wolf JM. Trigger digits: Principles, management, and complications. The Journal of Hand Surgery. 2006;31(1):135–146. doi: 10.1016/j.jhsa.2005.10.013.
- Park I, Lee Y, Kim H, Lee J, Roh Y. Multiple etiologies of trigger wrist. Journal of Plastic Reconstructive and Aesthetic Surgery. 2016;69(3):335–340. doi: 10.1016/j.bjps.2015.10.030. \
- Marti T. Schnellendes Handgeienk und karpal tunnel syndrome. Schweizerische Medizinische Wochenschrift. Journal Suisse de Medecine. 1960;90:968–988.
- Eibel P. Trigger wrist with intermittent carpal tunnel syndrome: A hitherto undescribed entity with report of a case. Canadian Medical Association Journal. 1961;84(11):602–605.
- Desai SS, Pearlman HS, Patel MR. Clicking at the wrist due to fibroma in an anomalous lumbrical muscle: A case report and review of literature. The Journal of Hand Surgery. 1986;11(4):512–514. doi: 10.1016/S0363-5023(86)80186-1.
- Leunam S, Kosiyatrakul A, Neti A. Acute tru trigger wrist following partial extensor carpi radials brevis tendon rupture. Musculoskeletal Surgery. 2011;95:241–244. doi: 10.1007/s12306-011-0107-x. [7. Vekris MD, Lykissas MG, Beris AE. Median nerve compression secondary to lipoma arising from flexor tenosynovium: A case report. Hand Surgery. 2007;12:83–86. doi: 10.1142/S0218810407003444.
- Parmaksizoglu F, Cansu E, Unal MB. Trigger finger at the carpal tunnel level: Three case reports. Acta Orthopaedica et Traumatologica Turcica. 2013;47(1):65–67. doi: 10.3944/AOTT.2013.2659.
- Patil AA, Bhandari P. True trigger wrist and carpal tunnel syndrome: A case report and review of literature. Journal of Trauma and Orthopaedic. 2014;9(4):15–18.
- Ogino T, Kato H, Ohshio I. Trigger wrist induced by finger movement, pathogenesis and differential diagnosis. Handchirurgie, Mikrochirurgie, Plastische Chirurgie. 1994;26(1):3–6.
- Carvell JE, Mowat AG, Fuller DJ. Trigger wrist phenomenon in rheumatoid arthritis. Hand. 1983;15(1):77–81. doi: 10.1016/s0072-968x(83)80040-0.
- Lemon RA, Engber WD. Trigger wrist: A case report. The Journal of Hand Surgery. 1985;10(1):61–63. doi: 10.1016/s0363-5023(85)80248-3.
- Iqbal QM. Triggering of the finger at the flexor retinaculum. Hand. 1982;14(1):53–55. doi: 10.1016/s0072-968x(82)80041-7.
- Yesilada AK, Sevim KZ, Sucu DO, Dagdelen D, Sakiz D, Basak M. Combined triggering at the wrist and fingers and severe carpal tunnel syndrome caused by macrodystrophia lipomatasa. Case report and review of literature. Acts Chirugiae Plastic. 2013;55:23–25.

ULNAR TUNNEL SYNDROME

Guyon Canal syndrome which is also known as Ulnar Tunnel Syndrome is a relatively rare peripheral ulnar neuropathy. Guyon canal syndrome is also known as ulnar tunnel syndrome or handlebar palsy. It is defined as a compression of the distal ulnar nerve at the level of the wrist as it enters the hand through a space called ulnar tunnel or Guyon canal. The clinical presentation can be purely sensory, purely motor or both depending on the location of the nerve compression.

Gaskell L. Musculoskeletal assessment [Internet]. Musculoskeletal Key. 2017.

Clinical Description

Cubital tunnel syndrome (CBTS) is a peripheral nerve compression syndrome. It is an irritation or injury of the ulnar nerve in the cubital tunnel at the elbow. This is also termed ulnar nerve entrapment and is the second most common compression neuropathy in the upper extremity after carpal tunnel syndrome. It represents a source of considerable discomfort and disability for the patient and may, in extreme, cases lead to a loss of function of the hand. Cubital tunnel syndrome is also often misdiagnosed.

Peripheral nerve compression syndromes are characterised by chronic irritation and pressure lesions on the sites where nerves have to pass through narrow anatomic spaces and fibro-osseous structures. The main clinical manifestation of this type of compression are paresthesia, sensory impairment and paresis.

Cubital tunnel syndrome can also be caused by traction, pressure or ischemia of the ulnar nerve which passes through the cubital tunnel at the medial side of the elbow. Pain or paraesthesia in the fourth and fifth finger and pain in the medial aspect of the elbow, which may extend proximally or distally, is caused by compression of the ulnar nerve. There is only limited evidence that proves the effectiveness of nonsurgical and surgical interventions to treat cubital tunnel syndrome.

Pearls & Oysters

Ulnar nerve neuropathy can be due to multiple etiologies. Differential diagnosis should be kept in mind while evaluating patients with ulnar neuropathy. Thorough knowledge of the motor and sensory distribution of the ulnar nerve is critical in evaluating patients with ulnar neuropathy and to identify the site of pathology.

One in eight patients may find that their symptoms recur after surgical decompression. Insufficient decompression has been the most frequent cause of revision surgery.

Symptoms may worsen before they improve.

Injury to the medial antebrachial cutaneous nerve of the forearm is a common complication with cubital tunnel release and can be painful.

Despite the significant amount of literature devoted to the diagnosis and treatment of cubital tunnel syndrome, optimal treatment often requires two very simple components of treatment - time and rest. While surgical intervention can greatly ease symptoms, successful lifelong management of cubital tunnel syndrome also demands education and a dedicated effort at activity modification. Hopefully, with better environmental work conditions and early detection, can the expenses involved, the time spent in rehabilitation and most importantly the pain and disability patients experience decrease with the help of the patient, employers and the medical management team.

Bottom Line Statement

Ulnar tunnel syndrome could be broadly defined as a compressive neuropathy of the ulnar nerve at the level of the wrist. The ulnar tunnel, or Guyon's canal, has a complex and variable anatomy. Various factors may precipitate the onset of ulnar tunnel syndrome. Patient presentation depends on the anatomic zone of ulnar nerve compression: zone I compression, motor and sensory signs and symptoms; zone II compression, isolated motor deficits; and zone III compression; purely sensory deficits. Conservative treatment such as activity modification may be helpful, but often, surgical exploration of the ulnar tunnel with subsequent ulnar nerve decompression is indicated.

Medico-Legal Traps

Misdiagnosis or Confusion with Carpal Tunnel Syndrome

- Ulnar Tunnel Syndrome is often mistaken for the more common carpal tunnel syndrome due to overlapping symptoms. Misdiagnosis may lead to ineffective treatment, such as unnecessary carpal tunnel release, which would not relieve ulnar nerve compression. This can expose clinicians to claims of medical negligence for failing to properly diagnose and treat the condition.
- **Thumb Rule Consideration:** Always differentiate ulnar tunnel syndrome from carpal tunnel syndrome by thoroughly evaluating sensory and motor deficits specific to the ulnar nerve (fourth and fifth digits).

Failure to Identify Compression Zone

- The ulnar nerve compression can occur in one of three zones within Guyon's canal, each with different symptoms (motor, sensory, or both). If the clinician fails to localize the compression zone, treatments may be ineffective, leading to prolonged symptoms or unnecessary surgeries, which could result in a malpractice claim.
- **Thumb Rule Consideration:** Use a precise clinical evaluation to identify the affected compression zone and tailor treatment accordingly.

Inadequate Decompression During Surgery

- Surgical decompression is a common treatment for ulnar tunnel syndrome, but inadequate or incomplete decompression can result in persistent symptoms or recurrence. This can lead to a need for revision surgery and potential legal claims for surgical negligence.
- **Thumb Rule Consideration:** Ensure complete nerve decompression during surgery by carefully evaluating the nerve's course and performing the procedure in a way that fully relieves compression.

Ignoring Coexisting Pathologies

- Patients with ulnar tunnel syndrome may also have concurrent conditions like cubital tunnel syndrome or other peripheral neuropathies. Failing to diagnose and address these conditions can lead to incomplete treatment and persistent symptoms, potentially leading to claims of mismanagement.
- **Thumb Rule Consideration:** Evaluate for coexisting conditions like cubital tunnel syndrome and ensure they are addressed during diagnosis and treatment planning.

Complications from Surgical Intervention

- Complications such as injury to the medial antebrachial cutaneous nerve during ulnar nerve decompression can lead to chronic pain and functional deficits, which may result in legal claims for surgical injury. Post-surgical symptom worsening, especially when unanticipated, may also lead to dissatisfaction and legal action.
- **Thumb Rule Consideration:** Discuss the potential risks, including nerve damage and postoperative symptom exacerbation, with the patient before surgery and use meticulous surgical technique to avoid complications.

REFERENCES

- Lowe JB, Maggi SP, Mackinnon SE. The position of crossing branches of the medial antebrachial cutaneous nerve during cubital tunnel surgery in humans. Plast Reconstr Surg. 2004 Sep 01;114(3):692-6.
- Palmer BA, Hughes TB. Cubital Tunnel Syndrome. J Hand Surg. 2010; 35(1): 153–163.

- Han HH, Kang HW, Lee JL, Jung S. Fascia Wrapping Technique: A Modified Method for the Treatment of Cubital Tunnel Syndrome. The Scientific World Journal. 2014; Article ID 482702, 6 pages.
- Cutts S. Cubital tunnel syndrome. Postgrad Med J. 2007; 83(975): 28–31.
- Assmus H, Antoniadis G, Bischoff C. Carpal and cubital tunnel and other, rarer nerve compression syndromes. Dtsch Arztebl Int. 2015;112(1-2):14-25; quiz 26.
- Lund AT, Amadio PC. Treatment of cubital tunnel syndrome: perspectives for the therapist. J Hand Ther. 2006;19(2):170-8.
- Rinkel WD, Schreuders TA, Koes BW, Huisstede BM. Current evidence for effectiveness of interventions for cubital tunnel syndrome, radial tunnel syndrome, instability, or bursitis of the elbow: a systematic review. Clin J Pain. 2013;29(12):1087-96.
- Feindel W, Stratford J. Cubital tunnel compression in tardy ulnar nerve palsy. Can Med Assoc J. 1958;78:351.

VULVODYNIA

Vulvodynia is a vulvar pain of at least three months' duration without a clear identifiable cause. It is a diagnosis of exclusion and is considered an idiopathic pain disorder. Vulvodynia can cause pain that is severe, debilitating, and devastating to the patients suffering from it.

Vieira-Baptista P, Lima-Silva J, Pérez-López FR, Preti M, Bornstein J. Vulvodynia: A disease commonly hidden in plain sight. Case Rep Womens Health. 2018 Oct;20:e00079.

Clinical Description

The current International Society for the Study of Vulvovaginal Disease (ISSVD) definition of vulvodynia is a vulvar pain of at least three months' duration, without a clear, identifiable cause, which may have potential associated factors. It is a diagnosis of exclusion and is an idiopathic pain disorder. The cause of vulvodynia is not known. Research is being done to learn what contributes to the condition. Possible contributing causes include injury or irritation to the nerves that transmit pain from the vulva to the spinal cord, an increase in the number and sensitivity of nerve fibers in the vulva, elevated levels of inflammatory substances including cytokines in the vulva, abnormal response to environmental factors, genetic susceptibility, and pelvic floor muscle weakness, spasm or instability.

The anatomy of the vulva and vulvar vestibule is very important to understand vulvodynia.

The vulva and vulvar vestibule: the vulva is the external female genitalia, which includes the mons pubis, labia majora, labia minora, clitoral hood, clitoris, and vestibule. The vulva is innervated by the anterior labial branches of the ilioinguinal nerve, genitofemoral nerve, and branches of the pudendal nerves. The pudendal nerve divides into three branches near the medial aspect of the ischial tuberosity:

(1) the dorsal nerve of the clitoris,

(2) the perineal nerve which innervates the labia majora and perineum, and

(3) the inferior rectal nerve which innervates the perianal area. The pudendal nerve also innervates the external anal sphincter and deep muscles of the urogenital triangle.

Pearls & Oysters

Research on the topic of vulvodynia is ongoing. Twenty-five percent of adult Americans suffer from a chronic pain condition. Patients in pain are often

neglected and under-treated. This pain condition is severe and debilitating and can be devastating to the patients suffering from it. The scientific level of evidence for almost all treatment regimens is poor, with very few randomized controlled trials having been performed. Treatment outcomes vary in the studies we have, but the majority of women improve with treatment. Practitioners should be encouraged to take their patients seriously and remember that this condition exists. If the practitioner is uncomfortable treating the condition or does not have the education and experience to treat the condition, they should query the National Vulvodynia Association and find a practitioner who does.

Bottom Line Statement

The cause of vulvodynia remains unknown and hence its treatment remains unsatisfactory. Treatment requires an interprofessional treatment approach. It is important to believe that the woman has pain.• In many cases, the woman has been struggling for a long time in silence, or she has seen many practitioners and no one has helped her. Different practitioners may be involved in the care of this patient. When a patient finds the correct practitioners they may include a gynecologist with a special interest in vulvovaginal disease health usually involved in the societies International Society for the Study of Women's Sexual Health (ISSWSH) and ISSVD, a dermatologist, nurse practitioner, a neurologist, a pain management specialist, a urologist, and/or a physical therapist who specializes in women's health. Unfortunately, despite adequate treatment, the pain is recurrent and seriously affects lifestyle and interpersonal relationships.

Medico-Legal Traps

Failure to Diagnose Vulvodynia as a Chronic Pain Condition

- Vulvodynia is often misdiagnosed or dismissed as a psychological issue due to the absence of visible physical abnormalities. Many patients go undiagnosed for long periods, leading to prolonged suffering and potential legal claims of medical negligence.
- **Thumb Rule Consideration:** Always take patient complaints of vulvar pain seriously and consider vulvodynia as a differential diagnosis after excluding other conditions.

Insufficient Documentation of Diagnostic Efforts

- Vulvodynia is a diagnosis of exclusion, requiring careful elimination of other possible causes of vulvar pain, such as infections, dermatological conditions, and neurological disorders. Failing to document these exclusions adequately can expose clinicians to claims of inadequate medical investigation.

- **Thumb Rule Consideration:** Maintain thorough documentation of all diagnostic steps, including tests conducted and conditions ruled out.

Inadequate Multidisciplinary Treatment Approach

- Vulvodynia often requires an interprofessional approach for effective management, including input from gynecologists, neurologists, pain specialists, and physical therapists. Neglecting this approach can result in ineffective treatment and ongoing patient suffering, which could lead to malpractice claims.
- **Thumb Rule Consideration:** Involve a multidisciplinary team in the management of vulvodynia, especially in cases where initial treatments fail.

Failure to Recognize Psychological Impact

- Vulvodynia has a profound effect on a patient's mental and emotional health, often leading to anxiety, depression, and relationship issues. Failing to address these psychological impacts can worsen the patient's condition and may lead to claims of incomplete treatment.•
- **Thumb Rule Consideration:** Assess and document the psychological impact of vulvodynia and refer patients for psychological support or counseling as needed.

Overlooking Informed Consent for Invasive Treatments

- Some treatments for vulvodynia, such as nerve blocks or surgical interventions, carry significant risks. Not adequately informing patients of these risks and obtaining clear consent can lead to legal claims for lack of informed consent if complications arise.
- **Thumb Rule Consideration:** Provide patients with comprehensive information about the potential risks and benefits of all treatment options, especially invasive procedures, and document informed consent thoroughly.

REFERENCES

- Vieira-Baptista P, Lima-Silva J, Pérez-López FR, Preti M, Bornstein J. Vulvodynia: A disease commonly hidden in plain sight. Case Rep Womens Health. 2018 Oct;20:e00079.
- Henzell H, Berzins K, Langford JP. Provoked vestibulodynia: current perspectives. Int J Womens Health. 2017;9:631-642.
- Dias-Amaral A, Marques-Pinto A. Female Genito-Pelvic Pain/Penetration Disorder: Review of the Related Factors and Overall Approach. Rev Bras Ginecol Obstet. 2018 Dec;40(12):787-793.

- Bornstein J, Goldstein AT, Stockdale CK, Bergeron S, Pukall C, Zolnoun D, Coady D., consensus vulvar pain terminology committee of the International Society for the Study of Vulvovaginal Disease (ISSVD). International Society for the Study of Women's Sexual Health (ISSWSH). International Pelvic Pain Society (IPPS). 2015 ISSVD, ISSWSH, and IPPS Consensus Terminology and Classification of Persistent Vulvar Pain and Vulvodynia. J Sex Med. 2016 Apr;13(4):607-12.
- Rosen NO, Dawson SJ, Brooks M, Kellogg-Spadt S. Treatment of Vulvodynia: Pharmacological and Non-Pharmacological Approaches. Drugs. 2019 Apr;79(5):483-493.
- Coady D, Kennedy V. Sexual Health in Women Affected by Cancer: Focus on Sexual Pain. Obstet Gynecol. 2016 Oct;128(4):775-91.

WINGED SCAPULA SYNDROME

In a patient who has a winged scapula, the medial (or in some cases, lateral) aspect of the scapula appears to be protruding from the back. As the name of the condition implies, it can create a winged appearance. This abnormal position of the scapula can lead to many physical functional disabilities such as pain, decreased strength, and range of motion disruptions. The ranges of motion that are most commonly affected are abduction and flexion of the affected upper extremity.

Saied GM, Kamel RM, Dessouki NR. The effect of mastectomy and radiotherapy for breast carcinoma on soft tissues of the shoulder and its joint mobility among Egyptian patients. Tanzan Health Res Bull. 2007 May;9(2):121-5.

Clinical Description

The most common etiology of a winged scapula is usually due to damage or impaired innervation to the serratus anterior muscle. The nerve that innervates this muscle is the long thoracic nerve. Sometimes, this nerve can be damaged or impinged, leading to malfunction of the serratus anterior muscle. Some patients may also complain of an inability to raise the affected arm above their head. This dysfunction results in the medial border of the scapula giving a winged-like appearance. The impingement or damage of this nerve leads to the winged appearance because the serratus anterior muscle attaches to the medial aspect of the scapula and holds it against the posterior rib cage. Less commonly, the scapula can wing laterally due to damage to the trapezius or rhomboid muscles, which are innervated by the spinal accessory nerves and dorsal scapular nerve, respectively. The scapula will move laterally due to unopposed muscle strength attributed to the trapezium or rhomboid paralysis or weakness; this occurs because the function of the trapezius muscle is to elevate, retract and rotate the scapula.

Pearls & Oysters

There are two main categories of complications associated with winged scapula syndrome. The first is damage to the shoulder due to the functional disability caused by the syndrome. This may include weakness, pain, and difficulty moving the shoulder and arm. The second category of complications is the failure to recognize that the cause of the winging of the scapula is not an isolated lesion of the long thoracic nerve of Bell, but rather a part of a larger neurological problem.

Winged scapula syndrome can be difficult to treat and early removal of the cause of nerve entrapment can allow for rapid recovery of nerve function and improvement in pain and shoulder dysfunction. It is important for healthcare providers to carefully search for other causes of winging of the scapula before attributing this neurological finding to winged scapula syndrome.

Bottom Line Statement

An interprofessional healthcare team providing care to a patient with scapular winging is crucial in ensuring the best health outcome of the individual. The integrated postoperative care given to the patient can determine whether the patient will make a full recovery or to what extent. When the patient is under post-operative management, all interprofessional team members, including the nurse and physical therapist involved in patient care, should be made aware of scapular winging as a potential complication. Thus, nurses who work closely with the patients can monitor and know what to look for to alert the medical team. The pharmacist should educate the patient on pain management, and the physical therapist should recommend the relevant exercises. That way, early and effective intervention can commence before the patient presents with symptoms. Prevention of this condition will clearly lead to the best outcomes for patient care. Interprofessional care can lead to the best success in the planning and evaluation of patient progress in recovery. Interprofessional collaboration is guaranteed to result in a better prognosis and outcome for the patient as an integrated approach to care.

Medico-Legal Traps

Failure to Recognize Nerve Damage

- The most common cause of winged scapula syndrome is damage to the long thoracic nerve, leading to paralysis of the serratus anterior muscle. Failure to identify the correct nerve involved, or assuming the problem is muscular without investigating the neurological causes, can delay treatment and worsen the patient's condition.

- **Thumb Rule Consideration:** Always assess for nerve damage (long thoracic, spinal accessory, and dorsal scapular nerves) when diagnosing winged scapula syndrome to ensure correct treatment.

Misdiagnosis as a Muscular Issue

- Due to the winged appearance of the scapula, clinicians may incorrectly diagnose the condition as purely a muscular issue without recognizing the underlying nerve dysfunction. This can lead to inappropriate treatment such as physical therapy focused solely on strengthening the muscles, which could exacerbate the problem.
- **Thumb Rule Consideration:** Include a comprehensive neurological examination in the workup to rule out nerve entrapment or paralysis before attributing symptoms to muscular weakness alone.

Neglecting Early Surgical Intervention for Nerve Compression

- In cases where nerve compression is causing the scapular winging, failure to perform early surgical intervention to relieve nerve entrapment may result in permanent damage and loss of function. Patients may later claim negligence for delaying appropriate care.
- **Thumb Rule Consideration:** Consider early referral to a neurologist or orthopedic surgeon when nerve compression is suspected, especially if conservative treatments fail to show improvement.

Inadequate Post-Surgical Care and Monitoring

- Post-surgical patients may experience complications like incomplete recovery or recurrence of winging. Failure to provide a well-coordinated rehabilitation program, involving physical therapists and other specialists, can lead to prolonged recovery or disability, potentially resulting in legal action for inadequate care.
- **Thumb Rule Consideration:** Ensure interprofessional collaboration for post-operative care, with ongoing monitoring by physical therapists, pain management specialists, and nurses to optimize recovery and prevent complications.

Lack of Informed Consent and Risk Communication

- If surgery is required, patients must be fully informed about the risks of nerve damage, post-surgical complications, and the possibility of incomplete recovery. Failing to provide a thorough explanation of these risks can lead to legal claims if the outcome is not as expected.

- **Thumb Rule Consideration:** Clearly communicate the risks, benefits, and possible outcomes of surgery and other treatments, ensuring that informed consent is obtained and documented.

REFERENCES

- Saied GM, Kamel RM, Dessouki NR. The effect of mastectomy and radiotherapy for breast carcinoma on soft tissues of the shoulder and its joint mobility among Egyptian patients. Tanzan Health Res Bull. 2007 May;9(2):121-5.
- Lung K, Lui F. StatPearls [Internet]. StatPearls Publishing; Treasure Island (FL): Jul 25, 2022. Anatomy, Thorax, Long Thoracic Nerve.
- Didesch JT, Tang P. Anatomy, Etiology, and Management of Scapular Winging. J Hand Surg Am. 2019 Apr;44(4):321-330.
- Krzesniak-Swinarska M, Caress JB, Cartwright MS. Neuromuscular ultrasound for evaluation of scapular winging. Muscle Nerve. 2017 Jul;56(1):7-14.
- Srikumaran U, Wells JH, Freehill MT, Tan EW, Higgins LD, Warner JJ. Scapular Winging: A Great Masquerader of Shoulder Disorders: AAOS Exhibit Selection. J Bone Joint Surg Am. 2014 Jul 16;96(14):e122.
- LURJE A. Concerning surgical treatment of traumatic injury of the upper division of the brachial plexus (Erb's-type). Ann Surg. 1948 Feb;127(2):317-26.
- Kauppila LI, Vastamäki M. Iatrogenic serratus anterior paralysis. Long-term outcome in 26 patients. Chest. 1996 Jan;109(1):31-4.
- Pallara T, Del Buono R, Marangi GF, Langella M, Toto V, Persichetti P. Outcomes of traditional cosmetic abdominoplasty in a community setting: a retrospective analysis of 1008 patients. Plast Reconstr Surg. 2013 Nov;132(5):863e-864e.

XIPHODYNIA

Xiphodynia is a term used to describe an 'uncommon' syndrome with a constellation of symptoms ranging from upper abdominal pain, chest pain, sometimes throat and arm symptoms which are referred from the xiphisternal joint or the structures attached to the xiphoid process.

Chiropr Osteopat. 2007; 15: 13.

Clinical Description

Xiphodynia is a condition involving referral of pain to the chest, abdomen, throat, arms and head from an irritated xiphoid process. The literature over a 60 year period reveals 12 citations relating to the terms xiphodynia and xiphoidalgia, with only 5 of these in English. The papers published between 1979 and 1998 present 10 cases of xiphodynia, all treated by localized injection. Lipkin et al published what appears to be the first 'modern' paper on the hypersensitive xiphoid in 1955. They reported on 24 cases observed over a seven year period where gentle pressure on a hypersensitive xiphoid reproduced all or most of the patients' presenting pain. Lipkin et al note that the earliest report of disorders of the xiphoid was recorded in 1712.

There are no clear data relating to the incidence or prevalence of xiphodynia. Most authors say that it is an uncommon disorder while Lipkin et al found the syndrome present in about 2 percent of the population of a general-hospital ward and stated that it is "far more common than is generally appreciated". They went so far as to suggest that examination of the xiphoid should be part of the routine examination of any patient presenting with upper-abdominal or chest pain.

Pearls & Oysters

One of the major challenges in the care of patients with xiphodynia is the possibility of underlying serious pathology, such as tumors or other abnormalities in the thorax or upper abdomen. It is important for healthcare providers to thoroughly evaluate patients with xiphodynia to rule out these potential underlying causes.

Injections of the xiphisternal joint may be used as a treatment for xiphodynia. However, there are potential complications associated with this treatment, including pneumothorax (collapsed lung) if the needle is placed too laterally or deeply and invades the pleural space, and infection if strict aseptic technique is not followed. Trauma to the contents of the mediastinum (the space between the lungs) is also a potential complication of injection of the xiphisternal joint.

To minimize these risks, it is important for the clinician to pay close attention to accurate needle placement.

Bottom Line Statement

Xiphodynia is a musculoskeletal disorder that can be responsible for extremely distressing and disabling upper abdominal, chest and/or throat symptoms. It is simple to diagnose and simple to treat. Given the principal author's experience, which concurs with Lipkin et al, it may be that xiphodynia is under-considered. Lipkin et al went so far as to suggest, "palpation of the xiphoid area be done in most general physical examinations and certainly in patients complaining of pain in the chest or upper abdomen". A short course of non-invasive treatment such as low-level laser or ultrasound may be worth considering before more aggressive injection treatment is utilized.

Medico-Legal Traps

Failure to Rule Out Serious Pathologies

- Given that xiphodynia can mimic symptoms of more serious conditions like tumors, thoracic, or upper abdominal abnormalities, a failure to thoroughly investigate these underlying causes before diagnosing xiphodynia could lead to misdiagnosis and delayed treatment of life-threatening conditions.
- **Thumb Rule Consideration:** Always perform a thorough diagnostic evaluation, including imaging if necessary, to exclude serious conditions before attributing pain to xiphodynia.

Inaccurate Diagnosis Leading to Mismanagement

- Xiphodynia's varied symptomatology, including chest and upper abdominal pain, can easily be mistaken for cardiac, gastrointestinal, or musculoskeletal conditions. Misdiagnosis could result in unnecessary treatments or surgeries, leading to further complications.
- **Thumb Rule Consideration:** Include xiphodynia in the differential diagnosis for unexplained upper abdominal or chest pain and confirm through clinical examination by palpating the xiphoid area for tenderness.

Inadequate Needle Placement During Injection Therapy

- Injection therapy is a common treatment for xiphodynia, but poor technique or incorrect needle placement can cause severe complications, such as pneumothorax or trauma to the mediastinal contents, increasing the risk of malpractice claims.
- **Thumb Rule Consideration:** Use ultrasound-guided injections to

ensure precise needle placement and minimize the risk of pleural space invasion or other anatomical complications.

Neglecting Aseptic Technique in Injections

- Infections from injections are a known risk, especially in treatments involving sensitive areas such as the xiphisternal joint. Failing to use strict aseptic techniques could lead to infection, which may cause further complications for the patient.
- **Thumb Rule Consideration:** Always adhere to strict aseptic techniques during injection procedures to reduce the risk of infection and related legal complications.

Overlooking Conservative Treatment Options

- Aggressive treatments such as injections might be recommended too early, overlooking simpler, non-invasive treatment options like low-level laser therapy or ultrasound. This could expose the clinician to liability for unnecessary invasive procedures.
- **Thumb Rule Consideration:** Always explore and exhaust non-invasive treatment options before recommending more aggressive treatments like injections or surgeries.

REFERENCES

- Speed C. Therapeutic ultrasound in soft tissue lesions. Rheumatology. 2001;40:1331–1336. doi: 10.1093/rheumatology/40.12.1331.
- Demir H, M P, Kirnap M, Calis M, Ikizceli I. Comparison of the Effects of Laser, Ultrasound, and Combined Laser + Ultrasound Treatments in Experimental Tendon Healing. Lasers in Surgery and Medicine. 2004;35:84–89. doi: 10.1002/lsm.20046.
- Koren W, Shahar A. Xiphodynia Masking Acute Myocardial Infarction: A Diagnostic Cul-de-sac. Am J Emerg Med. 1998;16:177–178. doi: 10.1016/S0735-6757(98)90041-9.
- Howell J. Xiphodynia: a report of three cases. J Emerg Med. 1992;10:435–438. doi: 10.1016/0736-4679(92)90272-U.
- Sklaroff H. Xiphodynia – Another Cause of Atypical Chest Pain: Six Case Reports. Mt Sinai J Med. 1979;46:546–548.
- Lipkin M, Fulton L, Wolfson E. The Syndrome of the Hypersensitive Xiphoid. N Eng J Med. 1955;253:591–597.
- Waldman S. Atlas of uncommon pain syndromes. Philadelphia: Saunders; Elsevier; 2003.
- Gray H. Anatomy of the Human Body. 1918; Philadelphia: Lea & Febiger; 2000. http://www.bartleby.com/107/27.html Accessed: 4/11/06.
- Mackenzie J. Some Points Bearing on the Association of Sensory Disorders and Visceral Disease. Brain. 1893;16:321–352. doi: 10.1093/brain/16.3.321.
- Kellgren J. The Anatomical Source of Back Pain. Rheum & Rehab. 1977;16:3–12.

www.ingramcontent.com/pod-product-compliance
Lightning Source LLC
LaVergne TN
LVHW060542061126
851857LV00017B/1868
* 9 7 8 8 1 9 9 8 4 7 6 8 2 *